So, what is this book about—and why do authorities believe it is an important reference for you and your family?

More people than ever have medical limitations that make them dependent on physical assistance from others. Today's hospital patients are being discharged earlier to recuperate at home. Others with life-long disabilities are living longer with active lifestyles.

There are three primary sources of help providers, and this is the only reference that tells you how to work in harmony and take maximum advantage of each one.

The majority of this personal help comes from family caregivers. While the love and caring of these family members may be unlimited, their personal energy and stamina understandably have human limitations. Statistically, many family caregivers are over worked, chronically fatigued, and headed for depression. Consequently, most will welcome the variety of topics in this reference for finding and hiring the outside relief help they need and deserve.

Agencies offer a valuable, second source of help providers to tired family caregivers as well as help recipients who are unable or unwilling to manage their own aides. Some agencies offer very competent services, while others fall quite short of their claims. Specialized chapters of this reference will enable you to identify the better ones and avoid the others.

When you personally employ your own aides (also known as personal assistants or PAs), you can control the quality of *help* you receive because you first control the quality of *help providers*. Your own PAs provide help each day according to *your* personal schedule, and not an agency's—and at a cost of less than half an agency's rate.

You will be interested in what people are saying about DeGraff, his previous publications, and this new reference—

"A fantastic resource for people to use in managing their care... (DeGraff's book) is a clear, concise manual designed to take the mystery out of self-managed care. Written by someone who clearly understands the process, the book leaves nothing to chance, providing step-by-step advice aimed at simplifying and bullet-proofing the process of hiring and managing personal aides. *Caregivers and Personal Assistants...* is destined to become the bible for anyone wishing to gain independence through managing their own care."

> —**Cliff Bridges**, Editor, *Total Access Magazine*, Canadian Paraplegic Association

"I sure wish I had this reference 22 years ago when I broke my neck. It is very detailed and should keep readers from making the early mistakes I made."

> —**Don Krebs**, President, *Access to Recreation, Inc.*, and quadriplegic

D0089060

"Mr. DeGraff provides a valuable in-depth survey on the complexities, intricacies and multi-faceted aspects of the caregiver-care-recipient equation. His treatment of the evolving dynamics of roles, expectations, and outcomes should be of keen interest not only to caregivers, families and recipients, but also to educators, policy makers, administrators, clinicians and other stakeholders involved in the supportive care arena. Mr. DeGraff's knowledge is first hand and first rate."

> —**Rick Rader, M.D.**, Director, Morton J. Kent Habilitation Center, Orange Grove Center, Chattanooga, TN and Editor-In-Chief, *Exceptional Parent Magazine*

"Accurate…well organized…a comprehensive approach to dealing with care recipient needs and caregiver responsibilities"

> —**Evelyn Rosen-Budd**, Resource Editor, National Family Caregivers Association

"Al DeGraff is the leading authority on managing home care. His books and advice columns have been followed for decades because his advice is savvy, grounded, 'tried-and-true.' Back when the medical model was in vogue, DeGraff was there at the leading edge, lecturing and promoting the sage reminder that the person with the disability is the authority of his or her own personal care. This new book is a synthesis of intelligent, practical problem solving. It is intended to empower people with disabilities, to keep families intact and wholesome, and to find and create ways for people with disabilities to stay and live fully at home.

"Like DeGraff's other books, this one is a must for health professionals, for families of youth who are recently disabled, and for aging individuals and their families who are gradually discovering home care needs. This book is about health and empowerment; it is chock full of practical 'how to's'—and ultimately, which may be its greatest gift, it is about grace."

> —**Margaret A. Short, Ph.D., OTR, FAOTA**

"Step by step, this book develops the big picture of personal home care. For those involved in providing or arranging for these services for the first time, the task seems insurmountable. And after beginning, you become certain that it's impossible. It was at this point that I found (DeGraff's) book. There I found the benefit of decades of point-on experience, confirmation of what I had learned the hard way, and suggestions of where to go from there. How much wear and tear could have been avoided if only I'd found this book sooner!"

> —**Diane Rehner**, Family caregiver for over 25 years

"DeGraff's passion is to revolutionize PA management…a whole set of strategies help family caregivers avoid…overwork, fatigue, and depression. DeGraff was writing on this subject when nobody else was, and the first two editions of this book were ground breaking"

> —*New Mobility Magazine*

"The book's…practical recommendations make the caregiver/help recipient relationship a positive one."

> —**Anita L. Abrams**, CSW, Manager, Case Management Department, Sunnyview Rehabilitation Hospital

"A must read. Everything you need—and more. This book…has the potential to be a bible for people who must depend on others to get through the day."

> —**Richard Holicky**, Author, researcher, and paraplegic

"If all families—regardless of whether they have a member with a disability—followed (DeGraff's) suggestions for assessing family health, they would be a lot healthier! In addition to caregivers, family members, and help recipients, students in health care professions and professionals, themselves, should read this book to see what it's like 'on the other side'."

> —**Anita Bundy, Sc.D., OTR, FAOTA**, Professor, Colorado State University

"Excellent resource for finding quality care for loved ones. Chock-full of answers to caregiver concerns. A great survival tool when caring for someone you love."

> —**Elaine Tillman**, Community Resource Specialist, Missouri Division of Developmental Disabilities and Mental Retardation.

"Well organized…I like the state-of-the-family meetings…offers the opportunity to communicate effectively…such a good point—don't burn out family caregivers on physical ADL needs."

> —**Tina Tapply**, Administrator, New Mercer Commons Assisted Living Center

"I have lived with muscular dystrophy for 40 years. Tom, my cousin, has been my faithful family caregiver for over 20 years. While he has unlimited love for me, we have each recognized there are understandable limits on his time and stamina for helping me. We spend a lot of time together. Learning to give each other space is very important.

"DeGraff's book has provided us with new planning strategies for deciding which of my help needs he might assist, and which to assign to outsiders. We now have more quality time for ourselves and each other! A very valuable, recommended reference."

> —**Lori Hinderer**, (National) Vice-President, Muscular Dystrophy Association

"I haven't been out of bed in twenty years. I need help daily. For me, personal assistance is key to my living independently in my home. Yet questions abound. Al answers the many questions about who, what, why, where, and how. Especially the how!

"Al's books are The Guide—The Standard for comparisons.

"They have helped me—and thousands of others. If you have a disability and need help with your activities of daily living, then *you need this book.* Period."

> —**Fred Fay, Ph.D.**, Chair, Justice for All; Co-founder, Boston Center for Independent Living

CAREGIVERS AND
PERSONAL ASSISTANTS

CAREGIVERS AND
PERSONAL ASSISTANTS

HOW TO FIND, HIRE AND MANAGE
THE PEOPLE WHO HELP YOU (OR YOUR LOVED ONE!)

ALFRED H. DEGRAFF, M.A., S.E.A.

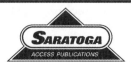

SARATOGA ACCESS PUBLICATIONS, INC.
FORT COLLINS • COLORADO • USA

Saratoga Access Publications, Inc. • P.O. Box 1427 • Fort Collins, CO 80522-1427 • USA
Web site: www.saratoga-publications.com • E-mail: caregiver@saratoga-publications.com

© 2002 by Alfred H. DeGraff • All rights reserved. No part of this book may be used, reproduced, stored in a retrieval system, or transmitted in any form or by any means without written permission from the author except in the case of brief quotations embodied in critical articles or reviews. Cover design and illustration by Lightbourne Images, © 2002.

Printed in the United States of America • Printed on acid-free, partially recycled paper

First edition, 1978 Boston, Massachusetts
Second revised edition, 1988 Saratoga Springs, New York
Third, completely revised edition, 2002 Fort Collins, Colorado • 10 9 8 7 6 5 4 3 2 1

Publisher's Cataloging-in-Publication

DeGraff, Alfred H.
   Caregivers and personal assistants : how to find, hire
and manage the people who help you (or your loved
one!) / Alfred H. DeGraff. -- 3rd ed.
   p. cm.
   Includes bibliographical references and index.
   LCCN 2001117773
   ISBN 0-9621106-1-2

   1. Home care services. 2. Home nursing.
  3. Caregivers. I. Title.

RA645.3.D44 2002   649.8
                QBI01-700719

Warning—Disclaimer

This book has been written to provide information with regard to its subject matter. It is sold with the understanding that the publisher and author are not engaged in providing medical, legal, accounting, personnel, or tax counseling services.

If medical, legal, accounting, personnel, or tax-counseling expertise is desired, the reader should enlist the services of a competent professional in those fields.

The topic of managing home health aides is not an exact science. The methods, strategies, procedures, and advice found in this book have been successfully used by many people; however, they are not infallible.

There is no guarantee—expressed or implied, regardless of any text that seems to state certainty or assurance—that a technique or advice will succeed. The reader agrees to take full, personal responsibility both for deciding how to use the information in this reference and for the consequent outcomes.

Every effort has been made to make this book as accurate as possible; however, there may be mistakes in both typography and content. Neither the author nor publisher shall be responsible or liable to any person or entity for any damage or loss caused or alleged to be caused, directly or indirectly, by the information contained in this book.

Ordering This Book

Please see details at the end of this book about ordering additional copies.

Contents—

About the Author—

Alfred H. "Skip" DeGraff is a spinal-cord injured, C 5-6 tetraplegic (quad) from a diving injury incurred when he was 18 years old.

After finishing graduate studies, he became the founder and first director of the Department of Disabled Student Services at Boston University, a post he held for 10 years. He then served as the CEO and director of two independent living centers for developmentally and physically disabled adults. Next, he founded Saratoga Access and Fitness, Inc. and spent 13 years designing, manufacturing, and marketing accessible aerobic fitness equipment, including the well-known Saratoga Cycle. He recently sold that corporation to dedicate his full attention to promoting and teaching skills in help provider management.

His highly independent and active lifestyle has resulted from his using a motorized wheelchair, driving a wheelchair-accessible van, and hiring and managing daily help from personal assistants (PAs) for more than 30 years. During that time, he has personally employed more than 350 PAs after interviewing over 1,500 applicants. He has also provided one-on-one counseling to help recipients, family caregivers, and paid providers; taught formal 16-week courses in PA management; and hosted magazine columns. His first and second books on this topic were published in 1978 and 1988. This is his third, completely revised edition.

In accomplishing these goals, he has learned a variety of approaches for recruiting, hiring, and managing help providers in a variety of settings. These settings have included—

- His mother's home, by using family caregivers for the year between his initial hospital discharge and moving to his first college campus
- A local community college, by using fellow students for commuting transportation and on-campus personal needs
- Three residential university campuses, by hiring dormitory roommates as live-in student aides
- Large urban apartment complexes (while pursuing careers) by recruiting live-in roommates to provide help in exchange for their room and utilities
- Extensive business and vacation travel by car and air, by using help from aides, friends, and caregiver-relatives in exchange for their transportation, room, and board
- Inpatient hospital stays (for many brief illnesses as well as lengthy surgeries), by instructing and managing the physicians and nursing staff for his routine disability-related needs, and accepting their instruction and care for the new, temporary acute needs

- In his private home, while married, by balancing help from his caregiver-wife (for a minimum of private-time needs) and from salaried outsiders (for the majority of his needs)
- In his private home, before and after marriage, by combining live-in and salaried help

His injury occurred just eight days after high school graduation. In order to attend college and pursue careers, he began to learn—solely from trial and error—how to hire PAs in this variety of settings. Although he took maximum advantage of his initial 14 months of inpatient rehabilitation in the 1960s, he found no formal instruction for managing the help providers he would use every day.

Even today, more than 30 years later, most formal rehabilitation programs still use quite informal attempts to equip patients with these essential PA management skills. A few rare facilities offer instruction and experiential learning environments where soon-to-be-discharged patients can practice recruiting, hiring, and training outside providers.

Most newly disabled people still rely primarily on the common-sense, trial-and-error approach to learning the RISHTMP skills for recruiting, interviewing, screening, hiring, training, managing, and parting ways with their help providers. Even with the advantages of the strategies in this reference, living with a disability and a physical dependence on PA help is a difficult and tiring lifestyle.

> *It takes an enormous amount of daily energy, year after year, to find, hire, and work in mutual respect with the people who help you while controlling the quality of help they provide. Thousands of us are managing people from 6 A.M. to after 10 P.M. every single day. Your physical dependence never takes a vacation. As exhausted as you often become, you have no choice but to keep up your continuous "waterdance" (a concept defined in the video by that same name).*

> *Routinely managing assistance, even in a familiar setting with trusted providers, requires enormous effort. However, you will also often have to devise new methods for finding and managing PAs in new settings and situations. I hope this reference of management methods and personal coping strategies will enable you to stay ahead of the game.*

> *I believe that all of us who have a disability, and share these unique concerns, also have a responsibility to support each other. We are socially responsible for routinely sharing the solutions that make life a bit easier for the next person.*

> *I have spent more than 30 years taking notes—from my experiences and from interviewing others—on which PA management strategies have worked and which have failed. This reference is one of my primary life contributions to us. Please use it to maximize your personal independence and productivity, so you, in turn, can share your own contributions.*

Preface: My Injury Wrote This Book for You

"Give me a fish
and I eat for a day,
Teach me to fish
and I eat for a lifetime!"
—Author unknown[1]

For the '60s Generation, it was the Summer of Love. The morning of July 4, 1967 was hot and muggy. I was 18 years old and had graduated from a parochial high school just a few days before. Instead of hanging with hippies in the Haight or educating America's political conscience in Berkeley, I was working for the summer on the east coast on Martha's Vineyard, Massachusetts.

The Vineyard is that well-known resort island about seven miles southeast of Cape Cod. As are most islands, it is surrounded by beautiful ocean beaches.

That Fourth of July was a holiday for me from my clerking in a clothing store, and in the early morning I sprang out of bed and pulled on my swim trunks. I was in great physical shape and thoroughly enjoyed bicycling the five miles to the Vineyard's South Beach. I planned to spend the day tanning, swimming, and boosting my social life.

After an hour of tanning, munching on apples purchased from the local A&P Supermarket, and listening to the AM-radio '60s rock of WBZ (Boston) and WABC (Manhattan), it was time to cool off in the Atlantic. Around ten o'clock that morning, I paddled my bare feet through the hot sand and climbed up onto a concrete bunker that nosed out into the crashing, cold surf. Standing tall at the front edge of the bunker, I looked out toward the huge waves rolling toward my toes.

---

1. Although this quotation appears too frequently in some literature, it aptly expresses the spirit behind learning as many independent living skills as possible, and minimizing one's dependence on others.

As many of us teenagers had done on previous days, I curled my toes tightly around the front edge of the pier, leaned forward like a cat about to spring toward a mouse, and dove headfirst into the bluish-green curl of a huge, incoming wave.

That simple dive would change the rest of my life, and make possible this reference book.

I felt the cold, refreshing splash of salty ocean slap my face as I entered the water—and then I heard a "snap." Regardless of the large appearance of that wave, I had apparently dived the 15 vertical feet downward into a 5-foot depth of low tide. My forehead hit the sandy ocean floor, my neck snapped at the C-5/6 level, and my body was instantly and painlessly paralyzed below the level of my broken neck.

A surfer saw me floating face-down and pulled me from the water before I had used my initial deep breath of air. Still very conscious and cracking jokes, probably as a defense against my body's traumatic state of shock, I was eventually flown by air ambulance to Massachusetts General Hospital in Boston.

As I felt the small plane touch down on the big city runway, I sensed that my new lifestyle had just begun.

My acute care at MGH began with 10-1/2 hours of cervical fusion surgery, followed by several weeks of lying prone on a Stryker frame with a 35-pound cervical traction anchored to my skull.

My widowed mother temporarily left her upstate New York home and moved into a summer sublet among "all those '60s hippies" on Boston's Beacon Hill. With the patience only mothers have, her daily stays at my hospital bedside began the essential psychological support that my adjustment required. It was the closest time that my mother and I had or would spend together. Thank you, Mother, I love you.

My medical situation stabilized after two and one-half months, and I was then transferred to the Sunnyview Hospital in upstate New York for an additional eleven months of rehabilitation.

I was then, and remain, paralyzed below the chest with neither motor control nor sensation. Medically, I am classified a quadriplegic or tetraplegic, because all four limbs are partially or totally affected. Typical of other "quads," I have partial use of my wrists and arms but no finger movement.

This situation may sound depressing to able-bodied folks, but I discovered early on that I could minimize depression simply by minimizing thoughts about my inabilities. Perhaps when carried to an extreme this is classic denial; however, I quickly learned to avoid teasing myself with wanting to do things that were beyond my new set of abilities.

Instead, I learned to concentrate on my abilities, set some realistic goals, and get back on life's track. The first step was to learn all I could about living as independently as possible from my cabinet of rehabilitation advisors at the hospital.

As with so many types of physical disabilities, the objective of my inpatient rehabilitation was not a "cure" or return to able-bodiedness. Instead, it meant receiving authoritative advice from highly trained medical professionals on making the most of my remaining physical abilities. Surgeons, rehab physicians, nurses, aides, physical and occupational therapists, social workers, and psychologists each had separate areas of expertise for training people with various disabilities in accommodating their limitations. Over the next few months, I tapped these specialists for all the rehab skills they could offer me.

As I progressed through the specialists, I noticed one serious void that no one could address in much detail—even now, more than 30 years later.

I realized that most people who have significant physical disabilities will require routine physical assistance from others to accomplish daily activities. Some folks will require very little help; some will need a lot. According to the duration of the disability, the need for help might be temporary or lifelong. For me, these activities include the assistance I need with activities of daily living (ADL), household upkeep, and pursuing goals of education, career, recreation, leisure, and even sex while living life to its fullest.

The state of the art for learning help provider management skills then was much what it is today. Few health professionals or reference texts adequately address how help recipients with a disability should best manage their aides who provide that physical assistance. Most "aide/nursing" books in bookstores teach methods for performing nursing procedures to the attendants or aides who provide the help. Others coach loving family caregivers in how to cope with and maintain their own emotional and physical health while providing unending assistance to a family member. In contrast, very few teach the person who receives help how to manage the quality of that help while working harmoniously with the providers.

If you require help from others, you are indeed the owner and president of a lifelong small business. When you find, hire, train, and manage the paid aides (here called "personal assistants" or "PAs") who fulfill your needs for routine help, you are operating your own small business. When family caregivers provide your help, your management concerns shift from employment to human relations.

Unlike your other career or job, if your PA business goes into a slump or you get tired of managing it, you cannot choose to change careers or go out of business. You have no choice with this one. Your dependence on physical help from others is as lifelong and permanent as your disability. Your PA business must always be a thriving and smashing success.

It is easy to see the parallels between a traditional business and one in which you manage PAs. Let's say you have designed a better mouse trap and want to market it. A brief listing of the steps to launching this small business would include:

- *Identifying and describing your customer*
  Who will be interested in buying your mouse traps?

- *Deciding where to advertise the traps*
  Which newspapers, magazines, posters, or notices are read by people who have rodent problems?

- *Deciding how to advertise*
  What benefits do "moused" people want from your traps, and how should advertisements be worded to attract customers?

- *Planning the step-by-step procedure for responding to customer inquiries*
  How will you describe how your mouse trap works? How do you suggest that the caller needs a dozen of them? How do you arrange for the caller to see a demonstration of your trap?

- *Making decisions about improving your efficiency*
  How can the advertising be improved to save money while increasing inquiries? How can your overall procedures be improved to increase sales and do it better next time?

- *Developing guidelines on keeping your customers happy*
  How do you show them appreciation so they will stay with you, buy more mouse traps, and recommend you to future customers?

It is interesting that these steps can sound so very MBA, businesslike, logical, and based in common sense. Now, let's look at highlights for finding and hiring the PAs whom you routinely use:

- *Identifying and describing your customers (the PAs)*
  Who, in your community, will be interested in providing you with assistance?

- *Deciding where to advertise your PA positions*
  Which newspapers, magazines, posters, or notices are read by people who like to help others?

- *Deciding how to advertise*
  What benefits do "helping people" want from your position, and how should advertisements be worded to attract your future PAs (customers)?

- *Planning the step-by-step procedure for responding to customer inquiries*
  How will you describe the duties of your position? How do you suggest that the caller would enjoy working with you? How do you arrange for the caller to see a demonstration of your routine while checking applicant references?

- *Making decisions about improving your efficiency*
  How can the advertising be improved to save money while increasing inquiries? How can your overall procedures be improved to increase successful recruiting (sales) and do it better next time?

- *Developing guidelines on keeping your PAs (customers) happy*
  How do you show them appreciation so they will stay with you, continue to provide you with quality help, and recommend you to future customers?

See—you *do* run a business!

If that sounds pretty serious, it is. Because your PA business cannot be allowed to fail, it should be operated as efficiently and cost-effectively as possible.

Hospitals and rehab centers have traditionally assumed that the patient will live primarily at home, and that caregiver-relatives will be the main source of personal assistance. If not family caregivers, it is assumed that home health aide agencies will provide plenty of employed and well-trained aides. In a third instance, rehab centers hope that their most motivated patients, who want to move away from home and into the public mainstream, will also be sufficiently motivated to figure out for themselves how to employ help directly.

In truth, even today's most dedicated rehab staff usually lacks the knowledge and resources for adequately teaching of comprehensive PA management skills. This situation has traditionally represented a serious void in the educational services they should be providing to their most motivated patients in preparing them for discharge.

The good news is that more and more of today's progressive rehab centers are at least providing pamphlets that introduce patients to basic resources for finding help providers. Some of these centers offer occasional lectures on the subject presented by social workers or experienced help recipients.

Disability-related magazines often offer one or two articles annually that outline common problems encountered by family caregivers and help recipients. In most articles, a series of introductory problem scenarios is somewhat answered by remedies and preventions that have been compiled by interviewing several experienced help recipients. Editorial letters also occasionally appear from readers who want to share a few beneficial PA management tips they have devised. Within the last 10 years, a handful of helpful guidebooks and references have been written by social workers, caregivers, and help recipients. These guides typically address the basics about placing newspaper ads, interviewing applicants, training new PAs, and paying them.

This gradual development of expertise for ADL-dependent people to learn PA management skills is a step in the right direction.

If asked to describe their most depressing nightmare, most people with disabilities would cite their impression—or, indeed, actual experiences—of daily life in a nursing home. The nightmare portrays a daily lifestyle where the quality of one's personal life is the consequence of a poorly planned, sloppily administered, understaffed, and underbudgeted residence situation. The clients' human needs are neglected—and their optimism and spirit are forsaken—as they submit to the decisions, schedules, and limitations imposed on them by the institution.

This depressing nightmare is, unfortunately, reality in many of today's residential health care facilities. It is common to receive a poor quality of assistance, provided on an undependable schedule, by uncaring or abusive providers. This frequently happens when an incompetent administrative staff half-heartedly hires uncaring providers who do not want to be providing assistance and should not ethically be doing so.

To be active and to maximize independence, you—or a trusted family representative—must be in control of the quality, type, and scheduling of help that you receive. If you are not in control of these factors and working in harmony with the people who provide assistance, then you have lost the freedom to choose your own lifestyle. To lose personal freedom is much worse than merely losing independence—it is losing one's spirit and soul!

Rehabilitation centers and patients with dependent ADL needs should both be placing the same importance on teaching and learning PA management skills as they now do about other self-care topics. As soon as a patient who is likely to have dependent needs after discharge is identified, the rehab staff should begin teaching these skills and encouraging the motivation that fuels a person's insistence on learning and using them. At this early stage—and not merely during the final days before discharge—the staff should be coaching patients toward being self-sufficient in their own PA management. Indeed, some model facilities are selecting patients and making them responsible for recruiting, hiring, training, and managing their own providers while they are still inpatients.

In addition to medical facilities providing this instruction in PA management skills, they should be advocating for changes in the way PA funding is provided. . Ironically, it is now easier to acquire funding for the expensive and less desirable life inside a *nursing home* than for the much lower cost of hiring help providers who are used in one's *own home.*

When funding is available for using help providers, the source usually stipulates that the providers must be selected, provided, and supervised by an approved health care agency. Funded clients are less frequently permitted to personally employ their own PAs. This requirement of using only agency aides is a significant impediment to help recipients who want to control both who provides them with help and the quality of help they receive.

Additionally, as this reference will show, the cost of agency help is usually two or three times the cost of personally employed help!

As you will see throughout this comprehensive reference, management skills are essential regardless of which of the three provider resources are used: family caregivers, agency aides, or personally employed PAs. Even if you use trained, agency aides, it will be you—and not an agency supervisor—who must know and routinely use skills for instructing, supervising, and keeping happy those aides who are meeting your unique needs. You—the help recipient—will be instructing, managing, and providing feedback each day to the provider who assists you. The two of you will seldom see an agency supervisor more than once each month.

If your disability requires you to use help from others, and you want to be as independent and in the public mainstream as possible, then you should have the skills for independently managing those help providers. You should be able to recruit quality help providers whenever and wherever you need them and use ongoing management skills to keep them for as long as possible.

Throughout your lifetime, you will be using the RISHTMP cycle two, three, or more times each year to get the help you need. *RISHTMP*, a term coined in this book, stands for recruiting, interviewing, screening, hiring, training, managing, and parting ways with the aides you use.

As mentioned, routine implementation of this management cycle is perhaps the most important small business skill that you will ever master. You cannot allow your PA business to fail, and efficiently operating it requires as much technical knowledge as does a traditional small business.

For more than 30 years now, I have hired and managed the attendants and aides who help me. My ability to hire and use help in a wide variety of settings has enabled me to enjoy a life rich in education, careers, and travel, even though I remain 80 percent paralyzed.

The foundation for all of these freedoms has been my ability—and insistence—to personally manage the people who provide me with physical assistance. From 30-plus years of experience, there is absolutely no doubt in my mind that if I were to lose control of the quality of assistance I receive—as well as the quality of people who provide that assistance—I would lose control of my lifestyle, quality of health, optimism, spirit, and perhaps my sanity.

I propose that if you are dependent on assistance from others, one of your most important life-sustaining skills is the ability to select and manage your *help providers*, as well as the quality of their *assistance*.

This comprehensive, indexed reference will enable you—as a person who uses physical help, or a family caregiver who coordinates it for a loved one—to work in harmony and mutual respect with help providers, while also being in control of the help they provide. Consequently, you can safeguard your personal freedom and be active in your chosen lifestyle.

Thousands of people in many countries have maintained control of their disability, lifestyle, and personal spirit through the management techniques in this book and its previous editions. These strategies have worked for me, for those people, and they should work for *you!*

Alfred H. "Skip" DeGraff

Dedications

This book was made possible, in part, by my experiences with family caregivers and personally employed aides.

To Peggy, my former wife: For more than 15 years, you provided me with some of the most responsible and dependable help I have known. You moved out because my need for help had consumed your living space, privacy, personal life, and finally your spirit. Please be assured that your personal pain and sacrifices were neither unnoticed nor forgotten. This reference provides detailed strategies for avoiding caregiver burnout by reserving family members for their unique love, caring, and support. How I wish this book had been available 20 years ago when we desperately needed it.

To my personally employed PAs: Throughout these 30-plus years, each of you has taught me something about being a better manager. I have learned from strategies that worked well and from those that failed. I am grateful for the help you gave me and the skills you taught me. If you spot your first name used in this text's "how-to" discussions, know that a skill you taught me is now being shared with thousands of help recipients and providers throughout the world!

Publishing History and Acknowledgments

My first, 38-page book on this topic, *Attendants and Attendees: A Guidebook of Helpful Hints*, was published in 1979 by the College and University Personnel Association, Washington, DC. I am grateful for the assistance of Carole Sturgis and Janet Long, formerly consultants to CUPA, for their assistance with that publication. At that time, I was the Director of the Department of Disabled Student Services at Boston University.

The second, 350-page edition, *Home Health Aides: Managing the People Who Help You*, was published by my company, Saratoga Access Publications. I appreciated the assistance of my former wife, Margaret Short DeGraff, Ph.D., OTR.

This third, 512-page edition is being published in 2002, this time in Fort Collins, Colorado. My appreciation goes to Shannon Bodie and Gaelyn Larrick of Lightbourne Images, for cover design; to Brooke Graves of Graves Editorial Service, for copy editing and indexing; to Greg and Lisa Greisen of Grandin Graphic Design, for typesetting and formatting; and to Joseph W. Reid of Reid Communications, for editing.

The author is also appreciative of these authorities who provided content reviews and encouragement: Anita L. Abrams, Connie Arnold, Sarah Babbitt, Mark Beck, Micki and Rick McMillan-Blacker, Cliff Bridges, Anita Bundy, Josie Byzek, Susan Charlifue, Steve Collins, Barry Corbet, Shirley L. DeGraff, Darrel Tom Eagan, Tony Fabriello, Fred Fay, Joe Flemming, Betty Garee, Kenneth A. Gerhart, Mickey Ginsburg, Millie and Clark Gittinger, Lori Hinderer, Richard Holicky, Ricky Hoyt, Dave Hudson, Marge Kolstad, Don Krebs, Bob Mackle, Wanda Mayberry, Sally Mather and Greg Mihalik, Suzanne Mintz, Joan Munson, Linda Norton, Kevin and Ken Oltjenbrums, Sherry Peterson, Pops and Woofy, Rick Rader, Diane and Hannah Rehner, Carol Ritchie, Evelyn Rosen-Budd, Jehanne Schweitzer, Peggy Short, Rob Sireno, Carol Sowell, Carol Sturgis, Tina Tapply, Margaret Tarter, Elaine Tillman, Carolyn Wojcik, and Kenneth Yoder.

Statement of Lack of Gender Bias

Statistically, the population of family caregivers as well as paid help providers is predominately female, whereas help recipients are mostly male. However, throughout this text, I have attempted to prevent gender bias by using gender nouns, pronouns, and possessives randomly and with approximately equal frequency.

Introduction

Why This Reference is Important to You: Your Freedom and Control

You have the right to maintain control over your own lifestyle and daily schedule—your quality of life. You enjoy and hold sacred the freedom of doing what you wish, when you wish. You recognize that your disability has imposed some limitations on this freedom; however, you strive each day to enjoy life to its fullest—to seize the day (*carpe diem*).

This means avoiding situations where you might lose this freedom. You carefully guard your health and minimize the chances of losing it to illness. Your mobility aid and other special equipment, on which you are very dependent, are carefully maintained to prevent unnecessary breakdowns. You protect your possessions against loss, theft, and other violations. You learn to be assertive and state your opinions and needs, and avoid being passive to prevent others from making decisions for you. You also prefer to choose the people who affect your life, and avoid those who negatively affect it or whom you do not trust. In short, the quality of your daily lifestyle is maximized when you are in control of making choices.

When you have a temporary or long-term disability, you often require physical assistance from others. When this happens, you must be in control of the quality of person who provides the assistance as well as the quality of assistance you receive. These are additional factors that contribute to your quality of life.

Not having control over who provides the assistance can result in working with people who arrive on an undependable schedule, whom you dislike or do not trust, or who might violate you or your possessions. In addition, you might be assigned an aide who is chronically angry and has a bad attitude for personal reasons that have nothing to do with you (even though you might assume so). As a result, you might not look forward to the daily arrival of certain aides, because they do not want to be providing you with the help you need.

Losing control over the quality of assistance can also result in having someone refuse to provide that assistance by the methods you prefer. The PA might also dictate which of your needs he/she prefers to assist, leaving other needs unfulfilled. In a third example, the PA might ignore your daily time schedule of when you need help, and instead arrive for work when he/she feels like it. Consequently, you are unable to participate in the career, education, or leisure activities that are important to your lifestyle.

Whether you get outside help from an agency or you personally employ your own, you need management skills to work in harmony with those providers while controlling the quality of their help.

Outside of using family caregivers, paid providers can be acquired through an agency or found by personally employing your own PAs. Some people would like to believe that when one contracts with an agency, the aides who are assigned will be thoroughly experienced and trained. Some believe that agency aides will arrive on the first day and know exactly what a specific client needs, as well as how and on what schedule the help should be supplied.

Computers can be programmed; health aides cannot be. Whether the aides come from your efforts or an agency's, they will arrive that first day and make the same request, "Please tell me what help you need, as well as how and when you need it."

> *If you are not making the decisions about who helps you and the quality of help they provide you, then someone else is making those decisions—and you have lost control over your own lifestyle.*

The person that can provide this detailed information is not the agency supervisor who has spoken briefly with you to list your primary needs. Instead, the extra details and day-to-day monitoring must come from you or your representative. Regardless of whether the aide has formal training, you are the only person who can express your individual needs and provide ongoing feedback and evaluation. So, regardless of the source of your aides, you should have adequate skills for managing them.

From that first day, if you cannot make the decisions and provide the aides with details of the what, how, and when for your needs of help, they will have no choice but to make those decisions for you. If you cannot manage the help that you need to maintain your chosen lifestyle, the aides will begin to manage your lifestyle by choices that they make.

It is a very simple, but powerful fact that if you are not in control of the help you receive, and consequently your own lifestyle, then someone else will take advantage of that control. At the point when someone else takes control of your lifestyle, you have lost your personal freedom. This can promote a conflict-of-interest situation between you and your controlling aides. The fox is now in charge of the henhouse!

Can this actually happen? Ask the residents of many nursing homes whether they believe they are in control of their daily lifestyle and have the freedom of doing what they want, how and when they want to.

Why is this book so important to you?

- If you have a disability that requires you to get assistance from others, this reference will empower you to be in control of both the quality of people who provide help and the quality of help they provide. You will know how to find quality help—where and when you need it—and how to keep it longer. You can live where you wish, how you wish, and either alone or with whom you wish—*as you wish!*

- If you are a family caregiver, and you are overworked and perhaps depressed, you will be better able to find relief or replacement help so that you can regain your own freedom of lifestyle and health.

- If you are experiencing a progressing disability or age, and worry about having to leave your home for a care facility, you will learn how to manage help providers while still at home, to delay or avoid relocating.

- If you are a professional, paid help provider, you will be better able to understand the concerns of help recipients, family caregivers, and supervisors—and both you and they will also better understand yours.

- If you are the administrator for an agency or health care facility that provides nurses and home health aides, you will be able to improve your recruitment and retention programs so that you can enlarge your staff, manage it more efficiently, screen out poor quality or abusive providers, and keep the quality providers longer.

- If you are a counselor, therapist, or instructor who instructs others in managing help providers, you will have a comprehensive, authoritative, and easy-to-use reference for your one-on-one and classroom needs.

This reference offers you the help-management skills you need.[1]

---

1.   For an annotated tour of this book's parts and chapters, please see
📖 "A Tour of How to Use This Reference."

Definitions of Titles and Terms Used in This Reference

- **You**
- **Caregiver, Personal Assistant (PA), Aide, and Other Providers**
- **Activities of Daily Living (ADLs)**
- **The RISHTMP Cycle**
- **Disability, Handicap, Impairment, Challenge, Gimp, Crip, Invalid, and Other Terms**

You

Throughout this reference, I have usually addressed the reader as *you*. Of more importance is that I have intentionally meant this person to be the recipient of help.

There are several reasons for this. First, this reference has been written by a help recipient for the ultimate benefit of other recipients. Use of the phrase "ultimate benefit" is meant to note that many readers will be representatives of recipients, such as family caregivers or a health care agency.

The primary objective for this reference is to offer strategies to help recipients for working in harmony with help providers. It is my hope that learning provider management skills will also enhance empowerment and independence.

The premise that has served as the ethical foundation for this reference is that help recipients should be directly managing and in control of both who helps them as well as the consequent quality of the help they receive. For people who are dependent on assistance from others, having direct authority in decisions about the quality of their providers and assistance enables them to maintain the quality of their health, lifestyle, and optimism.

Recipients should be making as many of these decisions as they are willing and able to make. If willing and able to be managers, they will require the management skills that enable them to do so. This means they either have been able to research and acquire the skills on their own, or have been taught adequate skills by rehabilitation professionals. This text is worthy of serving as the reference for either situation.

With these philosophies in mind, it should be clear why I have intentionally addressed help recipients throughout this reference. It is because the quality of their health and lifestyle is a consequence of the quality of their providers and assistance, that giving them first option on managing these factors becomes an ethical issue.

If recipients are unwilling or unable to manage, the family usually should be offered the second option for representing their interests. When the family also is unwilling or unable to manage, a health care agency or facility is the third choice.

In these situations where recipients are not the direct, daily manager, they next should be offered as much of an advisory role as possible. Their representatives will use the recipient's preferences, on issues ranging from daily lifestyle to dying and death, as guidelines in making daily decisions on their behalf. When representatives act on behalf of recipients in using this text, they become the party addressed by the author.

It is because of these ethical objectives of maintaining help recipients as either the direct or indirect manager of their providers and quality of help, that the *you* throughout most of this text appropriately refers directly or indirectly to help recipients!

Caregiver, Personal Assistant (PA), Aide, and Other Providers

Historically, household help providers were initially *attendants*. To *attend* was "to care for, to take care of, to wait on and serve," as a nurse *attending* a patient. The assistant to a nurse or physician was (and is today) an *aide*. This was the era of the medical model, when the people needing such help were *patients* whose role was to be sick, unable, passive, obedient, and *patient* to the unquestioned directives from medical authorities.

As the conservative medical model waned, *patients* became *clients* and *consumers* who stopped being passive and began making their own decisions about medical treatments and mainstreamed lifestyle. Advanced medical technologies enabled people with disabilities to survive initial traumas and get into the mainstream. In the 1960s, paraplegics and quadriplegics (tetraplegics) were among those with disabilities who started to appear on college campuses in more durable manual wheelchairs, as well as in the first motorized wheelchairs.

Ed Roberts, one of the first quads to have attended college classes in a wheelchair and a founder of the Berkeley Center for Independent Living (BCIL), began using the term *PCA* to mean *personal care assistant, attendant,* or *aide.*

More recently, *caregiver* has been adopted by most consumers, the media, and society to denote a help provider. This term is especially prevalent because, according to the National Family Caregivers Association (NFCA), more than one quarter (26.6%) of the adult population has provided care for a chronically ill, disabled, or aged family member or friend during the past year (1999–2000). Based on current census data, that translates into more than 54 million family caregivers. These unpaid providers, usually spouses, relatives, or close friends to a help recipient, provide about 90 percent of all long-term care services. These volunteer services are worth an estimated $196 billion a year.

According to the NFCA, a *primary* caregiver is a recipient's main source of direct help, as well as the coordinator of unpaid or paid help from others. In addition to *family* caregivers, who provide the traditional help within a household, there are *long-distance* caregivers who provide support and coordinate services for loved ones who live many miles away.

Suzanne Mintz, a family caregiver and the president and co-founder of the NFCA, notes that society has unfortunately developed the habit of referring to *formal* and *informal* caregivers. Formal caregivers are usually paid for their services, and the term has been used collectively to refer to nurses, home health aides, therapists, and even ministers. The implication of *formal* is that these are trained professionals. Informal caregivers are the family providers who provide the long daily hours of comprehensive help from their sense of caring, love, support, and duty. Mintz views the label as demeaning, as there is nothing informal about the extensive responsibilities that *caregivers* or *family caregivers* (the terms that she prefers) unselfishly assume.

> *For ease of readership throughout this reference, the two main categories of help providers will be termed—*
>
> <u>*Caregiver*</u> *or* <u>*family caregiver*</u>
> *= Unsalaried, volunteer help providers from within or close to a recipient's family*
>
> <u>*Aide*</u> *or* <u>*PA*</u> *(personal assistant, aide, or attendant)*
> *= Paid help providers from the outside community, obtained through agency or personal employment*

Indeed, as a help recipient for many years, I have found few—if any—paid help providers to be as comprehensively skilled, and willing to work the long hours, as a typical family caregiver.

In some other cultural circles, the term *PCA* (personal care assistant, attendant, or aide) has been revised to be *PSA* (for "personal service…") or, more simply, *PA* (for "personal…"). By the way, the actual *services* performed by a personal assistant are sometimes termed *personal service assistance (PSA)* or *personal assistance services (PAS)*.

In parts of today's politically correct society, this replacement of PCA with PSA or PA has become popular with some people who wish to avoid the image of being "cared for."

So, in millions of families, there are caregivers and help recipients who enjoy the comforting concept of providing care and being cared for. Other people, in other lifestyles, enjoy their image of personal independence and empowerment, and prefer to avoid the concept of receiving care.

The primary reader, to whom most of this text is addressed, is the help recipient. However, this reference is intended to empower both recipients and providers of help to be in maximum control of their desired lifestyle.

Regardless of personal agreement or disagreement with any of these philosophies or political viewpoints, the author respects each concern. Indeed, regardless of terminology, this reference is intended to teach skills of independent living and to empower people—both providers and recipients of help—to control their own lifestyles.

With respect to both philosophies, the terms *caregiver* and *family caregiver* will be used when reference is made to unsalaried, family providers. The terms *PA*, *aide*, or *assistant* will refer to the paid providers from the outside community who are obtained through agency or personal employment. The terms within each of the two categories will be used interchangeably in the interest of variety, brevity, clarity, and ease to readers.

Occasionally, additional terms will be used in reference to other types of paid help and service providers:

- Physician's Assistant (PA), Nurse Practitioner (NP), Registered Nurse (RN), or Licensed Practical Nurse (LPN)
- Medical technologists (techs)
- Certified nursing assistant/aide (CNA)
- Home health aide
- Personal assistant/attendant/aide (PA)
- Personal service assistant/attendant/aide (PSA)
- Personal care assistant/attendant/aide (PCA)
- Companion, Personal Companion (PC), or Personal Care Provider (PCP)
- Homemaker
- Household maintenance provider
- Housekeeper
- Transportation driver
- Domestic cook

Activities of Daily Living (ADLs)

As the primary reader for whom this reference is written, you typically have some type of disability that requires you to receive help from others. Your specific disability is one or more of the wide variety known and unknown to medical circles. Consequent to the type and extent of your disability, your current or upcoming need for help might be quite light or extensive. Unfortunately, with few exceptions, your dependence on help from others will probably only increase in the future.

Additionally, you probably need several kinds of help. Although a variety of kinds of help are discussed throughout this book, one is primary.

Your primary help need is for your routine, day-after-day *activities of daily living*, or ADLs. Included in this most inner circle is assistance with some or all of the following:

- Urinary collection device or self-catheterization supplies
- Bowel program
- Bathing or showering
- Getting dressed and undressed
- Transfers among bed, wheelchair, commode chair, car
- Food preparation and eating

- Taking medication
- Wound care

These are the hard-core needs for which you require hard-core, rock-solid, dependable, and continuous help providers. Volunteer help is essential for many needs, but usually not appropriate for ADLs. This help will come from family caregivers, agency-employed aides, or personally employed aides.

The RISHTMP Cycle

This is the seven-part process that you will go through with each new aide or group of aides. RISHTMP is my acronym for the steps of recruiting, interviewing, screening, hiring, training, managing, and parting ways with the providers who help you.

If you use agency-employed aides, you will be *recruiting, interviewing, screening,* and *hiring* the agency that supplies your aides. You will then be *training, managing,* and *parting ways* with each of those aides. If you personally employ your own aides, or PAs, you will be going through all seven steps directly with your aide applicants and employees.

Disability, Handicap, Impairment, Challenge, Gimp, Crip, Invalid, and Other Terms

Ah, the evolution of what we call ourselves—and what others call us! This continues to be simultaneously empowering and degrading, albeit usually amusing.

I have attended many week-long conferences about disability-related topics. It is common for the hotel that hosts such a conference to perform special, advance planning for best accommodating the special needs of that week's large population of guests with a variety of impairments.

A focal point for such planning is always within the restaurant and dining areas. Some hotels do strategic planning around seating, and find innovative ways of providing wheelchair seating at dining tables that respects both the wheelchair users and other forms of traffic flow.

As my former wife and I approached a restaurant entrance at one conference, we waited obediently at the reception desk to be seated. The wait staff asked for the number in our party, whether we wanted the smoking or non-smoking area, and then casually pressed a key on her computer keyboard before disappearing for a moment to arrange table space for my wheelchair.

While we briefly waited at the reception desk, I glanced at the computer screen. It was blank, except for two words: INVALID ENTRY.

This was the early '80s, before typical computer terms were commonly known. To most of us today, the computer term *invalid entry* simply means that some keyboard character that has been entered is inappropriate and not understood by the software.

However for me in 1980, the Macintosh had not yet been born. I saw the screen-displayed term INVALID ENTRY and was both impressed and a bit insulted. I gestured to Peggy, and said, "Look, this hotel apparently has a very sophisticated seating system. When you and I approached the wait staff, a special command must have been entered to indicate to the staff where we could best be seated. However, I think it is unfortunate that some insensitive software programmer decided to refer to a person with disability as an *invalid!*"

Indeed, entire books have been written about respectful, politically correct ways to refer to people who happen to have an impairment—or instead, should I be saying, "who are not able-bodied" (commonly abbreviated as *ABs*)?

I have spent many years in traveling around the country, lecturing on a wide variety of disability-related topics. Soon after arriving in yet another lecture city, I would often speak with some local people who had disabilities to ask about their locale's acceptable and unacceptable disability-related terminology. During my initial years of performing this ongoing sociological survey, I had the naive expectation of mapping out the country with locale-by-locale symbols of the good and bad terms for each area. After two or three years, I gave up. I found too many variables, often among different social, economic, and educational cultures within the same city.

Without engaging in a chapter-long justification for my choices, I will be using the following terms interchangeably throughout this reference. If my selections offend you, the reader, please accept my apology. However, at the same time, I urge all readers to become less sensitive; concentrating on differences in terminology can both divide us and waste our collective energy and time. Instead, please join me focusing energy on the objectives that we have in common in this reference— becoming more empowered, more in control, and more independent by learning to manage the people who provide us with the help we require.

When people refer to you with a less-preferred term, before you get angry or correct their usage, perhaps ask yourself:

- Whether the term was used intentionally to offend you, or merely out of ignorance, and
- Whether your correcting those persons will result in their becoming more educated and appreciated, or in their feeling even more uncomfortable in the future when they encounter someone with a disability.

Here are the terms I have selected for use throughout this reference:

- Disability or impairment
- Person with a disability or impairment; the second-choice usage is disabled person
- Able-bodied person (also *AB*, or *A-B person*)

Two Types of Assistance Providers: Unpaid and Paid

There are several types of people who can provide you assistance. Your situation of personal needs and available finances will determine which type of provider or combination you will use. The primary factor that categorizes these people is whether they are unpaid or paid.

Unpaid Providers

Unpaid providers include family caregivers, most respite and day-care help, and volunteers. The term *caregiver* originally referred primarily to spouses, relatives, and close friends who provide a loved one with unpaid, extensive assistance. Additionally, the media and society have found the term to be handy as a collective descriptor that can be expanded to include most types of providers.

Respite help refers to temporary relief assistance intended to give routine caregivers time off to fulfill their own personal and private needs. The majority of respite help is unpaid; however, there is a growing population of commercially available respite services and centers.

Volunteer help comes from formally organized groups as well as individual good Samaritans. Almost every community has organizations of volunteers who are the backbone and foundation of community-wide projects, as well as help providers to meet brief needs of individuals. In helping individuals, they provide a wide variety of services, including the brief, one-shot, informal help often provided by strangers while one is out in the public mainstream. These are the people who hold open doors, pick up a package dropped in a shopping mall, or stop to change your flat tire.[1]

Paid Providers

Paid providers come from two primary sources. They are employed either by the person receiving help or by some type of agency. Many people who have used assistance on a long-term basis have directly recruited, interviewed, screened, trained, terminated, and paid each aide. Regardless of whether personal or outside funding covers the salaries, in this case the recipient of help has been fully in charge as the supervisor and employer.

---

1. For more detail and cautions on how to use volunteer help appropriately, please see chapter 2, "Volunteer Help: Don't Wear Out Your Friendships."

In other situations, an agency employs the aides. Its representative meets with you to assess your needs, and then schedules its aides to provide you assistance. Commercially, the employing agency could be a health care facility, a home health aide firm, or an employment service. In addition, the agency could be a branch of a state, county, or city government.

It is equally common for a help recipient to use just one type of assistance or a combination of several types.

> *Most people use a combination of different types of unpaid and paid providers.*

Three Examples

Joe experienced a stroke after retirement at the age of 67. He comes from a tightly knit group of loving family and friends. His wife insists on being his primary, unpaid caregiver. Other family members take on supplementary caregiver duties to spell Joe's wife. Nearby friends from a church group chip in with respite relief, and offer afternoon or evening companionship to Joe while family members take a break.

In contrast, Sally received a spinal cord injury during a skiing accident when she was 19. Consequently, she is a quadriplegic, with paralyzed arms and legs, and uses a motorized wheelchair. When she initially came home from a seven-month rehab hospital stay, her assistance came from caregivers in her family. Because her disability is traditionally considered long-term, and Sally saw her family caregivers showing signs of chronic fatigue, she decided to supplement the family help by hiring some outsiders.

Sally was not eligible for outside funding, and all attendant expenses came from her pocket. Consequently, she decided to save the extra expense of agency fees by directly hiring her own help.

It is now 29 years later, and Sally has earned three college degrees, lived in several cities for several professional careers, traveled extensively, and now lives with her husband in a purchased home. To accommodate her very active lifestyle, she uses several types of providers. She keeps her romantic life as separate as possible from her disability needs. Her husband rarely provides unpaid caregiver help; 99 percent of her needs are accommodated by a team of four directly paid, personal assistants (PAs) who are local college students. One PA lives in an in-law cottage next to the house; this PA lives rent-free in exchange for providing half of Sally's help. The other three PAs are not live-ins, and help her on a salaried basis. In addition, she is dependent on volunteer help.

As examples of the brief help from volunteers, a co-worker sometimes helps Sally carry a stack of reports to the corporation board meetings she chairs; a parking lot attendant recently picked up the car keys she dropped in the snow outside a dinner restaurant; cashiers are routinely glad to carry her groceries or dry cleaning to her car.

In a third example, Margaret was recently in a car accident at the age of 46. She broke the radius of her right arm and the femur of her left leg. Upon discharge from the hospital, she required several weeks of home-based assistance for her activities of daily living (ADL). Her insurance company required that she used certified home health aides. Consequently, the hospital's discharge office lined up Margaret with a local home health aide agency. The agency employs, schedules, and trains the aides she will use for the next two months.

To summarize: Joe uses only caregiver and respite help. Sally's different lifestyle requires an occasional pinch of caregiver, liberal doses of directly employed PAs, and a sprinkling of volunteer help. Margaret uses only agency-supplied home health aides.

Regardless of the types of help Joe, Sally, and Margaret use, each of them has benefited from the strategies of this reference. Regardless of whether help comes from family caregivers, untrained college students, or certified home health aides, the provider always greets Joe, Sally, or Margaret on initially meeting them and says, "Hi, I'm glad to help you if you will simply tell me what you need done and how to do it."[2]

---

2. For more detail about the pros and cons of using unpaid and paid help, as well as whether to use hired help from agencies or personal employment, please see chapter 📖 1, **"Beyond Family Caregivers: Options and Settings for Finding Outside Assistance."**

A Tour of How to Use This Reference

This handbook has been designed to teach you, the person receiving assistance (or your personal representative, often a family caregiver), the skills required to manage the people who provide you (or your loved one) with assistance. It differs from other books that instead teach nursing techniques to help providers. This reference is jam-packed with strategies that have worked for me and for many, many others—they should also work for *you!*

For your convenience, this reference is divided into eight easy-to-use parts, and each part contains three, four, or five specialized chapters. After reviewing the discussions of this chapter, you might want your next stop to be **"Your Quick Start Guide—Five Topics to Get You Going Today!"**

Part I *Identifying Your Options for Assistance*

The chapters in Part I introduce you to types, sources, and settings for help providers that are typically available outside of the home. The options and settings for finding paid providers will be of as much interest to family caregivers who need relief or replacement as they will be to help recipients. Using volunteer help in appropriate ways from valid sources is essential; however, when it is used inappropriately it can quickly kill long-standing friendships. Live-in aides can actually be a free source of very dependable help, and another chapter tells you how that works. The last chapter on settings provides tips on using providers anywhere outside the home, from day trips within the community to residence on a college campus.

📖 1 **Beyond Family Caregivers:**
Options and Settings for Finding Outside Assistance
Your family caregivers might need relief or replacement help to relieve their chronic fatigue. You—and this reference—can help them by knowing the options for finding the additional assistance you need: at your home (agency-employed aides or personally employed PAs), within the community (respite day care or weekend relief), or at a community residence facility (independent or assisted living center, or nursing home).

📖 2 **Volunteer Help: Don't Wear Out Your Friendships**
On the one hand, your use of help from volunteers is probably essential to your everyday independence. On the other hand, you can easily see when your request for a favor is no longer welcome, or when some of your more extensive needs are exceeding the volunteers' intentions. When, where, and from whom is it okay to ask for favors; when is it not; and when does federal law actually require volunteers to help you?

📖 3   **Live-In Aides and Other Residence Options**

Live-in aides can benefit your safety, security, and budget. In sharp contrast, they can also threaten your safety, steal your possessions, and become an inescapable nightmare. You will find out how live-ins can provide you with free help, and how to evict them when their help is no longer wanted. For aides that live nearby, those who live closest to you often will be the most reliable, dependable, and punctual. Residence options are outlined to give you ideas about increasing the odds that your PA will be at your door at six o'clock sharp tomorrow morning.

📖 4   **Settings Where You Use Help**

You are familiar with using help providers at home, but your daily lifestyle probably brings you to many additional places. Learn how to use help for community meetings, appointments, and errands; for overnight business travel or vacations; and at college campuses. Special strategies are also outlined for making sure that the staff at hospitals, rehab centers, and residential living facilities provide you with adequate help in ways that accommodate *your* needs, not only theirs.

Part II *Three Ten-Step Plans for Getting the Help You Need*

Part II is the nucleus of this reference. These three ten-step plans address the three primary sources for help providers, with a specialized game plan for pursuing each one. Most recipients combine at least two sources to accommodate their variety of needs.

📖 5   **Ten Steps to Getting All or Some of Your Help from Family Caregivers**

📖 6   **Ten Steps to Getting All or Some of Your Help from Agency-Employed Aides**

📖 7   **Ten Steps to Getting All or Some of Your Help from Personally Employed Aides**

Okay, you have read through these preparatory topics and now you are ready to tackle the recurring RISHTMP cycle—recruiting, interviewing, screening, hiring, training, managing, and parting ways with help providers. There are three primary sources for providers: family caregivers, agency-employed aides, and personally employed aides or personal assistants (PAs). Here, you will find three original ten-step procedures for getting help from each source. Introducing each chapter are strategies and comments from experiences of both the author and scores of help recipients and providers. Special attention is warranted for the advice to family caregivers on how careful planning can minimize their chances of overwork, burnout, and depression.

Part III *More Topics on Getting the Help You Need*

The chapters of Part III are supplements to the three ten-step plans of Part II. Although some details apply to all three of the provider sources, most apply to recruiting, training, managing, resolving problems, and parting ways with personally employed PAs (personal assistants).

📖 8   **Where and How to Advertise for Your Own PAs**

To hire the best PAs, you will want to attract a maximum number of the best applicants. This chapter details the strategies of professional, commercial advertising firms and applies them to the question of where and how to attract desirable PA applicants. Included are the five primary parts of any successful advertisement; special ways to make your PA ad, poster, or Internet notice attract attention; and the best places to advertise for aides in a typical community.

📖 9   **Initial Training and Ongoing Management of Aides and PAs**

Once you have recruited and hired quality PAs, training them is next. Agency and personally employed aides both require training. This chapter is packed with ways to clone the skills and good habits of your current, best aides into the new ones. You will learn how to train new PAs by using a three-step procedure that uses your current PAs, and saves you time and energy. You will also find an efficient, three-way teaching method of citing what help you need, along with how you would like to receive the help, and why your preferences are important. This method, when coupled with routinely expressed appreciation, will significantly accelerate the learning curve for your PAs and help you to keep them longer.

📖 10   **Recognizing and Resolving Your PA Problems, or Parting Ways**

Once you have hired and trained your PAs, you will want to keep them as long as possible. Tips in this chapter will help you recognize problems early and resolve them quickly, to prevent unnecessary aide resignations. When problems cannot be remedied, more tips will help you to recognize when PAs are ready to resign—often before the PAs themselves are aware of it. You will know why, how, and when (in a work shift) PAs typically resign, so you can be prepared to react appropriately and then smoothly replace them. In the rare instance when you must fire an aide, you will know how to deliver the news while safeguarding yourself and possessions against repercussions.

Part IV *Taking Control of Your Help Needs*

This part provides you with strategies for identifying, listing, and conveying to providers your needs for help. With these chapters, you begin by evaluating whether all your initially identified help needs are appropriate for requesting assistance from providers. Next is a chapter of assurance that your preferences in what, when, and how you want help provided are, indeed, very important—regardless of the feedback you might occasionally receive from angry providers. With that foundation in place, it's time to define your final list of needs and preferences, and then be ready to describe them to PAs. The last section addresses the clear, direct, assertive way you should use to communicate with aides to increase the chances that your needs will be understood and fulfilled.

11   When It Is, and Is Not, Okay to Ask for Help

If you have a wide variety of needs for help, you request many tasks each day. Your requests are usually granted, until you get "that look" from a PA that says you have stepped over the line and asked for something that does not feel right. Where is that fine line that separates what is and is not okay? This chapter proposes three types of inappropriate requests, and a list of negative consequences of your making them. There are also four sets of factors to help you decide when it is, and is not, okay to make a request.

12   Getting It Done—Your Way!

You have preferences in the what, how, when, and why for the ways that you receive help. Be assured about how important these are, and why they are important. Also be aware of strategies for getting the help you need—provided your way.

13   Defining and Describing Your Help Needs

Your clear list and schedule of needs are as important to you and PAs as a set of blueprints is to an architect and construction crew. In addition to a list of needs, sometimes it is helpful to create a job description that includes the nature of the work, your expectations of the qualifications and qualities of aides, and comments about the salary. A sample list and schedule of needs plus a job description are illustrated. In addition, right now, could you ad lib a short, 30-second and a more detailed, 5-minute description of your PA job and work routine? If you advertise the job and speak with PA applicants, you will be narrating both versions, for different reasons, hundreds of times over the next few years. Your first impression to applicants should be of someone who is reasonably organized, intelligent, and clear-thinking. Like most of us, you might want to outline and then rehearse your descriptions once or twice before your phone rings with that first inquiry.

14   Say It, Ask for It, and Act—Assertively!

Perhaps you have heard complaints from PAs that you are making too many demands. Others might tell you it is not *what* you are requesting, but *how* you are making requests that irritates your helpers. This chapter should clarify what PAs are trying to tell you. It advises you how to get what you want by using clear, direct, and assertive communication and behavior, while avoiding passive, aggressive, and passive-aggressive habits.

Part V *Strategies for Being a Good Manager*

The first chapter provides you with commonsense "how-to" details on being the first-class PA manager for whom quality aides want to work. The next discusses the strategy and advantages of dividing your needs among several PAs. Here, you will find strategies on deciding how many part-timers to employ, and then how to have PAs self-assign their work shifts during monthly staff meetings. Next, if you want PAs to work efficiently, you must provide an efficient work area with sufficient supplies, and this chapter tells you how. Finally, the help providers upon whom you are so dependent are also the people who routinely fail to satisfy their commitments to you. The most common crisis situations are listed along with strategies that you can use for coping, reacting, and surviving.

📖 **15   Your Qualities and Strategies as a Good PA Manager**
You will find guidelines about how to be an in-charge manager who is also caring and appreciative—a person for whom help providers *want* to work extra hours. You will learn why routinely expressing appreciation is essential to retaining the quality PAs, as well as when, how, and how often to most effectively express it.

📖 **16   Dividing Your Needs, and Assigning Work Shifts, Among Several PAs**
It costs no more to employ several part-time aides than just one, for the same total of hours. More than a dozen listed advantages include having instant backups and subs when a scheduled aide suddenly cannot work or quits; making the job more attractive to applicants; and avoiding the chance of abuse or unfair advantage that a one-and-only PA can exert over you. This is one of the most important strategies for managing help providers.

📖 **17   Setting Up Efficient Work Areas and Maintaining Adequate Supplies**
Your PAs prefer and require work areas that are reasonably clean, efficiently organized, and adequately supplied. Here are strategies for setting up, stocking, and maintaining favorable work areas, while staying on top of supply inventories.

📖 **18   Coping with and Reacting to PA Failures**
It is a fact that the people upon whom you are most dependent are those who too often fail to satisfy their commitments to you. They might fail to show up for a morning work shift, while you lie in bed wondering how to summon the help you need to get up. At the time you hire them, other PAs might vow a minimum employment commitment of nine months, and then quit three weeks later to move to a higher paying job. Or perhaps you discover that your most trusted aide has been stealing your medications, petty cash, or girlfriend. This chapter advises you about how to react constructively in order to survive the current ugly situation, while reducing the chance for future ones.

Part VI *The Costs of Your Personally Employed PAs*

The bottom line of the first chapter is to help you realize the costs of hiring PAs and then keeping them happy. Next, you will find details about the cash, non-cash, and combination ways of paying PAs, and which will work best for you. The third topic is about your tax obligations and how to keep your tax bill as low as is legally possible. The strength of these chapters lies in helping you to calculate the costs, keep financial records, and realize the basics about tax obligations. Regrettably, there are few details about potential funding sources, because there are currently not many sources to list.

□ **19   Your Costs of Recruiting, Training, and Keeping PAs Happy**
This chapter begins by listing and discussing what it costs you—in time and money—to advertise, interview, screen, and hire each new personally employed aide. A comparison is presented between the typical costs of using agency-employed aides and employing your own. Based on this comparison, you will discover the total annual savings of employing your own PAs over paying for agency aides from your pocket. Finally, you will again be reminded that the most effective, powerful incentive you can use to keep your providers happy costs you nothing—it is simply your routine expression of appreciation for the help your PAs provide.

□ **20   Paying Salaries: Cash, Non-cash, or Both**
Three types of salary are commonly used for paying help providers. This chapter discusses when to use a straight cash salary; a non-cash salary of live-in space, services, or goods; or a cash and non-cash combination. If you choose the cash option, you are shown a step-by-step bookkeeping system for calculating and recording paycheck amounts. In the United States, after you have paid salaries, you are required to file quarterly and year-end reports to various agencies and to pay employment taxes. You are coached on where to find the up-to-date requirements regarding these responsibilities, and on how to use a local accountant to research or routinely fulfill them for you.

□ **21   Tax Obligations, Deductions, and Publications for PA Employers**
Two approaches could be taken here. In one, I could provide a detailed listing of obligations, which forms to file, the calendar deadlines for each filing, and the current criteria used for calculating taxes. However, some of this printed data would be outdated and useless by the time you read it. Instead, this chapter introduces these obligations and then identifies the sources for you to use to get up-to-date information.

Part VII   *"I Understand How You Feel"—Concerns Heard from You,
as a Recipient, Family Caregiver, or Paid Provider*

This section is about increasing understanding, communication, and respect among
help recipients, family caregivers, and paid providers. Therapists tell us that the most
basic, twofold need that people have in any relationship is the desire to be heard and
understood. Here is an anthology of concerns from each of the three parties, so each
person can be better understood by the others while also gaining a fresh viewpoint
on his or her own realities.

To supplement these lists, I have published these concerns, along with needs
and typical remedies, in a separate publication.

📖 **22   A Bill of Rights for You, as a Help Recipient, Caregiver, or Paid Provider**
You and your help providers each have personal rights. The strongest and
longest-lasting recipient-provider relationships exist when each party
respects the rights of the other. As a PA manager, you are wise to work in
harmony with the people who help you. Relationships can be
understanding, respectful, and harmonious when each person reviews
the lists of his colleagues, and then reads his own list to better
understand himself or herself.

📖 **23   Your Personal Concerns as a Help Recipient**
Most of this reference book provides details so that you can better
understand others and be able to manage the help they provide you.
However, what about you and your concerns? Yours are equally
important, and usually only someone else with a disability can truly
understand them. It would be very helpful for the family caregivers and
paid providers who interact with you to better understand how you feel
about your abilities and inabilities, your being dependent on assistance
from others, your having to ask for that assistance, and the feedback that
you feel when asking them for help. This chapter hears you, and lists
many of your concerns so both you and others can better understand
them.

📖 **24   Your Personal Concerns as a Family Caregiver**
When a family member experiences a disability that requires help, some
other family members often become caregivers. These selfless people
typically abandon their own needs to provide whatever assistance the
recipient requires, whenever it is needed. However, because of their
forfeiture of personal needs, these caregivers soon become overworked,
chronically tired, and depressed. Few people fully understand their
concerns or needs, so this chapter attempts to bring them to light. Its
extensive listing of concerns helps caregivers better understand
themselves and be better understood by others.

📖 25 **Your Personal Concerns as a Paid Help Provider, plus
Ten Reasons Why PAs Quit and Are Fired**

Your paid profession is to provide personal help to others. Whether help
recipients are in a good mood or not, you have promised to fulfill their
personal needs—and to attempt doing so with a smile. You provide help
with the tasks that the recipient cannot do, that the family caregiver is
too tired to do, and that your supervisor refuses to do. How do you
maintain your desire for this tiring, day-after-day work while too often
receiving mostly complaints about your performance? This chapter
advises you, as well as those whom you serve and your supervisors,
about what situations typically become so intolerable that you must
resign (ten reasons why PAs quit their jobs). Also, it advises you about
what negative habits you should avoid in order to keep a job you like
(ten reasons why PAs are fired).

Part VIII *Parting Advice for You*

This closing part comes straight from me, your author. If you were learning management
skills by working with me in one-to-one counseling or in one of my 16-week formal
courses, these are some of the topics that typically would surface in the final few minutes.

📖 26 **When You or Your Help Provider Has—or Might Have—AIDS**

This chapter does not discuss how the HIV virus is contracted or what
precautions to take. Instead, it addresses the philosophical and ethical
question about whether either a help recipient or provider who is HIV-
positive is required to inform the other. We can assume the usually
negative consequences when one party does inform the other, so this
chapter centers on opinions about when disclosure is necessary and
when it is not. The discussion is based on the premise that every one
of us probably has a relative or friend who is HIV-positive, regardless of
whether we are aware of it.

📖 27 **Medical Monitoring Services: Your Push-Button Lifesaver**

There is a growing population of people with disabilities who attempt to
live at home alone, but who would be wise to have a live-in aide or a
medical monitoring system. These folks might live with the risk of falling
and urgently needing help to get back up, or of suddenly falling victim to
a heart attack or diabetic coma. By wearing the transmitter contained in a
necklace or wristband, these people can live alone while being able to
instantly summon help as needed. This chapter discusses these services.

📖 28 **Your Discretion, Privacy, and Confidentiality**

It is unfortunate that so many aides unavoidably know your intimate
thoughts, concerns, values, and beliefs. In return, you often know more about
their personal lives than they would prefer. While this exchange is probably
unavoidable, what should be avoidable is the sharing of these facts with the
outside world. This chapter provides examples as well as strategies to
minimize a "slip of the lip" for you or your PAs with outside friends.

📖 29 **Your Training Role and Objectives: Direction, Training, and Education**

Your PAs come in all shapes and sizes, with differing interests in the job you offer and different abilities to learn and benefit from working with you. Some have a pint-sized capacity for absorbing only the basics of your brief directions, others have a quart capacity for remembering your more detailed instructions, and a rewarding few are working for you on their way to a therapy or medical degree. The third group is eager for an education from you. This chapter helps you recognize the difference among these three types of PAs, and how to gear your directions, instructions, and education accordingly.

Appendices

MiCASSA, Olmstead, and ADAPT

The mission of this book is to provide you the *skills* to manage your PAs; other people have concentrated their efforts on ensuring that you have the *funding and rights* to manage them. This appendix briefly outlines some of those legislative efforts and provides references for monitoring their progress and getting involved.

Selected Resource Bibliography

Although this reference is quite comprehensive in "how-to" strategies, it is far from exhaustive. I have provided a list of books, journals, magazines, small publications, and videos that can supplement the topics found in this book.

Your Advice Is Requested

Feedback from readers of the two previous editions made possible this third edition. You are invited to share what parts of this book worked well for you, and which did not. Your own innovative strategies and management tips are also welcome.

How to Order Additional Copies of This Reference

Would you like to gift a copy of this reference to a friend? It's easy.

Index

Your Author

Your Quick Start Guide—
Five Topics to Get You Going Today!

You say you have skimmed through this reference's table of contents, the previous chapter, "How to Use This Reference," and yet you still feel a bit overwhelmed and unsure of where to start?

Not to worry!

Here is a Quick Start Guide to identifying your needs, identifying the source(s) for your help providers, and then recruiting those providers and keeping them longer.

❶ Examine your help needs.

(a) Create your list and schedule of needs.

You will find these chapters helpful—

(b) Be sure all the help needs on your list are valid,
and then be ready to describe that list to prospective aides.

You will find these chapters helpful—

❷ Examine your finances.

Calculate the cost of hired help providers,
and identify a funding source.

If you currently intend to use only unpaid family caregivers, this is still a valid planning exercise, for now or later. Statistically, most help recipients eventually hire outside providers for at least some of their needs when tired caregivers require relief help.

You will find these chapters helpful—

❸ Identify a source for your help providers and the setting where you will use them.

You will find these chapters helpful—

❹ Pursue one or more of the three primary sources for help providers.

You will find these chapters helpful—

❺ As questions and concerns occur around the following common topics, know that these specialized chapters are ready to serve you.

(a) Training and educating help providers (agency aides included!).

You will find these chapters helpful—

(b) Facilitating communication and better understanding the concerns of others and yourself.

You will find these chapters helpful—

(c) Being a quality manager.

You will find these chapters helpful—

(d) Setting up efficient work areas.

You will find this chapter helpful—

(e) Expressing your needs; dividing and assigning needs among
several part-time PAs.

You will find these chapters helpful—

(f) Recognizing, coping with, and resolving problems,
or parting ways from providers.

You will find these chapters helpful—

Part I

Identifying Your Options for Assistance

Part I

Identifying Your Options for Assistance

Before identifying the trees, let's examine the layout of the forest and the directions of the main roads. Before pursuing a specific type of help provider, it is wise to decide whether to use volunteer or paid people, home-based or community-based help, aides who live with you or nearby, and agency-employed or personally employed helpers. In addition, you should be aware of how to obtain help in different settings, including home, college campus, office, health care facility, local appointments and meetings, and long-distance travel for vacations or business trips.

Whether you are on your own or use family caregivers, sooner or later you will probably be looking for outside (of family) help providers. If you use family caregivers, you would be wise at the initial stages to complement—and safeguard—those caregivers with auxiliary help. In several places of this reference, you will find lists and discussions of the advantages of giving family caregivers a break by relieving or replacing them with outsiders. In contrast, if you are on your own, without the benefit of family help, you will be seeking outside help as soon as you develop help needs. In either situation, the first chapter, 📖 **1 "Beyond Family Caregivers: Options and Settings for Finding Outside Assistance,"** will introduce you to the forest of help provider types, sources, and settings.

📖 **2 "Volunteer Help: Don't Wear Out Your Friendships"** explores the dos and don'ts of using free help. Your ability to be independent each day in the public mainstream is dependent on your wise use of volunteers, when appropriate, and your wise insistence on using paid providers for heavy-duty, at-home needs. Indeed, few of us could financially afford to have salaried providers follow us around all day, so we routinely use Good Samaritan passersby for opening doors or picking up the car keys that we drop in a parking lot. In addition, U.S. federal law now requires public facilities, retail stores, and hotels to provide us with help in many situations. Some of the help is free, and some is offered with the provider's expectation of a tip. In still other situations, attempting to use volunteer help is clearly not wise. You would seriously jeopardize your ability to meet your busy daily schedule if you expected volunteers to get you out of bed each morning at 6 A.M. or to assist with your bowel and shower routine each night. Sound confusing? This chapter provides all the guidelines you need to avoid wearing out friendships.

Did you know that by wisely using live-in PAs, you can get some—or all—of your daily help for free? It is true, and chapter 📖 3, **"Live-In Aides and Other Residence Options,"** tells you how to arrange it. The chapter discusses the pros and cons of live-ins, and how to calculate the amount of monthly help that a live-in aide would agree is fair. If live-in help is not feasible for your residence situation, you should next favor hiring PAs who live nearby. In some settings, an aide's dependability and punctuality are directly related, at least in part, to how close or far from you she lives.

Few people spend the entirety of their lives solely within their residence, and if they require assistance at home, they will also need it when they are out and about. Chapter 📖 4, **"Settings Where You Use Help,"** provides strategies for using assistance at home, during local errands and appointments, for overnight travel on vacations and business trips, at a college campus, and at hospitals and other types of health care facilities and residences.

Having accomplished the introduction to provider options found in Part I, you are next invited to examine the three primary provider sources: family caregivers, agency-employed aides, and personally employed aides. The chapters of Part II offer you a well-coordinated balance of easy-to-follow numbered steps and in-depth, supplementary discussions. The three ten-step plans of Part 2 form the core of this book.

Part II: Three Ten-Step Plans for Getting the Help You Need

📖 5 Ten Steps to Getting All or Some of Your Help from Family Caregivers

📖 6 Ten Steps to Getting All or Some of Your Help from Agency-Employed Aides

📖 7 Ten Steps to Getting All or Some of Your Help from Personally Employed Aides

Chapter 1

Beyond Family Caregivers: Options and Settings for Finding Outside Assistance

Congratulations. You, or your family caregivers, have wisely decided to arrange for outside (of family) help with your routine activities of daily living (ADL) needs. The first common questions are:

- "What kinds of help are out there?"
- "Is any of the help free, and if so, why do most people use hired help instead of volunteers?"
- "If hired help comes primarily in two flavors, from an agency or personal employment, which source better meets my needs?"
- "If I decide to get my help from an agency, where do I start my search and how do I shop for it?"
- "If I decide to employ my own providers, what is the best way?"

This chapter outlines alternatives for using at-home as well as community services. The options outlined here are often sought by tired family caregivers who want relief or replacement help. They are also important to help recipients who want an alternative to their current use of family caregivers only, or who need outside help because they do not have family caregivers.

To create their own help source, individual caregivers often band together in informal, home-based day-care or respite networks. These volunteers take turns, spending some days enjoying off-duty time while others provide group care. More formal alternatives include using licensed, community day-care and respite centers where professional staff provides paid help. These commercial centers are often located within assisted living centers, filling unoccupied residence rooms with day-time and weekend clients.

Beyond the short-term relief provided by day-care and respite services, some family caregivers—or help recipients—seek replacement help because the daily, routine responsibilities have caused caregivers to become chronically fatigued or depressed. Those who want at-home assistance might find it in the paid providers who are available either through agencies or personal employment. Also, when a recipient's needs have advanced beyond the attention that can be supplied at home, community-based services are available by relocating one's residence to an independent living center, assisted living center, or health care center (nursing home).

Besides discussing this variety of options, this chapter explores the pros and cons of using an agency or your own personal employment as a source of aides.

At-home services

Three primary kinds of outside help are available for your disability needs:

- volunteers
- agency-employed aides
- personally employed aides (PAs).

Volunteers

You probably already receive several kinds of help from volunteers. For your special concerns there are at least five functional types of volunteers beyond family caregivers:

- friends and neighbors
- strangers and passersby
- employees of retail stores
- employees of hotels, motels, restaurants, and other service-oriented businesses
- members of volunteer service organizations.

Asking for free help from others can be a very delicate negotiation, and yet your appropriate use of help from volunteers is essential to your independence. The good news about volunteers is that they are usually very dedicated, dependable people who want to serve and be needed by others. So why not use a group of volunteers for your day-to-day disability needs?

Generally, the day-to-day help that you need in your activities of daily living (ADLs) is rarely the type of help that they are interested in or willing to provide. By the way, please note that our discussion of volunteers does not include the unique caring provided by family caregivers. The use of a caregiver network to provide informal day-care and respite services is separately examined in a later section.

It is not reasonable to expect most volunteers to be at your apartment each morning at 6 A.M. to help with your "get up" routine. For any recurring or extensive day-after-day, week-after-week, personal or medical assistance, volunteer help is rarely the answer. The punctuality, dependability, type, and duration of help that you routinely need usually requires either a very dedicated family caregiver or a salaried provider.

However, once you are dressed, up, and ready for the day, these categories of volunteer help can, and should, be used appropriately and routinely. Knowing whom to ask for what kind of help, is indeed an art.[1]

So, for daily assistance, you really do need to hire outside help, and you have the choice of letting an agency hire and coordinate the help, or personally employing your own aides or PAs.

Agency-employed aides

This type of help is provided by professionals who are employed and supervised by an agency. Agencies can supply several categories of staff. The titles for these staffers may vary among agencies, but here are the three primary types:

- companions (or personal care providers, PCPs) who have minimal, non-medical training
- home health aides (or certified nursing assistants, CNAs) who have usually completed at least one, six-week training course on basic medical details
- nurses, registered (RN) or licensed practical (LPN), who have completed at least two years of formal medical training and state licensure.

In many communities, there are also three main categories of agencies:

- commercial agencies found in most telephone Yellow Pages
- government-sponsored agencies found in some public, state, county, or city health departments
- nonprofit agencies that may charge minimal fees on a sliding scale to cover basic expenses.

> *Agencies provide essential services for people who need them and who can afford them.*

An agency's role is to recruit, interview, train, schedule, pay, and otherwise manage aides on behalf of the actual recipient of services. Agencies perform an essential set of services for people who:

- are unwilling or unable to manage their own care
- prefer agency help because their needs are temporary, and therefore they have no desire to take the time to learn management skills

---

1. For a complete discussion, please see chapter 📖 2, "**Volunteer Help: Don't Wear Out Your Friendships.**"

- receive funding for services and are required by the funding source to use assistance only from certain approved agencies

- are new to a community, have an immediate need for help, and are as yet unaware of where to personally recruit PAs within the new locale

- have a personally employed PA who suddenly quits, and require immediate fill-in help from an agency until their personal recruiting is again successful

- eventually intend to personally employ PAs, but currently need agency assistance while they ready themselves to begin personal recruiting.

Personally employed aides

These are the PAs (personal assistants), PCAs (personal care assistants), or aides whom you personally recruit, interview, screen, hire, train, manage, and eventually part ways.[2]

This approach requires that you be able and willing to directly manage and otherwise employ the assistance you need. These skills are covered throughout the topic-by-topic information in this reference. Beyond these textbook details, PA management abilities are fine tuned—as within any field of management—through years of trial, error, and practice. Many folks have found that the advantages of being a self-sufficient manager in complete control of the PAs they use are well worth the effort.

If you need assistance, and want to remain living in the comfort of your own home, then look over the following list of comparisons before deciding whether to use agency-provided or personally employed help.

At-home comparisons: agency vs. personal employment

If you have wisely decided to employ outside help for some or all of your routine needs, beyond the help of family caregivers, the next question is probably, "Should I use agency-employed aides, or employ my own?"

The following section will provide comparisons to help you with your decision.[3]

A main attraction to using agency aides would seem to be the saved effort. True, agencies theoretically do the recruiting, interviewing, screening, (very) basic training, scheduling, and payroll paperwork instead of you. However, do agencies do a better job than you could? Could you take more care during your searches, and wind up with higher quality aides?

It boils down to this question: How hard are you willing to work at providing yourself with quality providers? Some of us will go through an agency every time, because we cannot imagine doing all the work. Others of us have never used an agency throughout 20, 30, or more years of disability, because we want to be in the firmest possible control over the who, when, where, how, and how much of the help we require.

---

2. For details about the different titles of providers, please see the Introduction's **"Definitions of Titles and Terms Used in This Reference."**

3. If you have already decided, and want to skip to the step-by-step "how-to" procedures for recruiting, hiring, and training providers, please see chapter 📖 6, **"Ten Steps to Getting All or Some of Your Help from Agency-Employed Aides,"** or 📖 7, **"Ten Steps to Getting All or Some of Your Help from Personally Employed Aides."**

Overall, your decision about using either agency or personal aides will be based on these concerns:

- cost
- ability and willingness to manage
- control
- training
- flexible range of duties for aides
- scheduling
- authority to replace undesirable aides
- insurance provision
- payment of salaries, maintenance of records, and payment of taxes.

Cost. Are you using outside or personal funding? If you are eligible for outside funding for the aides you use, that funding source usually requires the use of agency aides. In contrast, if you will be using personal funds, can you afford the extra cost of agency aides?

The cost of agency providers is often two to three times that of personally employed help. That is acceptable if you receive outside funding. However, if you are paying for help from personal funds, the savings of employing your own aides year after year can be significant.

For example, when the aides actually receive an $8 hourly salary, the bottom-line agency billing to you or your funding source typically ranges from $18 to $25 per hour or more. In contrast, the typical hourly total when you personally employ your own aides (at an $8 hourly rate, and for 40 hours weekly or 2,000 hours annually) will be in the ballpark of $10 per hour (see *Figure 1-1*). When these hourly costs are projected on an annual basis, and a personal budget is used for funding, the savings from personal employment can be significant (see *Figure 1-2*).

Figure 1-1: **Hourly cost comparisons of using personally or agency employed aides**

Hourly cost of personally employed PAs—	
The hourly salary that you pay the PA	$8.00
+ Social security (FICA) employer contribution example $8.00 x 7.65%	0.612
+ Typical state unemployment tax $25/year example: $25/1,560 annual hours of help	0.016
+ Workers' compensation insurance (if required), $500 to $1,500/year, example: $1,500/1,560 annual hours of help	0.962
+ Filing of quarterly reports & annual income tax by your accountant, example: $350/1,560 annual hours of help	0.224
+ Newspaper advertising for recruiting example: $300/1,560 annual hours of help	0.192
= Typical hourly total	~$10.01
Hourly cost of agency-employed aides—	
The salary the agency pays its aides	$8.00
+ Employment taxes, insurance fees, administrative and operational costs, & profits	$10.00–17.00
= Typical hourly total	~$18.00–25.00

Figure 1-2: **Annual costs and savings of using personally or agency employed aides**

• Personally employed PAs— average hourly costs	$10.01
estimated annual cost for 1,560 hours	$15,609.72
• Agency aides— typical hourly cost	$18.00–25.00
estimated annual cost for 1,560 hours, $21.50 hourly	$33,540.00
• Est. annual savings, 1,560 hours, personally employed over agency employed aides	$17,930.28
• Est. hourly savings over 1,560 hours	$11.50

An agency will send you or your funding source billing statements that include four types of costs:

- the salary that the agency pays to its aides
- the employment taxes and insurance fees that are linked to those salaries
- the overhead costs of operating the agency
- profit.

It might seem to some that the extra cost of agency aides is worth the simplified agency billing, as opposed to juggling the extra paperwork of employing your own providers. In contrast to receiving this simple periodic billing from an agency, there are several tasks and additional costs to financially managing your own aides. Cost categories include advertising, paying salaries, and then calculating, reporting, and paying employment taxes. However, if a personal budget is the funding source, the annual savings of personal employment usually far outweighs the extra paperwork and effort.

Ability and willingness to manage. Are you able and willing to personally employ help, or would you much prefer to have an agency routinely perform all the duties with providers?

Many folks are willing but unable to manage assistance. They lack the emotional stability or cognitive ability required, first for assessing their own needs and then for the overall, day-after-day management of providers.

Others are able but unwilling to be managers. For those undergoing a short-term, homebound recovery from a hospital surgery or ailment, sometimes there is an understandable lack of desire to learn and practice management skills for such a temporary need. For others with a longer-term or lifelong disability, sometimes refusing to become a self-sufficient manager is consistent with their refusal to coordinate their own care, and often many other responsibilities. Still others simply want an agency to take care of the details of their needs; the personal employment alternative seems to be too much trouble. In any of these cases, an agency's coordination and management of professional help are essential.

However, if you have a long-term or lifelong need for assistance, and you are able, willing, and desirous of being in control of that assistance, then you should strongly consider personally employing the aides who help you. In an upcoming chapter, this book provides you with the step-by-step detail that you will need.

Figure 1-3 compares the primary tasks of managing help providers with using agency or personal help.

Figure 1-3: **Comparing management functions—
agency-employed and personally employed aides**

Routine Function or Concern	If Agency Employs	If You Employ
Create newspaper ad and advertise for aides	Agency does it	You do it
Receive and screen ad inquiries	Agency does it	You do it
Do face-to-face interviewing and screening of applicants	Agency does it	You do it
Check employment references	Agency does it	You do it
Make ultimate decision about who helps you, including each aide's personality and the quality of work	Agency decides	You decide
Hire new aides	Agency does it	You do it
Supervise aides; who is recognized by aides to be their supervisor, and the person who is "in charge"?	Agency is	You are
Calculate and pay salaries	Agency does it	You do it
Calculate, report, and pay quarterly employment taxes	Agency does it	You or your accountant do it
Identify the what, how, and schedule of the help you require	You do it	You do it
Determine which duties an aide will or will not perform	Agency policy	You and your aide agree
Train new aides by describing and demonstrating your help needs	You do it	You do it
Provide daily, face-to-face management of aides: performance feedback, evaluation, and appreciation	You do it	You do it
Receive aide resignations	Agency does it	You do it
Fire an undesirable aide	Agency does it	You do it
Establish, implement, and manage a backup replacement system when a scheduled aide is unable to work (or fails to appear for) a shift	Agency does it	You and your aides do it
Pay the costs of advertising, salary processing, employment taxes, liability insurance, etc.	Agency does it	You do it
Total hourly costs billed to you or your funding source (approximate, based on an $8/hr. actual salary)	$18–$25 or more	$9–$10

Some efficient agencies provide excellent services and truly do take care of your concerns. However, other agencies provide administrative services and aides of a quality that falls far short of this expectation.

There are several factors that vary considerably from one agency to another. When deciding between using agency or personal aides, or which specific agency to contract, you should include the following in your criteria:

- The agency's administrative services—whether the agency staff is thorough, prompt, and courteous in responding to your individual concerns.

- The agency's operating policies—whether the agency's overall customer service routinely provides customer satisfaction, or customer frustration.

- The quality of the aides the agency employs—whether the aides assigned to you will be of high personal and professional quality, be dependable and punctual to meet your schedule, and consistently be the same people (or frequently changed).

- The total costs of using the agency—and whether the costs are entirely covered by your outside funding source.

The bottom-line decision about your ability and willingness to be a manager is decided by which of the three management roles best describes you. A review of these traits can be found in *Figure 1-4*.

Figure 1-4: **Your three choices of management styles as a help recipient**

Role One—	You can independently manage the people who help you.
	You have the desire, cognitive (memory, problem-solving, and decision-making) ability, and functional abilities to manage and use your choice of family caregivers, agency-employed aides, personally employed PAs, or any combination there of.
Role Two—	You can independently manage the people who help you, after you accommodate a secondary impairment to your doing some of the management tasks.
	You have the desire and cognitive (memory, problem-solving, and decision-making) ability; however, you have a speech, hearing, sight, or learning disability; a limitation on physical writing or computer interfacing; or other impairment to your independent accomplishment of some functional management tasks. You have already developed ways to accommodate this impairment in your daily lifestyle, and you do so again (and fully manage the people who help you) by:
	• doing the tasks in innovative ways
	• using technology and special equipment to do the tasks
	• using extra help from these same help providers.
	Consequently, you can manage and use your choice of family caregivers, agency-employed aides, personally employed PAs, or any combination there of.
Role Three—	You require someone else to remember your routine, make decisions, solve problems, and manage the people who help you.
	You lack the desire and/or cognitive (memory, problem-solving, and decision-making) ability to personally manage the people who help you. Consequently, you require a family caregiver or an agency to make decisions, employ, and manage your help providers.

Control. Is it important to you to be in maximum control over the quality of providers who help you, as well as over the what, how, and when of the help you receive? Can you live with decisions from agency policies, or are you a hands-on person who habitually insists on making his or her own decisions? Besides wanting to make your own decisions, are you also comfortable in being assertive in communicating and supervising their implementation?

The third consideration in your decision of using agency or personal help is one of control. Personal employment provides you with more control, specifically in the following areas:

- deciding who helps you
- setting the schedule of available help
  to best match your personal schedule
- training aides in what help you need,
  as well as in how you prefer the help to be provided
- monitoring the quality of help that is provided,
  and having the direct power to evaluate that quality
  because you—and not an agency—are in charge.

An agency recruits, interviews, screens, trains, schedules, supervises, and sometimes replaces providers on behalf of the actual recipients of services. The agency, and not you, creates guideline policies and makes decisions that determine who assists you, their qualifications, their schedule for arriving and departing from your home, and whether poor performance will be repeatedly tolerated or promptly considered grounds for replacing the aide.

How important is it for you to be in maximum control of these factors? Can you accept the decisions made by an agency? The tradeoff, of course, is that while personally employing means more control, it also means more work. More details about topics involving control are discussed in the following sections.

Training. Is it important that your aides already have previous training in generic care procedures, before you additionally instruct them about your specific needs? Regardless of whether your PAs come from an agency or your own employment, and regardless of whether they have extensive training and experience, it will ultimately be your responsibility to instruct them, supervise and guide them, and keep them happy with appreciation.

If you use an agency's help, in theory some of the staff will have been trained and certified to the extent required by the title the staff member holds. All nurses must have years of extensive training and be licensed by the state in which they practice, whether they work for an institution, an agency, or an individual. A home health aide or certified nursing assistant (CNA) employed by an agency is supposed to have completed at least one six-week course of basic medical training. At a third, lowest level are companions or personal care providers (PCPs), who receive very little, if any, formal training.

So, each level of staff is allowed by the agency to perform very specific duties that are appropriate to their particular level of skills. Some agencies will provide this training for aides, or will subcontract the task to a school. Other agencies merely require that new employees provide documented proof of having completed training and certification on their own.

If you decide to employ your own assistants, but you believe that the agency-required training is important, then you can still tap into help providers who have completed that training and certification. The recruiting that you conduct can attract responses from trained aides. These folks may be working part or full time for an institution or agency, and may be willing to work additionally for you in their spare hours. You would be using the same trained providers who would be supplied by an agency, but your financial savings would be considerable.

However, if personally employing your own aides appeals to you, how important is the generic training that agencies require of the aides they employ?

The vast majority of PAs you employ will not have received any previous training. Many of us have successfully employed untrained and inexperienced providers for years from the general community or the students of a nearby college campus. We have seldom used previously trained aides, and have simply recruited inexperienced help and instructed them about how to fulfill our particular needs.

What few people realize is that, whether agencies employ your providers or you do it, there is a common step when your one-to-one instruction and management of each aide—without the benefit of any agency supervisor or instructor—begins. It is the moment when each new agency aide or personally employed PA walks through your front door for his or her temporary stay in your disability lifestyle. From this moment, your role and management duties are essentially the same toward both agency and personal aides.

Typically, it is not important that the PAs you directly employ be trained, certified, or experienced. The exception would be for any complex medical needs that only a nurse or other trained professional should provide.

Indeed, whether your aides come from agency or personal employment, and whether or not they are trained and experienced, you (or your representative) will still need the skills provided by this reference for PA training and management. In the long run, using agency-trained help will yield very few—if any—advantages that have the potential to reduce the time and effort in either your initial instruction or your long-term, daily management.

Despite their previous training or experience, and regardless of how well they have been briefed by the agency staffer who met with you, each new aide will greet you on the first day of work by saying, "Hello, I'm April, please let me know what help you need, and when and how you want me to provide it. Also, as I work with you each day, please be sure to let me know how I am doing." This is the same greeting you will hear from a new PA whom you have personally hired!

Flexible range of duties for aides. Agencies have strict guidelines about the types of help that different types of their providers are permitted to perform. In contrast, you can request a wide range of duties from the PAs you employ, and in return, they have the right of refusal.

If you have a wide range of needs for help, you may be frustrated to discover that agency providers are not allowed by the agency to perform certain duties. Your wide range of help needs might include certain medical needs, getting your nails trimmed, housecleaning, doing laundry, help in stores with shopping, providing transportation, and simple household maintenance. In some cases, two or three types of providers must be hired through an agency to cover the entire range of duties. In other cases, when funding or other restrictions prevent hiring two or three types of help, some of your needs will go unfulfilled.

This strict hierarchy of duties is due, in part, to the agency's responsibility to its malpractice insurance carrier. As we have seen, each type of service provider from an agency has theoretically completed a level of formal training appropriate to his or her title. The agency must guarantee the insurance carrier that each provider is sufficiently trained for the duties being performed. In addition, some agencies and the funding sources do not want to pay an aide for duties that they consider to be beyond your basic medical needs, despite the importance of those tasks are to you.

In contrast, if you directly employ the assistance you use, there are few restrictions on the types of duties that a provider can perform for you. You can ask your own PA to do almost anything. However, in answer to your requesting, "Would you help me with such-and-such?, an aide always has the right to say, "No, I would rather not." Refusals are rare, as long as you have respected the following:

- The type of work that the PA expects to be doing. When you initially describe to each PA applicant the types of tasks, be specific and comprehensive. Do not hide some of the less attractive duties. This is full disclosure time.

- The schedule and duration of help. Again, be specific from the beginning with each aide. What each initially agrees to do is what you can later request.

- The physical, cognitive, and mechanical abilities of each PA. You should match an appropriate category of provider with an appropriate category of duty. For example, it would be a waste of the high level of training and high hourly salary of a registered nurse to ask her to wash, dry, and fold laundry or to mop floors and wash windows. However, these would be appropriate duties for a less expensive aide whom you employ. In another example, your wheelchair might need some minor mechanical repair. If you personally employ more than one PA, you could best review who is mechanically inclined and who is not, and then select someone who knows which end of a wrench to use.

- The personal values of each PA. Each PA comes with a set of personal values, based partially on his or her own culture, religion, and upbringing. If you have been totally candid about describing the nature of the work, then each aide will know in advance about the commitments. Regardless, each has a right of refusal, based on personal values, regarding each task.

With these limitations in mind, the PAs you directly employ can be requested—but not ordered—to do almost anything. In return, their right to refusal must be respected.

Scheduling. Agencies sometimes have difficulty matching your personal schedule with the availability of their providers. In addition, you often share an aide with other agency clients. Sometimes your aide's arrival will be delayed if the routine for the client before you has required extra time. If you employ your own aides, you have direct control over scheduling, and you are spared having to share your aides with other help recipients.

If you are unable or unwilling to manage and directly employ assistance, the agency's scheduling of your aides is essential. You inform the agency of the ideal frequency and time schedule for which you need help. The agency checks its listings of nurses and aides and does its best to assure that a nurse or aide will arrive somewhat on schedule at your home. Sometimes the availability of aides does not exactly match your desired schedule, and you are notified by the agency about adjustments that you must make.

You should also realize that an agency usually schedules a service provider to visit several recipients each day, one after the other. This cost-efficient system works well until one of the recipients on a provider's list has an unexpected need that takes extra time (for example, a bowel accident).

Agency-supplied service providers have been known to handle the situation in one of three ways:

- to leave the recipient on schedule, perhaps with some tasks unfinished

- to finish all scheduled details, and perhaps be late for each of their next appointments

- to call their agency supervisor for an on-the-spot decision regarding one of the two previous choices.

In the first instance, each recipient receives assistance on schedule, but one recipient is left for the day without all of her scheduled needs fulfilled. In the second case, the provider takes the extra time required to complete all expected duties, but is consequently late for each subsequent appointment that day. If you are fourth or fifth on your aide's list, the aide might arrive at your house an hour later than expected. Consequently, your arrival at your day's activities and appointments will also be delayed. In the third case, agency supervisors make a decision based on factors such as their opinion of the importance of the request, whether the staffer with the client is trained and qualified to accommodate the special need, and whether the availability of staff that day will allow extra time with this client. Your request for a favorable decision is dependent on several variables.

Special needs are certain to happen, so if your daily schedule is important to you, you will want to discuss a prospective agency's policy about these situations.

In addition, it is not uncommon for a scheduled service provider to be sick or otherwise unable to provide expected help. Some agencies have readily available replacements, and others do not. Sometimes the supply of available aides is not sufficient, or an agency simply may not maintain an adequate list of backup aides. Thus, some agencies have trouble staffing even initial client requests.

When a routinely scheduled first-stringer is suddenly sick, some agencies cannot provide replacements from their own staff. That agency might then start calling a list of freelance aides with the hope of finding a fill-in. This task becomes additionally difficult because these floating aides are often not employed on a full-time basis by any single agency, and therefore, they often register for work with several agencies. Consequently, few agencies can count on a substitute being available for unexpected work when needed.

If you are considering the use of a particular agency, ask in advance about how promptly sick-time replacements are routinely made, and if there have been circumstances when no replacement has been possible. If you employ your own PAs, and divide your needs among several part-timers, you should usually have readily available substitutes whenever necessary.

Authority to replace undesirable aides. Most agencies are very interested in hearing any complaints about the personal quality or work quality of their aides. When significant problems arise, most agencies will do their best to resolve the issue or replace the aide. In contrast, some agencies are not ideally responsive. If you employ your own PAs, you have direct control to hire or fire as needed.

Many agencies operate within a geographical area where there is a shortage of available aides. If an agency has difficulty in initially filling your schedule, and has additional difficulty in promptly finding sick-time replacements, then it will also have difficulty in replacing an aide with whom you are not satisfied. Your dissatisfaction may arise from a poor quality of work, a frequently poor schedule of arrival and departure times, an inability or lack of desire of an aide to follow reasonable instructions from you, or even unethical behavior.

Here, though, you are not the direct employer and you lack the authority that the agency possesses, because it alone is the source of the aide's paycheck. You can complain to the aide about problems, but if the aide ignores complaints, you must plead your case to the agency. Some agencies are prompt to remedy a problem situation and replace an aide if necessary, and some are not.

If you are the direct manager and employer of the assistants that you use, you have more authority and control over each of these situations. You are in a position to insist that one of your PAs changes bad habits or finds another job.

Of course, controlling all these factors is a considerable responsibility and requires careful management. It is doubtful that even an experienced manager will always be successful, but the personal employer will have more of an opportunity than agency clients. Most PA managers will agree that having as much control as possible over the quality and schedule of the help they receive is well worth the effort that personal management requires.

Providing insurance. Agencies are required to maintain at least three types of insurance in relation to their employment of aides. If you employ your own aides for private use in your own home, you will usually be required to carry all these except malpractice.

The three types of insurance that agencies provide are malpractice (liability) insurance, worker's compensation and disability benefits insurance, and unemployment insurance.

Malpractice insurance is provided by most agencies for their employees to protect the agency against a lawsuit in case an employed aide causes harm to a client. As an agency client who is injured as the result of negligence by an agency-employed aide, you could sue the agency in an attempt to collect financial compensation for your injuries.

As a private employer of PAs, if one of your own PA's negligence were to cause you harm, you could try to sue the PA. However, PAs rarely can afford to carry their own malpractice insurance. Consequently, most would not be much of a financial target to sue. If a personally employed PA causes you harm through negligent behavior, the most you can usually do is fire her. Instead, you minimize the chance for their actions to harm you by carefully instructing and supervising them in safe methods of doing their work. Subsequently, you are usually working face-to-face with the PAs who help you, so you can constantly monitor how safely they work. In addition, you should be very quick to correct poor habits. You also have the authority to fire and replace any PA who repeatedly performs duties in a hazardous way, or who at any time attempts to perform duties while under the influence of drugs or alcohol.

Worker's compensation insurance pays an employee medical benefits and a portion of his or her salary for the duration of an illness, or an injury that is caused by their job or occurs on the job site. Agencies are required to provide this insurance for their aides. If you personally employ your PAs in your private home, many states have not historically required you to provide it. However, state regulations seem to be shifting more toward including your aides under their mandated protection, so check with your state department of labor. Many renters or homeowners will find that limited workers' compensation coverage is included (or can be included at an additional charge) in their renter's or homeowner's insurance coverage. As an alternative, if your state department of labor requires you to carry worker's comp insurance, ask the department if it has a list of insurance companies that offer the coverage. Here, you would be contracting for worker's comp insurance with an insurance company, much as you now contract for car or homeowner's policies. The annual cost of specially contracted worker's comp can typically run from $250 to $2,000 or more.

Unemployment insurance is required by both federal and state governmental departments, and both agencies and private employers are required to pay for it. Your relatively inexpensive premiums for these two coverages are paid quarterly to federal and state revenue departments.

In this text, I could provide you with the current regulations, the annual due dates for making payments, and the percentage rates for calculating the insurance premiums. However, these details frequently change, and they would probably be out-of-date—and useless to you—by the time you read them here. Instead, I will advise you to check with your local accountant, or federal and state departments of revenue, for the current regulations and payment details.

Paying salaries, maintaining records, and paying taxes. Any employer must keep income and expense records, in part, so that employment and income taxes can be paid. If you use agency aides, the agency handles all these responsibilities. If you employ your own aides, either you can perform the tasks or you can contract with an accountant to have them done for you.

In the interest of keeping operations simple, as someone who personally employs PAs, you can share the same record keeping strategy used by most small businesses. Throughout the year, you maintain your own income and expense records on a personal computer, using a very user-friendly software program such as Quicken® or M.Y.O.B.® ("Mind Your Own Business").

Next, to complement your computer records, you could consult with an accountant at the end of each three-month calendar quarter and at year's end. The accountant, or CPA (certified public accountant), can initially advise you about the types of records to keep. Once your record keeping system has been established, the CPA can meet with you to receive each quarter's or year-end summary. From there, the accountant completes the state and federal forms required each term, informs you of any tax payments that are due, and mails everything to the appropriate government departments for you.[4]

Community services

Some people want help provided within their own home and decide to bring in either agency-provided or personally employed assistance. For others, having help and services provided outside the home, in a day-care or residential setting, is preferred. New options become available each year, but the basic types of today's typical programs include:

- respite and day care, at one's home or at a day center
- independent living, at a facility or private residence
- assisted living, at a facility or private residence
- skilled nursing, at a nursing home (also called a health care facility).

Today's family and personal lifestyles come in a variety of flavors and colors, and today's living alternatives at some facilities are just as colorful.

Details about some services are available in slick, colorful brochures that represent health care centers from a more traditional marketing approach. For other centers, you can click on the bell-and-whistle hyperlinks of a high-tech Web site. At these sites, it is becoming more and more common to comparison shop by taking a virtual, 3-D tour of the new health care centers.

This multimedia advertising and public relations style implies that the health care center is on the cutting edge of new operating philosophies, program innovations, high-tech equipment, and facility features. However, whereas some facilities are up to date, others are still operated from outdated philosophies that treat their clients quite poorly. Because the future quality of life for a loved one is at stake, and there is a wide range between the favorable quality of modern centers and the deplorable quality of antiquated ones, it is very important to visit, inspect, and evaluate each center.

---

4. For more detail about setting up your record keeping system and using a CPA, please see chapters 📖 20, "Paying Salaries: Cash, Non-cash, or Both," and 📖 21, "Tax Obligations, Deductions, and Publications for PA Employers."

Respite and day care

For a family caregiver, day-care and respite services provide essential help and off-duty time. When friends and neighbors volunteer to provide help as needed, this is the appropriate help to request.

In some circles, the terms *day-care* and *respite* services are used interchangeably. Other customs define *day-care* as lasting a few hours, whereas *respite* help refers primarily to overnight facilities that can be tapped for two days, a weekend, or even two weeks.

Whatever the definition, both services provide family caregivers time off from their constant feeling of responsibility and having to be available to do whatever is needed. These short-term services can enable a morning's shopping, an afternoon's walk along the beach, or an evening's dinner and theater. The overnight help can make possible a weekend or week-long getaway that relaxes, restores, recharges, and rejuvenates.

When caregivers form support groups for their own needs, often their first innovation is to begin a small network for respite day care. Most of these home-based co-ops begin when two or three family caregivers band together to assume rotating shifts. One or two will agree to provide a day of care and help, while the third gets the day off. These informal (and often illegal) day-care groups usually provide a hassle-free, quick fix to satisfy basic caregiver needs unless a client accident or death makes the news and introduces a liability issue. In a few instances, a state agency has shut down a co-op and brought lawsuits against all involved families.

In contrast, a formal, state-licensed network can provide free or fee-based services. The word about a good thing soon spreads among caregivers, and the initially small day-care group may quickly outgrow its original home base to require a community meeting place. As the group continues to grow, paid staff is enlisted. The group might be kept small and nonprofit, or might become commercialized and operated by an agency.

For simple, non-medical needs, agency-employed personal care providers (PCPs) or companions often provide the commercial services. The primary role of companions is to provide physical assistance, supervision, and social company within firm guidelines. The training for companion staff is minimal, relative to CNAs, home health aides, and the nurses who supervise them.

PCP tasks can include the following:

- meal preparation, assistance with eating, meal cleanup
- personal help with bathing, dressing, care of skin and teeth
- household cleaning and laundry
- assistance with pets
- help with grocery shopping, appointments, leisure activities (transportation supplied by the service recipient or public transport)
- companionship.

People needing a higher level of medical assistance are required to enlist help from an agency's certified nursing assistants (CNAs) or personally employed PAs.

The alternative to home-based services is a care facility or center. Volunteer organizations, nonprofit groups, government agencies, or commercial facilities often operate these. Indeed, an independent living or assisted living facility sometimes extends its empty rooms and available staff to offer day-care and respite services.

Independent living at a facility or private residence

Independent living provides a residence for adults for whom the tasks of private home upkeep have become overwhelming. Residents are usually physically independent for their ADLs, but are often dependent on a mobility aid of a cane, walker, or wheelchair.

Residents of a facility usually live in private apartments that are equipped with 24-hour call buttons. If a resident falls or needs urgent assistance, the call button will prompt the center to provide minimal physical assistance, to phone a local relative, or to summon 911 emergency medical help.

The facilities aim to provide flexible living, as evidenced by these commonly offered features:

- private and semi-private apartments, within a choice of configurations, that feature a kitchenette with microwave, refrigerator, and sink

- meal plans that range from a continental breakfast to three meals daily, served in a central dining facility

- weekly housekeeping that includes a cleaning of living quarters plus fresh towels and bedding

- complimentary washers and dryers

- daily local transportation, using the facility's sign-up bus, to medical appointments, local errands, and group outings

- recreational and social activities

- cultural and educational in-house programs as well as day-long outings

- exercise facilities and programs

- emergency call system.

Although routine, personal home health aide services are not available from facility staff, residents often privately contract for services with facility-connected or outside agencies. As an alternative to contracting agency help, some residents personally employ their own help providers.

Assisted living at a facility or private residence

Assisted living, sometimes called personal board and care, is the intermediate step between independent living and a nursing home.

An assisted living center provides a group living situation where residents have routine access to an in-house nursing and home health aide staff.

The role of onsite medical professionals in an assisted living facility is one of supervision, ADL assistance, medical monitoring, and protective oversight. (In a nursing home, the staff is more medically oriented, as evidenced by their higher level of training and assigned responsibilities.)

Each resident is assessed by the center's staff to determine the level of assistance required.

In comparison with independent living, assisted living facilities tend to offer smaller apartments with a more expensive room, board, and service package. However, costs are still not as high as in a nursing home.

The assisted living facility usually offers all of the (previously listed) independent living features, plus:

- medication administered and coordinated by staff
- ADL (activities of daily living) help from staff for grooming, dressing, and bathing
- call-light system to summon staff assistance as needed
- protective oversight from staff.

Some communities also offer the assisted living option within the homelike atmosphere of private housing. The landlords of these private residences are usually subject to most of the federal, state, and local regulations that apply to the larger facilities.

Skilled nursing at a facility

A nursing home is the facility that provides the highest level of supervision and medical help, second only to a hospital.

Types of living quarters and staffing structures vary, as do operating philosophies. To avoid their negative historical image, these facilities have sought a change of image through a change of name, from "nursing home" to "health care center." However, you would be wise to tour a facility and interview staff and residents to be sure that the new programs are consistent with the new names and warm-colored brochures.

The bottom line is that a nursing home is necessary for those dependent persons who require more supervision than is available through independent or assisted living. Compared to independent and assisted living, the living quarters for skilled nursing are typically the smallest, while by far costing the most for the room, board, and services package.

Although health insurance does not cover long-term nursing home living, special long-term care insurance for nursing homes has become increasingly available in many states.

Ten steps for selecting and moving to a community residence facility

As mentioned, residence facilities come in three basic types that address three levels of independence as well as needed help, care, and supervision: independent living facilities and assisted living centers, and nursing homes. Regardless of a facility's new-age title, slick-printed brochures, or glitzy Web site, it is still wise to do some careful shopping and follow some time-proven, logical steps.

❶ At some point, a formal decision must be made that commits the recipient of services either to stay at the family home or to move to an appropriate group living facility. This is an important, and often emotional, milestone in the help recipient's life that deserves formal recognition. If the circumstances allow, it is ideal for the recipient to make this decision about his own future. If the recipient is unable, unwilling, or just uncooperative about making an assertive decision, then the family will decide on behalf of the recipient.

❷ Identify which of the three types of facilities seem to provide the type of living that meets the recipient's needs. Some communities additionally offer choices of specific facilities within each care level.

❸ Call each facility with basic questions to determine which ones merit a visit. It will soon become apparent which physical and program features are important for a recipient. Facilities can be quickly evaluated by phone. For each semi-finalist facility, request that a brochure packet, including representative floor plans of residences and a price sheet, be mailed to you and the recipient.

❹ After you have evaluated the facility brochures, schedule a guided tour of each center to observe the facility, the staff and their philosophies, and the residents. If possible, the recipient should be included. During the tour, you will be comparing the ideals of what the recipient wants, needs, and likes with the reality that exists at the facility.

The factual information about the available services and programs is, of course, essential. However, it is equally important to weigh the personalities of both the staff and the other residents. Besides assessing the staff members as they discuss the facility, you should also take a few minutes to chat with a few of the residents about what they like and do not like about living there. Your feeling and intuition are very valuable assessment tools during these visits.

❺ If you are in doubt about whether a facility and its services match the recipient's medical and living needs, you would be wise to arrange an evaluation appointment between the staff and the help recipient. If you are representing a recipient who lives a long distance away, and who cannot meet with assessment staff, have the person and staff meet by phone (perhaps with you, in a three-way conference call). The recipient will be able to ask questions about the facility in the same phone call.

❻ Identify any personal equipment and services, besides those offered by the facility, that must be purchased, contracted, or hired. Determine the costs and sources. Examples often include contracting with outside home health aides for help with minor dependencies, a new kind of mobility aid (sometimes motorized), and phone and cable TV services.

❼ Review the available family budget, or level of outside funding, after totaling the costs of the facility and any extra equipment or services. Perform a projection for at least five years to determine whether family assets can cover the current level of expenses as well as predictable increases. If the recipient's functional abilities or health will predictably change, and require transfer to a higher level of care and more expensive facility, factor these increased costs into a second version of the budget.

If family resources will not cover these increases, identify any outside funding that can be tapped. If outside funding is to be used, research the eligibility criteria. Remember that a funding source often stipulates which facilities it will fund.

❽   Reserve and contract the living space, as well as any extra equipment or services. Ask the facility for a detailed floor diagram that includes room dimensions for the new living space; some people also take photos of each room's closet, cupboard, and pantry spaces. These graphics can later be a big help when looking around the current, home residence and deciding what to pack and move.

❾   Contract for cable TV, phone, outside home health aides, and any other services so they will be already up and running on move-in day. Arrange for service disconnects at the recipient's current address.

❿   Schedule and perform the move from home to the living facility. If the recipient will be traveling a long distance by airline, and there are too many last-minute personal belongings for the flight, divide the belongings between in-flight baggage and separate shipping by UPS or a similar express service.

Visiting care facilities—essentials to evaluate

If you are the help recipient, and the one who is coping with the concept of relocating to a group residence, here are some observations and considerations that might help the process. If you are visiting facilities and later reporting your findings to a recipient, these topics should also be helpful in illustrating what to look for.

During your visits to facilities, you will be comparing the many ways in which this new facility views and "treats" its clients, and consequently, how they will treat you. Regardless of the facility or level of care, there will be many significant changes between the previous, at-home lifestyle and this new, at-facility routine.

Much flexibility and compromise from you will be essential to your succeeding at the upcoming transition. While there will be some areas where compromise will be appropriate, there will be others where your preferences—as they are— cannot be compromised without affecting your safety or physical and emotional health. Your preferences here cannot be changed, so either the facility must compromise or a different facility should be found.

Facility and food

- Are both comfortable and warm, or cold and indigestible? Are the smell and appearance of each as they should be?

- As a stranger approaching the entrance of the facility for the first time, what is your first impression? Is it well maintained, reasonably warm, and attractive, or is it poorly maintained, old, and in need of repairs? Does it feel warm and welcome you, or does it feel like a cold institution that will be uncomfortable to visit for this next hour—and unbearable as a place to live?

- During your inside tour, are the features of the facility as well as your future apartment fully accessible to you?

- In the facility, can you negotiate the cafeteria-style food line of the dining room? Would staff help be readily available—or actually prohibited—if you needed it?

- Can you go the distance of the long hallways from your quarters to the dining room, mailboxes, laundry facility, hallway lounges, and assembly areas?

- Aside from wandering through lounges, you can usually request to eat a complimentary meal with your future fellow residents in the dining room. This will answer the essential question:"How good are the food and the company of your future fellow residents?"

Staff attitudes

- Genuine warmth, or hyped excuses?

- When you tour a facility, does the staff refer to residents in respectful and comfortable ways, or does the guide refer to the residents as "those people" and "them"?

- During the tour, when the staff guide meets residents in the hallway, is the encounter the warm, casual type that occurs between two old friends? Or does the staffer, in trying to impress you, greet the old geezer with an artificial, insincere howdy and hug with which the senior citizen is obviously surprised and uncomfortable?

Today's hospitals, rehab centers, and residence facilities are increasingly owned by large management corporations. When operating any business, a basic premise is to keep costs to a minimum. However, resident needs require expenditures. Some facilities are quite responsive to upgrading features and resident conveniences. In contrast, other centers will try to avoid spending money for equipment that their customers plainly need.

> *In a group residence, the people, programs, and facility will each contribute to your happiness—or depression.*

When touring a facility, it is very important that you note any comments that reveal the staff's attitude toward residents and their needs. In the following true story, you will see how an administrator's answer to a question revealed to your author the facility's poor attitude toward meeting its clients' needs.

A couple of years ago, I decided that it would be wise to relocate my elderly mother from a rural area to an assisted living center. I toured three or four centers, while comparing my mother's needs to each center's features, to find the center with the best match.

My mother had previously received knee replacements, so she could not get in and out of a tub shower. Instead, she required a walk-in stall shower. This was a preference that could not be compromised.

During my tour of one center, I asked to see an apartment with a stall shower. I was told that this older facility had only tub showers, and that the managing corporation had decided that changing the tub shower for stalls in several apartments would be too costly. Instead, each facility wing had been outfitted with a whirlpool tub. Once each week, at his or her scheduled time, each resident is escorted to the whirlpool tub room. An aide uses a lift to assist residents into the tub, where they sit for 20 minutes before being dried and returned to their rooms.

I then asked my tour guide, "So any residents who cannot independently use the tub shower in their rooms are limited to one, 20-minute, supervised whirlpool bath per week?"

Her reply to me was very revealing: "Well, we feel that when they get that old, too many baths each week can dry out their skin. Dry skin can cause bedsores, you know. So, given that we are always looking out for the long-term health of our residents, we believe it is in their best interests to limit them to one bath each week. We also discourage them from independently using their own tubs between weekly tub appointments. There are just too many injuries these days with these older people."

Her plastic answer revealed several facts to me:

- Since staff attitudes are usually adopted by all, beginning with the administration, I could probably assume that her subordinates felt the same way toward clients as did my guide.

- The staff had developed a "we-they" attitude toward residents—a very intentional distancing with probable consequences of poor communication and a lack of caring and respect.

- The administration was operating this facility with priorities that respected the financial bottom line and not the needs of residents. After refusing to spend money that would have improved the comfort, health, and safety of the clients, the unethical administration then created a lame excuse that attempted to justify its actions.

- This blatantly false excuse for unethical behavior was probably not merely a single, isolated incident, but instead the sign of routinely unethical operating policy. There were undoubtedly other unethical practices.

- As a person who has lived with a disability as well as with many incidents of bigotry, discrimination, and prejudice for about 35 years, I was now very uncomfortable in this facility. I certainly would not recommend it to my mother or anyone else.

Your future fellow residents

- How is their hair kept and how are they dressed? Are their clothes clean? Do they seem to care? Are they proud or ashamed with how they appear and who they are? How would you feel if you routinely looked like them, or had their attitude?

- Do they inspire you with an interest to know them better, or distress you with depressing moans, groans, and complaints?

You should also spend some time speaking with, or simply observing, the residents. Wander into a reading lounge, introduce yourself as a possible future resident, and ask one of your questions. Other residents will naturally join in with their opinions, particularly if they are especially pleased or angry with the place.

Your degree of comfort with other residents is essential to your future ability to seek happiness and avoid depression. While no longer living with your natural family, if you move here you will spend the first few days surveying residents and selecting your new "family." In doing today's quick survey of residents, are there some that are interesting and that you would like to know better, or are most of them dull, uninteresting, and depressing?

Typical costs, and considering long-term care insurance

Americans are living longer than ever before and are requiring professional help and care to do so. Each year, the costs of both at-home and community services are rising. Each year, more families are wiping out their life savings to ensure that their parents will receive professional care as long as they need it.

For a more complete accounting of the costs for care, see *Figure 1-5*. This chapter has introduced the following services, listed here with average costs in midwestern United States as of this book's 2002 printing date.

Figure 1-5: **Comparison of costs for listed services in year 2000**

Companion and home health aide help, at home, from an agency	$18–$25/hr.
Companion and home health aide help, at home, from personal employment	$10/hr.
Day care	$8.50/hr., $40/day
Respite care	$85–$100/day
Independent living facility, private apartment of 600–700 square feet, two meals daily, no aide assistance	$1,550–$1,750/mo.
Assisted living facility, private apartment or room of 400–650 square feet, three meals daily, aide assistance and medication coordination included	$1,950–$3,250/mo.
Nursing home (health care center), small private room, three meals daily, aide and nursing assistance included	$4,000–$5,000/mo.

Medicare pays for limited nursing home care (following a hospital stay) and limited home health care. Medicaid will consider nursing home care for the poor and those who have exhausted their life savings. People who qualify for a Medicaid residence should be aware that Medicaid-dedicated beds are limited in both number and geographic availability.

Long-term care insurance has been available since the 1970s and provides benefits in a variety of facility types. Many people with preexisting medical conditions and disabilities do not qualify. About 120 U.S. companies currently offer the coverage, which can cost between $900 and $8,000 annually, depending on the insured's age and desired benefits. The American Association of Retired Persons (AARP) offers a variety of publications that provide details about planning and budgeting for community residences and about long-term care insurance.

Chapter 2
Volunteer Help: Don't Wear Out Your Friendships

Your use of volunteer help can be very important to your being independent and active in the public mainstream. However, using it wisely—and not overworking family, friends, neighbors, office co-workers, and strangers in the process—can require some special skills and guidelines.

Perhaps you have learned to be cautious about generously offered help. Many very caring people often offer "to do you a favor anytime," and yet when you trust in their sincerity and try to cash in, their enthusiasm is replaced by hesitation and reluctance. Too often the originally unconditional offer suddenly develops some obvious, and yet undefined, conditions. When you cannot fully trust in a friend's offer of a favor, it becomes easy to question your trust in that friendship.

In truth, usually the friendship is not in question, but merely the friend's availability for fulfilling the offered favor. The friend's unlimited feelings of support, caring, or love for you have become confused with the limited availability of personal time and energy to fulfill favors.

So, when it comes to offered volunteer help:

- What offers can you trust?

- Who can you trust?

- When can you trust that offered help will actually be available?

- Are there any consistent guidelines? If so, what are they?

Volunteer help: essential when appropriate, abuse when not

First, do you need, and when should you use, volunteers? The temptation to maximize your use of volunteers, without the need for guidelines, is strong. It appears, at first glance, that volunteer help is always available, quickly and on-demand, and with significant financial savings. In short, volunteer help maximizes your freedom, and it is free!

However, is volunteer help really appropriate for all your needs? When is it safe to take advantage of a friend's offered favor, and when is it wise to politely decline it while expressing your appreciation?

You probably instinctively (and appropriately) use volunteer help for some of your brief, one-shot needs. If you are on your own and independent each day, you use brief volunteer help each time a stranger opens and holds a door into an office building, a cafeteria worker carries your tray to a table, or a grocery bagger loads your car. The only pay each expects is a simple "thank you." If only fulfilling all your ADL needs were this simple!

In another situation, some folks routinely and successfully use very dedicated, dependable help from organizations that recruit and maintain large pools of volunteers. Examples include volunteers who provide reading, tutoring, and occasional companionship during leisure and shopping events. Surely, using this type of volunteer help must be okay.

In yet another situation—emergencies—the volunteer help that we openly offer each other is essential. However, when you need general help, and you want to justify your desire to get it promptly from the nearest person, it is tempting to stretch the true definition of an emergency to mean urgent, important, or simply "want-it-now."

At what fuzzy point does your concept of a favor exceed the volunteer's intentions, and become the volunteer's concept of a burden?

As a beginning guideline, it is not reasonable to expect most volunteers to be at your apartment each morning at 6 A.M. to help with your "get up" routine. For any recurring or extensive need for personal and medical assistance, volunteer help is seldom the answer. These are your activities of daily living needs, or ADLs. Discrepancies too often occur between the frequency, length, punctuality, and dependability of your ADL needs and the volunteer's availability.

Generally, for brief and non-routine needs, volunteers can be essential for doing favors. However, for routine, personal ADLs, hired help is usually the best approach.

Again, we are not questioning here the dedication of volunteers, but merely the appropriateness of using them for certain needs. Indeed, there are thousands of agencies that routinely coordinate volunteer help. These organizations, from the Red Cross and Peace Corps to community church, school, and fire department auxiliaries, successfully depend on very dedicated, rock-solid volunteers. In addition, there are individuals without group affiliation who are more trustworthy in seeing through personal commitments than most salaried employees. Among these, only the best of paid aides will match the loyalty and self-sacrificing hard work that family caregivers and other volunteers routinely provide.

The theme of this chapter is to provide you with guidelines for recognizing situations in which volunteer help is not appropriate, and for which your help should be formally hired. In addition, there is a listing of at least six situations in which using volunteers is okay, expected, and welcomed.

After reviewing this chapter, you will seldom wonder whether it is okay to ask for a favor, and those stomach knots of guilt and uneasiness should be things of the past!

A real-life, college experience of overusing volunteer favors

It is so tempting to take advantage of occasional favors offered by friends, and then gradually increase your routine use and dependence on them until the situation gets out of hand. Consider the following, common example from my own college-campus experiences.

During my college years in the late 1960s, I lived for a time in a campus dormitory. I had one of the 75 two-person rooms in the three-story dorm, and easily became friends with many of the 149 other students who shared the same building.

I was a 19-year-old, spinal-cord-injured, C 5/6 quad (tetra) using motorized wheelchair mobility. When I arrived at the Illinois campus from New York, a formally hired, fellow-student PA greeted me at the airport. During the previous summer, while still in New York, I had placed a classified ad in the campus paper. Patrick, a junior, had answered the ad. By phone, I had described my needs, interviewed and hired him, and scheduled him to meet me at the airport. I was a naive, trusting adolescent who was burning to be free from small-town, upstate New York by becoming a college student 1,600 miles away. I was incredibly appreciative of Patrick's response to my ad, and he had fully met the stringent requirements I had set as my "PA ticket to college"—he was able-bodied and had a pulse!

I trained Patrick to assist me with dressing, wheelchair transfers, using the toilet, and showers. Just 18 months post-injury, I wanted as much as possible to deny my disability and my dependence on formal PA help. I had wisely arranged for Patrick, my sole PA, to be my roommate in our two-person dorm room. I reasoned, way back then, that if my only PA slept in the same dorm room, I would not need to worry about his availability each morning and night. At that time, no handbook on PA management, like the one you are holding now, was available. I was just taking one common-sense step at a time to fill my needs while trying to minimize personal risk.

As I now reminisce, I was ashamed of my disability and my dependence on the personal help that I required from Patrick. "Wheelchair students," "wheelies," "gimps," or "crips," as we then called ourselves, were not as common as today. Most were paraplegics who could live independently. In 1968, I was among the first generation of trailblazing quads. For coping with my more extensive limitations, I found peer role models to be rare. I was the only quadriplegic student in my dorm who got toilet and shower help from his roommate. I guess I resented—even as I regretfully accepted—the morning and evening help, and so I wanted my daytime lifestyle to be as able-bodied (AB) as possible.

I was also afraid to ask for too much help from Patrick by stating further needs during the day, between classes. He was my very first hired aide, and I denied myself imagining any possibility that he might resign because my needs for his help had become over-whelming to him. Like any one-and-only aide, Patrick held enormous power over me—and both of us knew it. After just a few days, he was already tiring of his morning-and-evening, 24/7, continual duties and lack of freedom. I knew that I would have a few undeniable needs for help during the day, but I sensed that assigning Patrick additional daytime duties would have pushed him beyond his tolerance. It would never have occurred to me to hire a second, daytime aide.[1]

Initially, the image of using formal PA help during the day would have made me feel too disabled and dependent. In contrast, my AB friends exchanged favors frequently, so for me also to accept favors was cool and within the AB image that I wanted to see—and have my colleagues see—in myself. In contrast, being dependent on meeting up with a salaried PA on a set schedule during the day would not have fit my image of freedom. If I were forced to have a disability with extensive, paid-PA dependence each morning and night, then I would strive to be able-bodied at other times—and need just occasional "favors."

Therefore, at the beginning of each semester, when we all made new friends, several students would typically introduce themselves to me and emotionally offer, "Skip, if you ever need anything, please be sure to call me. I will be so glad to help you!" I would then file that name and face away for future use.

When Patrick was not around, a book might drop on the floor in my room, my electric typewriter (remember—or ever hear of—those?) might not be plugged in when I wanted to type a report, or my urinary leg bag might need an empty before Patrick was scheduled to return. Consequently, I would often ask one of my dorm neighbors for just a tiny favor that would require just a second.

I usually tried to specially phrase a favor to trivialize it. As most people do, I would word each favor so it appeared to be small and brief. If you had asked me then, I would have justified my ploy as a scheme to make the request more acceptable and an easier sell to the volunteer provider. In truth, when I now remember the embarrassment, shame, and stress I felt when asking each favor, I now admit that my primary objective was to reduce my own guilt. My subconscious self knew that my overuse of favors was inappropriate; my conscious self was in survival-stage, disability denial.

---

1. For more detail about the disadvantages of using just one PA, please see chapter 📖 **16,** **"Dividing Your Needs, and Assigning Work Shifts, Among Several PAs."**

I did not have a monopoly on overusing volunteer help. Although I used a motorized wheelchair, some of my more disabled wheelchair buddies had come to the large campus with manual ones. Their limited physical ability, their desire to be active in the campus mainstream, and the mile-long campus would have all combined to make a motorized chair a wiser choice. However, their ego-fueled desire to deny their true limitations caused them to be stubbornly loyal to their manuals. While I independently whizzed by in my motorized, they would routinely be sitting at various points of the campus sidewalks, begging for a push to class, a push to the library, or a push to the pizza place downtown.

Trusting in the sincerity of our friends who had offered to do favors, we asked and were usually granted our initial requests. As we thanked them the first and second times, we received the standard volunteer-help pledge renewal: "Do not mention it. You are so welcome. Remember, call me anytime." However, there was noticeably less enthusiasm in these subsequent renewals than there had been in the original offers.

After the first week's series of granted favors, our AB dorm buddies no longer offered to do us favors. Gradually and consistently, they began to avoid us. However, since we still depended on them for help with certain needs, we learned from trial and error some of the even finer points of downright begging.

Each of us should have noted—as a warning flag—the attitudinal change in our dorm mates. Initially, they offered us favors; now, since they no longer offered favors, we were aggressively begging and tricking them into providing help. At that point, we should have realized that we were overusing and abusing the volunteer help. Our needs had become too numerous and frequent for favors from volunteers. We should have faced the extent of our disabilities and needs, and assumed justifiable responsibility for formally hiring PAs or obtaining appropriate mobility equipment. That current situation was costing us friendships with the unwilling volunteers, as well as our own self-respect and independence.

In becoming accomplished beggars, we learned how not to appear to be needing a favor. We used a sort of non-purposeful, unfocused body language that disguised the very carefully planned and choreographed, cat-and-mouse game that street beggars use.

If you look as though you are anxious to ask a favor from the next passerby, the next passer will avoid your eye contact or actually change direction to stay outside of your pounce-and-beg distance. In contrast, if you seem to be preoccupied and free of need, then passers will erroneously feel safe to approach you and occasionally even start conversation.

Much like fishing and sensing a bait nibble, we would often begin that conversation and then slyly slip in our unavoidable request:

"Hi, Jim, has this been a rough exam week for you? You don't say. Me, too. By the way, would you mind doing me a teeny, real-quick favor?" As we delivered that last line, and saw that Jim could not politely escape without performing the favor, we would feel a distinct "gotcha" smile of having hooked yet another live one.

After a semester or two, some of us realized that we were sacrificing the potential for many friendships as the cost of routinely asking for favors that were no longer offered to us. Sociologically, it was interesting that some of us decided to hire the help we needed and stop asking for favors. The friends who had been avoiding us soon started warming up to us again. However, others did not catch on. They continued to beg favors, and continued to encounter avoidance.

This is not to say that we smarter dudes have never again asked for another favor from anyone. No, I still today routinely depend on, ask for, and receive favors. However, what I learned—and am about to pass on to you—is the what, when, where, and from whom of asking appropriate and usually welcomed volunteer favors. If I have a routine help need, I formally arrange for a paid provider who is genuinely happy to provide the help—and my conscience is clear. No more shame, guilt, or stomach knots!

Reasons for preferring volunteer help, and overusing it, while denying the need for hired help

There is a common progression for first taking advantage of offers for friendly favors, and then gradually slipping into overusing and abusing them.

Able-bodied folks are mostly independent in their lifestyle, and they rarely need to ask for favors from friends. Consequently, ABs rarely get into trouble by asking for too many favors, or by asking for help with unsuitable needs. In contrast, if you have a disability, you are more dependent on help from others. Some needs are appropriate for volunteer favors, and some are not.

There are at least six situations in which you can feel comfortable using volunteer help. These are detailed near the end of this chapter. Some situations continue to be okay for asking favors.

Where, then, is that controversial area that gets so many of us into trouble by straining friendships in overusing the favors that are offered by volunteers?

Perhaps the primary difference between an AB's needs and yours is in your routine, day-after-day need for help with ADLs. In the most inner circle is the need for assistance with some or all the following:

- urinary collection device or self-catheterization supplies
- bowel program
- bathing or showering
- getting dressed
- transfers among bed, commode chair, wheelchair, and car

- food preparation and eating
- taking medication
- wound care.

These are the hard-core needs for which you require solid, dependable, and continuous help providers. The help for these ADL needs should not come from the impromptu volunteering of your friends; it should be hired.

Is asking for volunteer favors so tempting because the help is free? Actually, there are several reasons related to having a disability that make using volunteer help especially attractive.

Independence

First, you want to think of yourself—and be seen by others—as a strong person who does not need help from others. Regardless of whether you were brought up in the John Wayne era of films, it is natural for you to want to think of yourself as strong, self-sufficient, and independent. If you have a disability, your desire to be, as well as to appear, that way are even stronger. If your disability prevents the former, you can at least strive for the latter. In many ways, you must thoroughly believe that you are independent and in control to maintain the mindset and ability to live that way.

It does not seem fair that those of us with disabilities must be doubly firm about our mindset of pride, strength, and independence, and yet be forced by our physical limitations to ask humbly for help from others. Indeed, there is a lifelong lesson to be learned and practiced here regarding this balance of pride and humility.

After considerable life experience and personal reflection, we learn about the irony of having immense spiritual power and strength as a consequence of having significant physical weakness and paralysis. Indeed, the presence of a disability often requires us to routinely ask others for help. We are forced to develop the strength and courage to ask for help, and the humility to accept it.

Asking for help is not a sign of weakness but of strength. However, there are many, many people who are so weakened by their own pride and ego that they are actually unable to ask for help.

Denial

You want to believe that your dependent needs for help are so minor that formally hired help is unnecessary, and that mere help from occasional favors and volunteers will be adequate.

If asking for help has a negative image, and your disability requires you to do so, then your preference is to ask for favors from volunteers rather than pay for help from employees.

Again, you probably have an understandable desire to accentuate your strengths and deny your weaknesses—and your disability. You want to see yourself, and be seen by others, as strong and independent.

Informality

It is easy to fall into the volunteer trap because volunteer help is readily available whenever you need it—no muss, no fuss.

If you prefer not to think about your routine needs for help, then you will also prefer to spend a minimum of time and effort in getting that help. That means a preference for asking strangers for quick favors, instead of spending time recruiting employees.

Limitations
In contrast to having volunteer help available as needed, using hired help would require formally identifying, listing, and scheduling your needs, and then limiting the availability of help to that schedule.

To expand on the previous point, employing help requires time and effort in going through what I refer to as the RISHTMP cycle of recruiting, interviewing, screening, hiring, training, managing, and parting ways with providers.

In addition, employing help is admittedly a structured activity. Job applicants usually want to know what, when, and how you want help provided (how unfair and demanding of them!). This requires you both to create a structure and schedule of your needs, and then to live by that structure and schedule. In contrast, simply asking for favors from volunteers seems to provide so much more freedom!

Experience and skills
Also in contrast to using volunteers, perhaps you lack experience and the required skills—or simply prefer not—to formally recruit, hire, train, and schedule paid help, and then be committed to routinely performing this cycle.

Asking for favors from volunteers is so easy and requires few skills, except knowing how to beg from and con people. In contrast, the RISHTMP cycle requires learning the process for personally employing PAs, or finding a good agency to do it for you. In comparison, snagging favors from volunteers and passersby is a no-brainer.

Cost
Finally, in contrast to the free volunteer help, hired help costs money. The bottom (financial) line is that favors from volunteers are free, whereas hired help typically costs between $9 and $25 per hour. Wow, two hours of agency-hired help to do a laundry, take a shower, and get into bed could cost 50 bucks!

Signs of overusing volunteer help, and of needing to hire help
There are common warning flags that should signal the wisdom of shifting dependent needs from volunteer to hired help for your ADL needs.

- First, if you feel increasingly uneasy, stressed, and guilty about continuing to ask for favors.

Deep down inside, you feel stressed and your stomach knots up as you make your pitch to each potential volunteer helper. You brace yourself against most reactions which are too often refusals and rejections. Each time someone does agree to help you, you quickly change stress gears in your effort to make nervous conversation while you receive the help. The reason for your strained conversation seems to be divided between an effort to entertain the helper so he or she will not mind the time spent in assisting you, and to help the time pass more quickly (with reduced guilt and embarrassment) for you!

- Second, you sense that volunteers are no longer eager to do favors or provide help, and are trying to avoid contact with you.

You begin to know how a street panhandler feels. Friends who formerly went out of their way to greet you now try to avoid you. They quickly began to associate your approach, exaggerated smile, and "hi there" with your imminent request for a favor. You might also sense that they resent your friendliness as an insincere coverup for a favor request. You feel as though you are abusing friendships—you know it, and they know it.

- Third, you sometimes feel angry when your request for help is declined or granted with reserve. You initially believed you were angry with the volunteer, or your disability, for causing your needs. However, you now suspect that you are angry with yourself, both for denying to yourself the extent of your needs and for procrastinating in formally hiring help.

In the early stages, as discussed in the preceding section, you denied to yourself that your disability and needs were sufficiently extensive to merit hiring formal help. You wanted, and wanted others, to believe that quick little favors from volunteers were all you needed.

However after months of uncomfortable begging, jeopardizing friendships, and watching your needs actually increase, you cannot continue denying reality. You are not angry with the reactions of your friends; you are angry with yourself for the games you have played.

The time has come for you to admit your extensive need for routine help, to hire it, and to resume enjoying friends for their friendship.

Congratulations! You have succeeded both in achieving an advanced degree of accepting your disability, and in accommodating your limitations in a constructive, positive way. In addition, you have in your hands the best possible reference guide for taking that next step of efficiently hiring and managing your help. Read on.

Six sources, purposes, and guidelines for appropriately using volunteer help

To this point, we have been warning of the inappropriate use of friends and volunteers for routine ADL needs. These day-after-day personal needs include getting dressed, using the toilet, eating, recurring transportation, and frequent errands.

In contrast, remember that there are some situations in which it is okay to continue to ask for favors. Unless you are quite wealthy, it is usually not practical to have the constant accompaniment of hired help (or of chronically tired family caregivers) wherever you go.

Here is where you and able-bodied friends commonly share the brief, one-shot situations and needs for valid, volunteer help. However, for your disability lifestyle, your routine use of appropriate help is even more important than for your A-B friends. Taking advantage of this appropriate volunteer help is essential for your active and independent lifestyle. Indeed, you are quite dependent on it and should feel free to routinely use it from at least the six sources discussed in this section.

The primary caution in appropriately using volunteers is to understand the following:

- the sources of help
- the appropriate types and limitations of help available from each source
- how to take advantage of each source's help
- how to "reimburse" the volunteer help provider—
  always with appreciation and sometimes with monetary tips.

In some of the following situations, such as for store employees or members of volunteer organizations, there are clear guidelines for the intended type and availability of a source's help—what each is willing to do and how long or often you can depend on the favor. Where formal guidelines exist, respect them. Where they do not exist (and often they do not), as with family caregivers, friends, and neighbors, you should create your own conservative guidelines, discuss them, and then carefully monitor feedback.

Here are six sources and types of readily available volunteer help, with guidelines about using them.

Caregiver help

Suppose family caregivers have agreed to provide routine help for personal needs. Boundaries and guidelines are essential but often do not exist. As the recipient who appreciates their help, you should take responsibility for establishing guidelines and then periodically calling family meetings to review the family's welfare.

Just as there is "no place like home," there is also no equal to the caring, warmth, and love that comes with the help provided by family caregivers. Caregivers will often agree to do almost anything for you, and therein lies the caution about using their assistance. More than 50 percent of caregivers are chronically tired and depressed because they are overdoing without sufficient rest and time off.

As important as it is for them to establish and maintain limits on how much they do for you, most caregivers find it nearly impossible to say "no" to the loved ones whom they help. If you get help from your family, do them a favor. Be the one who establishes limits and then insists on formal, periodic family review meetings. A family-wide discussion—that includes you, family caregivers, and other family members—to review how things are going should be held at least once each month, and more often when problems or tempers surface.[2]

The agenda for family meetings should include a review of the following:

- How tired they are (yes, you can trust that they are tired).

---

2. For more details about caregiver concerns and yours, and considering outside help, please see the following chapters:

   📖 1 "Beyond Family Caregivers: Options and Settings for Finding Outside Assistance"
   📖 5 "Ten Steps to Getting All or Some of Your Help from Family Caregivers"
   📖 23 "Your Personal Concerns as a Recipient of Help"
   📖 24 "Your Personal Concerns as a Family Caregiver"

- What changes in duties and scheduling—for you, caregivers, and other family members—would make life easier for the family?
- Whether the family should consider hiring some, or more, outside PA help, especially for your ADL needs.

Friends and neighbors

People you know well or who live nearby have probably offered to do general favors or provide help with certain kinds of tasks. Realize what they cannot realize. Know that their true availability for favors is so limited, and so important, that they should be saved for only the most important events: crises and emergencies.

These volunteers are very similar to the college-student friends and neighbors from my earlier story. Without a doubt, their hearts are in the right place, but their true availability will be limited. Out of their care for you, they might promise you the sky. However, as with your family caregivers, it is your responsibility to set realistic limits on what favors you request and how often you do so.

A good rule of thumb for these volunteers is to save them for real emergencies, and to use formal volunteers from civic groups or paid PAs for routine needs. Your experience will tell you what limits you should set for their help. These people will give you 150 percent in the truly rare crises and emergencies, but not for routine, daily ones!

Their sincerity is not being questioned, but the depth of their commitment is a concern. Their offer to "help you anytime you need anything" is, indeed, an emotional testimony of their friendship, caring, and often love for you. However, compared to the carefully calculated commitments made by organizational volunteers, friends often first make an emotional, off-the-cuff offer… and then they start thinking about it.

These friends might be your neighbors, office co-workers, college campus colleagues, or acquaintances of a social group. Too often, their offer to help is not meant as an offer of assistance, but as a conceptual expression of their friendship and caring about your welfare and good health. You should interpret these friendship volunteer offers:

- primarily, as expressions of good will
- second, as valid offers of help for true emergencies
- third, not as help that is intended to be routinely tapped for ordinary needs.

Keep their phone numbers on a printed list and stored in the one-button speed dialer of your bedside phone. When an emergency occurs at 3 A.M., and your life or property is in danger, feel comfortable in knowing that these people are truly eager to help you.

Strangers and passersby

Those whom you encounter in stores and on streets can be tapped for brief, one-time help with simple needs. Feel comfortable in asking for help while respecting some simple concerns.

These folks fulfill a very special niche in your everyday independence in the public mainstream. If not for them, many of us would have to bring a paid PA wherever we went. These are the good Samaritans who:

- open and hold doors into public places
- pick up your car keys when you drop them
- spot your car breakdown along the highway and change your flat tire
- offer to carry your burger, fries, and drink from the fast-food counter to a nearby table in the shopping mall
- give you and your wheelchair an emergency push back to your car when a part breaks
- help you sit up straight again in your wheelchair when you lose your balance and fall forward.

Like your friends and neighbors, many of these folks would be thrilled to assist you in an emergency. Different from the friends and neighbors whom you see over and over, it is common that you will never again see the person who today held the door into the store for you. Because you are not repeatedly "hitting up" the same people, you can more frequently ask different strangers for one-shot help with brief needs.

When asked politely, told how important their help is, and thanked afterward, few strangers will refuse you if:

- the favor will not take them too far out of their way
- they are not already in a hurry and your need is brief
- they are physically able to provide the help
- the task is not too personal as to make them feel uncomfortable
- they do not believe their own possessions or personal safety will be jeopardized
- they do not have a private, personal reason or hangup for not helping you.

It is also interesting to note that additional bystanders are often observing your entire interaction with the good Samaritan stranger who helps you, from your initial request through the parting "thank you." Most of the onlookers have one or two of these three reasons for watching instead of helping, including:

- they are curious and will watch anything
- they are willing to help, and would eagerly add their assistance if it becomes necessary
- they are currently too uncomfortable to offer help to you, but if your interaction with the good Sam goes smoothly, they might decide to offer help to someone else in the future.

Each time you work with a stranger, you are simultaneously receiving help, educating the public, and changing attitudes. Improve the future for yourself and the rest of us by clearly expressing appreciation to the helping stranger, and so making a favorable impression with any onlookers.

Employees of retail stores

Employees of retail stores and other businesses have been formally designated to receive help requests, or to offer assistance as you enter a store. Feel free to ask for whatever help you need to have the same access to the store that able-bodied customers have. In the United States, much work went into the drafting and 1990 passage of the federal Americans with Disabilities Act (ADA); take advantage of these legislated rights.

In the United States before 1990, this offer of store assistance while shopping was a common courtesy. Now, after the passage of ADA, the offer is usually required by federal law. Help in reaching display items, getting them to the cashier, and loading them into your car is now considered a requirement for providing you with equal access to the store's facilities.

Monetary tips, by law, should neither be expected nor accepted by a store employee, and you should feel comfortable with this. Feel free to ask for whatever help you need in order to have the same access to the store that is enjoyed by able-bodied customers.

As mentioned, many retailers now routinely offer you help as you enter the store. Unfortunately, a few folks who have obvious disabilities, and a bad attitude, have a tendency to feel anger when clerks offer help, and to "blow them away" with an angry reply. There is no reason to get angry at innocent clerks who are simply doing their jobs.

Employees of service-oriented businesses

Employees of hotels, motels, restaurants, and other service-oriented businesses are often on a minimum salary because of the tips they get from the public. These employees are included within this section on volunteers because they offer assistance without requiring a monetary fee or charge. However, a financial tip for many services is a cultural expectation. Take advantage of their help, and provide them with verbal appreciation as well as the customary financial tip when they deserve it.

Yes, these businesses are also subject to ADA requirements. However, the culture in many countries has traditionally required a 15–20 percent tip—long before ADA—for the following:

- parking lot attendants, who park or watch over your car
- hotel bellhops, who carry luggage to your room
- hotel concierge, who provides you special services
- restaurant wait staff, who serve your meal, and can be asked to cut up food or otherwise arrange or prepare the food they serve to you
- hotel room service, who will deliver just about anything to your room
- taxi drivers, who also help you with luggage and your mobility aid

- home-delivery people, who deliver something to your home
- airport skycaps, for handling your luggage.

Tipping remains a cultural expectation for many services as an appreciation for customized, personal help. Although, each of these people routinely provides a traditional type of help, most are also glad to provide you with the extra accommodations your disability requires.

You should feel comfortable in asking for extra help; someone can always decline a request that is not appropriate. As a quadriplegic who uses a wheelchair, I have traveled alone extensively. I have learned to ask for help, and provide detailed instructions, for my special needs. In return, I have been especially appreciative when a provider deserves it.

I have always traveled within a reasonable budget, and so have learned that while extra services do merit an additional tip, the money need not be extravagant. However, everyone can be extravagant about verbally expressing appreciation.

Often, an airport skycap has helped me with a seat-to-wheelchair transfer, a push to the faraway baggage carousels, retrieving my baggage, getting me a cab, and help with a wheelchair-to-cab transfer. What retains their hour-long help and makes them eager to provide me with extra services? I sense each time they are tempted to leave, and fuel them with more appreciation, and then flash the largest bill of the money that I am holding in my hand for their eventual tip!

Without these willing service providers, much of your independence would not be possible unless you brought your own salaried help with you. I often consider how prohibitively expensive that would be when I am occasionally tempted to be stingy with financial tips. When the value of travel and other special services is calculated, tips are really an inexpensive way to ensure that these services are readily available, so that you and I can remain as independent as possible.

When people provide me with special help, I try to squeeze my budget and offer an above-average tip. However, for a truly lasting impression as I hand them the tip, I make firm eye contact, smile, and very assertively and warmly reinforce what I have appreciated: "Denise, thank you for your special help with my meal. This is for you."

If you return later to that same restaurant, and Denise is again your waitress, you could probably count on her remembering you and the special help that you need. If you asked her why, would she remember how much of a financial tip you gave her on the previous visit? Probably not. Instead, she will remember that you were "one of her nicest customers" because you took the time to tell her that she and her assistance were important to you.

By expressing your appreciation while you provide a tip, you make her feel special and important. You are indeed a statistically rare person—use it to your advantage!

Volunteer groups

Members of volunteer-service groups, hospital auxiliaries, centers for seniors and people with disabilities, meals-on-wheels groups, churches, and other civic organizations want to provide specific kinds of volunteer assistance. Because providing you with help is what they most want to do, you should not feel guilty about making volunteers feel good by accepting their services.

People who donate their time through an organization have made a carefully calculated commitment. From a sociological point of view, some folks are attracted first to join the organization and then to volunteer their help, while others first decide to volunteer help and then join an organization to do so.

Regardless of their personal priority, these people have joined an organization, become acquainted with other volunteers, and committed themselves both to the organization's guidelines and to volunteering. These people are in it for the long haul.

As mentioned before, volunteer organizations are a primary foundation of worldwide and community help. Society would probably collapse without it. You should feel free to research local volunteer organizations about the typical types of help they provide. Take advantage of the help they offer, and in return, offer to join a group to provide your own help to others, or to donate money to the organization. There are few experiences in life as rewarding as helping others.

The good news about volunteers is that usually they are very dedicated, dependable people who want to serve and be needed by others. Their services are free, except perhaps that donations are frequently "welcomed," though not required, by their sponsoring civic group.

So why not use a group of volunteers for your day-to-day, ADL needs?

In contrast to community-wide activities, the day-to-day help that you need for your ADLs is seldom on their menu. However, you might want to call several volunteer agencies and map out what volunteer help is available, from which agency, and for what kinds of needs. You might find that after your routine, hired help gets you out of bed and dressed, volunteer help might furnish you with meals or with transportation within the community.

This help often comes from people who have retired from work, but have not retired from their desire to help, to be needed, and to volunteer their services. These folks join a civic group that formally provides volunteer help of certain kinds. As someone needing help, you would contact the organization's office to get a clear understanding of the type and amount of available assistance. As long as you respect those guidelines, you should feel comfortable, and not guilty, about accepting the help of and making friends with some of the volunteers.

Universal tips for getting help from volunteers

With these six sources for volunteer help, and the guidelines for using it, keep in mind these universal suggestions when you ask for help. Smile, make direct eye contact, speak clearly and warmly, and be assertive, in order to:

- get a help provider's attention
- ask for the help you need
- provide clear, patient instructions about what you need and how you want it provided
- express sincere appreciation

For service-oriented restaurant wait staff and the like, provide the customary monetary tip, plus a bit extra if you can and they deserve it.

Politely accept a provider's occasional decline of your request and promptly look for another person.

Save friendships for having fun, and not for using the restroom

The moral to these very true and common stories is to keep to a minimum favors that you ask of volunteers, friends, fellow students, and co-workers. If the cool reaction that you get when asking a favor seems to say that you might be wearing out your welcome, then you probably are.

When this happens, start taking notes to identify the what, when, where, how, and how often regarding the favors that you have been overusing. Then schedule a hired PA who gets paid for doing you those favors.

And by all means, if you require a motorized mobility aid, get one. You may initially be concerned that you might look or feel "more disabled" if you use a motorized instead of manual wheelchair. However, it is almost guaranteed that you would be the only person who would feel that way.

A primary goal of independent living is going where you wish, when you wish, and with a minimum of physical dependence on others. You will appear to yourself, as well as to others around you, to be far more disabled if you are often begging pushes to destinations in your manual.

The alternative is to arrive independently, on schedule, and truly in the mainstream. Save your manual for exercise around the house and for bite-sized trips that match your strength and stamina.

Your friends and co-workers will not care what provides power to your four wheels, or who routinely helps you use the restroom, as long as it is not them! At the end of a social gathering, would you rather have your friends impressed by remembering your able-bodied wit and conversation, or the way you needed their help to transfer and use the restroom's toilet stall?[3]

---

3. For more detail on identifying, listing, and getting PA help for those face-to-face, setup, and remote needs, please see chapters 📖 11, "When It Is, and Is Not, Okay to Ask for Help," and 📖 13, "Defining and Describing Your Help Needs."

Chapter 3
Live-In Aides and Other Residence Options

If you have used help from family caregivers, you know the advantages of live-in assistants. When it comes time to hire outside PAs, you can still have the comfort of free, live-in help.

Live-in arrangements can provide especially dependable help, with financial savings, when carefully managed. This specialized chapter tells you about the advantages of using live-in help, how to calculate and negotiate it, and ways to stay in control of it.

In contrast, live-ins can also be an internal source of abuse and theft when not controlled. This chapter will also give you strategies for making a live-in arrangement work to your advantage while keeping it tamed, and when live-in aides cease to be desirable roommates, how to show them the door and have them use it.

When having a live-in aide is not possible, the salaried PAs you hire might live quite close by or a considerable distance from you. When you have to choose and hire one PA from two or three applicants, you should be aware of the advantages of having your salaried aides live as close as possible to you.

Two real-life examples
of exchanging live-in space for free live-in help

To introduce you to how you can negotiate a rental space in your home or apartment for free live-in help, here are two actual case histories.

In a first example, I was once a departmental director at a major university in Boston but could not afford the additional expense of salaried PA help. I rented a two-bedroom apartment and offered the second bedroom to two college-student aides. Instead of paying me with rent, various apartment mates provided me with "free" help— for nine years!

To recruit my PAs from students at the campus, I used a combination of posters and ads in the campus paper.[1]

---

1. Examples of using each format are shown in chapter 📖 8, **"Where and How to Advertise for Your Own PAs."**

With the room, I included only utilities and our common phone line. This meant that their toll calls appeared with mine on the phone bill I received. The disadvantage to this was my monthly accounting of finding their toll calls, running totals, adding taxes, and then hounding these guys until they paid me. Today, I would pay to have extra phone lines run to the apartment, and then make the aides financially responsible for arranging their own service and paying the bills that were addressed to them.

To have three guys living in a two-bedroom apartment was an adventure and a bit claustrophobic. For whatever reason, I ran dry of college students a couple of times and resorted to placing ads in the city-wide newspaper. These were the times when I had to work very hard to weed out the undesirable applicants. These included alcoholics who were running from bill collectors, druggies who were looking for a fresh dealing address that was not yet on the police observation sheet, and people of various sexual preferences and fantasies who were convinced that all people in wheelchairs were also looking for the same thing. With experience, I became increasingly skilled at sensing when the applicant on the other end of the phone wanted something other than what I was offering.[2]

In a second example, a high-level quad friend who lives near Denver has arranged perhaps the most desirable PA situation I have seen. Sam (not his real name) is a middle-aged professional who bought a unique residence. His residence consists of his main house surrounded by three smaller cottages on the same grounds. Two of the cottages provide private living quarters for two aides. The third cottage is larger and offers two shared semi-private living areas for two more aides.

Sam's mortgage runs about $1,250 a month. He could not afford this expense on his own, so he charges a monthly rent to each of the PAs who live in the two private cottages. After checking with a local realtor, he assessed that each PA in the private cottages would ordinarily be paying a monthly cash rent of $750, and each PA in the shared cottage would be paying $500. The two $500 PAs in the shared cottage are not charged rent, and live rent-free in exchange for their help to Sam. Each $750 PA in the two private cottages also receives the first $500 of monthly residence rent-free, but each then pays rent to Sam for the $250 extra value. By receiving this total of $500 in monthly rent, Sam's out-of-pocket mortgage expense is reduced to $750.

---

2. The interview and screening process that I consequently developed is the basis for the process outlined in chapter 📖 7, "Ten Steps to Getting All or Some of Your Help from Personally Employed Aides."

In addition, he receives $2,000 worth of assistance from the four PAs who live in the cottages surrounding his house. If the going rate in his living area for salaried PAs is $9/hour, then $2,000 worth of assistance entitles him to about 220 hours of help per month, about 55 hours per week, or about 13 hours per week per PA. As a well-educated professional, Sam is not a wealthy person, but he has good business sense. As we printed this book, his accountant was not sure of the tax implications for Sam or his PAs. Meanwhile, Sam's situation provides an excellent example of being innovative in employing PAs to your double advantage.

Advantages of live-in help

There are a number of benefits to having live-in assistance. Here are some of the most important to consider:

"No-cost" help

If you rent an apartment or buy a house, consider getting a two or three-bedroom and offering the extra space to live-in PAs. If you are using college students in an urban area where available housing is rare, you might even be able to have two PAs share one spare bedroom. Instead of paying you with rent, they pay you with help—and you pay them nothing.

Overnight help for emergency needs

Aside from emergencies at the residence, you might also be concerned about personal needs that occasionally occur. At 2 A.M., you awaken with a pounding headache because your urinary catheter has clogged and you need help in the next 10 minutes. Or you have a rare need for medication that is out of reach. Live-in help can be essential.

Security

If you are dependent on help for out-of-bed transfers, then you are also concerned with residence emergencies that might happen during the night. Imagine that you hear an intruder or smell smoke, or perhaps you awaken at 2 A.M. in a 50-degree bedroom because the furnace is malfunctioning. Having on-call, live-in help can be a great comfort over sleeping alone.

Reliability

If you need help each morning, and it comes in from the outside, there will be occasions when it does not appear on schedule. Causes can include poor weather or a PA oversleeping. If your morning help lives with you, you know it will be there.

Retention

In some circumstances, a live-in aide who is getting tired of the work will take longer to resign, because quitting a live-in job also requires finding another residence. An additional factor in keeping live-ins longer is the ease with which they "commute" to work.

Friendship and companionship

Some folks find that they get closer to live-in PAs than outside, salaried PAs. Some mighty fine friendships can occur.

Settings for live-in help

For live-in help, there are two financial plans. In some situations, the help shares your living area and there is no additional expense to you. Examples include your paying rent for a two- or three-bedroom apartment, and assigning the one or two extra bedrooms to one or two aides. If you reside in a house that has extra living space, again one or two live-ins will cost you nothing extra.

The second option occurs when you want live-in help, but must rent additional space. When traveling with an aide, if the aide shares your hotel room in a separate bed, she costs nothing extra; if she sleeps in an adjoining suite room, she does. Although the help is not free, it does provide the advantages associated with close proximity.

Logistically, live-in options include the following:

Live-in roommate—the same room within the same building as yours

This setting is usually a college campus dorm room or a one-bedroom apartment. You and one of the PAs share a bedroom as roommates. Some help recipients have found that bunk beds in a small bedroom like a college dorm can make it possible to have more than one PA roommate. Others find this situation to be much too crowded.

The primary disadvantage to you and the PA is a lack of privacy, quiet, and living space. As a group, you and your roommates are constantly sharing your living and sleeping space. Many compromises and sacrifices will be necessary to maintain smooth living relations. In addition, with PA help usually readily available, you must be very careful to resist the temptation of asking for instant assistance whenever the slightest need arises. The PA and you do live in the same quarters; however—for the PA's sanity—this cannot mean that the PA is on duty and a "butler-in-waiting" for whatever and whenever you might need something. Review your list of needs and stick to requesting assistance only during the times listed unless a really urgent, unscheduled need arises.[3]

Live-in suite mate—same building but separate room or quarters

For this setting, the PAs live in the same college dormitory building, apartment building, or house as you, but sleep in a different room or living unit.

For example, at a college campus you and your PAs might live in the same three-room dorm suite, but sleep in different rooms—or simply each live in separate private rooms within the same dorm building. If you have a two-bedroom apartment, you could occupy one bedroom by yourself and offer the second bedroom to be shared by one or two PAs. As a group, you share the bathroom, kitchen, and living room. An alternative could be the PAs living within the same apartment building, but in a different apartment, than yours.

---

3. Details on using live-in help, knowing when and when not to ask for help, and some key strategies for making valid requests are found in chapter 📖 11, **"When It Is, and Is Not, Okay to Ask for Help."**

The advantages over being roommates include increased privacy and living space for both parties. The PA is far enough away to provide this privacy, but close enough to provide assistance for urgent, unscheduled needs for help.

Good communication is the key to the success for this setting. If you live out of shouting distance from your PAs, you should share an easy-to-use electronic communication system that is free from audible communication noise and interference. Your telephone, cell phone, or pager system should have at least one station within your reach while you are in bed. The device is especially essential if, during the night when you are alone in bed, an urgent and unscheduled personal need for assistance occurs, a fire or medical emergency arises, or the PA does not awaken and arrive at your place on time in the morning. Ask your PAs to be sure the communicator is located where they will both hear it and be awakened by it if you have a 2 A.M. emergency.

Dependability increases as the commuting distance for live-nearby help decreases

When you are not offering live-in space, your PAs will be living in their own residences. There is a direct correlation between the commuting distance between your residence and the PAs', and their dependability and punctuality; that is, for showing up for scheduled work shifts and being on time.

If you are hiring a new aide, and have a choice among three PA applicants whose commuting distances vary, you are wise to examine the commuting distance and potential dependability of each candidate as an additional hiring consideration. If you need to choose one PA applicant, and other factors are equal, choose the person who lives closest to you.

The overall rule of thumb: The greater the distance—and commuting hassle—between your residence and a PA's, the greater the chance for no-shows, late arrivals, and the PA quickly tiring of commuting to the job.

The term *nearby*, regarding the distance between your residence and theirs, is defined in terms of geographical distance, commuting time, and commuting ease. In a densely populated urban area, an aide might live just two miles from you. However, let's imagine that she relies on public transportation, and the bus, subway, and walking commute takes her a half hour during the daytime. Additionally, her public transit does not operate from 1 A.M. to 5 A.M. each night when you might occasionally need urgent help. When considering whether to hire her, she does not live "nearby"! In contrast, if she drove her own car and you both lived in a less populated and trafficked area, and she could buzz those two miles in less than 10 minutes at any time, then she would, indeed, live nearby for your needs.

So in some circumstances, the distance between your residence and an aide's will most certainly affect the aide's dependability, punctuality, and desire to keep a job. Other factors influencing a PA's early-morning decision to come to work can include the city or country setting and its traffic density (densely urban or rural), the PA's age and stamina (college age or senior), the crime rate (within the commuting zone), and the PA's cultural mindset.

Consequently, with each increase in distance between you and the PAs, there is an increase in the wisdom of having additional backup PAs. This can mean dividing your needs among more than one part-time PA, and keeping everyone's phone number handy by your bedside for the occasion that a scheduled PA is suddenly unable to work.

Here are two more residence options for you to consider about PAs who live nearby, and their proximity to your quarters.

Live nearby—and in the same city

For this setting, you have your own private residence and the PAs have theirs. They could live within a block or so of your residence, or a couple miles away (hopefully) in the same city. This is the residence option that will apply to most of the PAs you hire: You have your place and (preferably) nearby, they have theirs. The closer their places are to yours, the better your chances of finding the PA dependable, punctual, and wanting to keep the job longer.

Combination—live-in and live-nearby help

With the combination approach, you hire more than one PA, and combine the use of live-in and live-nearby PAs.[4]

In hiring PAs, you might hire one or two live-ins as well as others who live nearby. Including at least one live-in PA is particularly wise for those who live alone and are dependent upon assistance for urgent, unscheduled needs or for evacuation help during a fire or sudden medical emergency. If, however, you live with family members, you will probably choose to hire only PAs who live nearby.

In summary, these are the primary types of live-in and live-nearby residence options, and you now have an understanding of how to use each to your advantage. You should assess which ones best fit your own needs for help, your desire for privacy, your need for physical help during emergencies, and your objective of hiring dependable and punctual PAs who live nearby and commute.

Calculating your amount of "free" live-in help

When using live-in help, the procedure for establishing a non-cash salary system (see *Figure 3-1*) is rather simple. The objective is for you to know, and be able to clearly explain to PA applicants who ask, how many weekly and monthly hours of help you can fairly expect in exchange for your non-cash salary of free room and board.

You should first determine the going hourly rate for PA assistance in your community and the monthly rental rate for your live-in space. Then you can "crunch the numbers" in our five-step calculation.

---

4. The advantages of diversifying your base of help providers are discussed in chapter 📖 **16,** "Dividing Your Needs, and Assigning Work Shifts, Among Several PAs."

Figure 3-1: **Calculating your amount of free help
from a non-cash salary**

In these steps, you can calculate the cash value of the help you need; the value of your live-in space; whether you need more help than the space is worth; and if so, how much cash salary you should additionally pay for the total help you need.

① Determine the hourly salary that you would otherwise offer a PA for providing assistance. For example, $9/hour.

② Determine the average number of daily, weekly, and monthly hours of help you need. For example, 20 hours weekly or 80 hours monthly.

③ Multiply the hourly cash salary you would be paying ①, times the monthly hours of help you need ②, to determine the total monthly cash salary you would be paying. For example, $9/hour x 80 hours monthly = $720 monthly salary.

④ Calculate the monetary value of the living space, utilities, and anything else that you could offer a PA. If necessary, consult a local realtor or the newspaper's classifieds to determine the room's value. For example, the second bedroom of a two-bedroom apartment ($900 total rent, divided by two apartment mates, equals $450 each) plus one-half the average $100 monthly utilities = a $500 value for the living space.

⑤ Calculate whether the value of the living space will adequately reimburse a live-in PA for the value of the help you need. If not, calculate how much additional cash salary you should pay the PA to make up the difference. Start with the $720 monthly value of the help you need ③, and deduct the $500 monthly value of the living space ④, and you will owe an additional $220 monthly cash salary.

If there is a balance, and the help you need exceeds the value of the living space, then the balance is the additional cash salary. In the example, $720–$500 = a $220 cash salary that you should additionally pay a live-in PA.

Please note that this example mathematically shows a help recipient receiving all of her help from one live-in aide. Although using just one live-in aide for all your needs might seem to be an ideal situation, it can also be quite risky. Instead of paying the live-in PA an extra $220 monthly to take care of all your needs, you would be wiser to hire a second, cash-salary PA who is not a live-in.

If you cannot afford any additional cash salary for a second PA, at least consider safeguarding yourself against domestic abuse, in case the live-in suddenly turns nasty, by establishing a small network of volunteer PA friends. The concept of establishing PA friends is discussed later in this chapter.

The caution about entrusting all your dependent needs within just one aide is discussed in the next section.[5]

Coping with and resolving live-in PA problems

It is rare for a paid aide to last forever. Almost every employed aide resigns sometime, including live-ins. Though live-in aides can offer unique, cozy advantages, their eventual departure can sometimes begin especially difficult times. When a friendly live-in announces the need to resign, there can be some additional depression or stress because you are losing both an aide and a valued part of your household.

In contrast, live-in aides occasionally become unfriendly or even nasty. When they resign and go quietly, your prayers are answered with an incredible relief; when they refuse to continue helping you while digging deeper into your space, your worst nightmare becomes reality.

Before we discuss how to get you out of this particular problem situation, let's acknowledge the one word that will protect you from having to experience it again: diversify.

If your current live-in PA is also your sole, one-and-only PA, start today to diversify. Establish a backup plan with either a second live-in aide or a second outside, salaried aide. You cannot be more vulnerable than to have entrusted all your needs to just one PA and to have that PA as your sole, live-in roomie. Many of us have been there, but we soon took steps to get out of that potential danger. With all due respect to family caregivers, please note that this can also be a problem if your only aide is a family caregiver who lives with you.

"Are you crazy?! My caregiving relative would never refuse to help me or cause me harm. Why should I ever think of such a possibility, or have any need to read further in this chapter?"

You are correct, to a degree. It is usually employed aides who might become unwilling to continue their help to you, and occasionally turn nasty. However, it is not uncommon for family caregivers to become unable to help, or even refuse to do so. Often through no fault of their own, caregivers sometimes get clobbered by the flu, break a leg, or become unable to provide continuous assistance to you.

---

5. For more details about different ways either to pay cash salaries by check, or to pay non-cash salaries by offering an exchange of services, items, or living space, please see chapter 📖 **20, "Paying Salaries: Cash, Non-cash, or Both."**

In addition, it is not unheard-of for a relationship with a sole, live-in family caregiver also to go sour. Family members certainly have disagreements, and those times can become intensified when you are dependent on those family members for caregiver help. Your heated disagreement with a parent or spouse can be incredibly humiliating when you must subsequently ask them for caregiver help. Indeed, there could be family disagreements that are so unreasonable and bitter that the caregiver would refuse—or be emotionally unable—to provide you with routine help if you could muster sufficient humility to ask for it. So, yes, there are potential situations in many families when a caregiving relative could become physically unable, or indeed refuse, to provide you with help. This possibility brings you back to square one—diversify.[6]

If all your help now comes from just one live-in PA, restructure your game plan toward two live-ins, or a live-in and an outside salaried PA, or a live-in and some PA friends.

Establishing "PA friends" as a safeguard

If your limited budget allows only your one live-in PA, and you cannot hire any hours of an additional, outside salaried person, then establish a network of at least three PA friends. The concept is incredibly simple, and can be a lifesaver. A *PA friend* is any current, close friend who formally agrees to provide some special help if you experience a crisis with your one paid or live-in PA.

The way to establish this is easy. Think about your close friends (who are not current aides) and identify three who would help you in a crisis. You want to establish at least three people, to increase your chances of being able to call and reach at least one person in urgent time of need. Each of these three buddies should have his or her own button on your phone's speed dialer.

You should not assume that they will help you in an urgent occasion. Instead, take a few minutes to explain what you might need from them and have them formally agree to be "on call."

These are people who would temporarily chip in if you get into a PA crisis. These are the "buds" whom you could call if your one-and-only, live-in or paid PA is suddenly unable or unwilling to provide you with help. Even more important, these are the people who would drop what they are doing and race over if your live-in aide has become physically abusive. What might you be asking them to do? Here are some examples:

- Help you get out of bed in the morning if your aide suddenly is unwilling or unable.

- Come to your apartment or house if an aide ever becomes abusive or threatens you.

- Help you think through a crisis and logically plan the steps of your action plan.

---

6. To understand the sharp disadvantages of using just one aide, and the benefits of two or more, please see chapter 📖 16, "**Dividing Your Needs, and Assigning Work Shifts, Among Several PAs.**"

- Provide you with a crisis hug when it seems to be unavailable
  from any other source.

- Help you feel empowered—merely by being available—so you know that
  you would not be facing a sole, abusive aide alone.

Resolving the current problem

Imagine that you and a sole, live-in PA have been sharing your apartment for several months. Last night, as the aide was helping you into bed, he announced that he is tired of the traffic noise that is constantly heard inside the apartment, of how much you hog the single phone line with your academic research on the Web, and of the early-morning and late-night shifts of helping you. Both of you were up until midnight while you tried to talk him out of leaving; however, he wants out and he got pretty angry about it. So what can you do now, the next morning, as an escape from the current problem situation? You have not slept much while your mind created every imaginable, worst-case scenario.

It almost always pays at least to attempt to discuss your concerns and get cooperation. Select a discussion time after the PA has helped you up for the day. If the discussion goes completely sour, and the PA walks out (yes, as in "out, out"), then this will happen while you are independent, functioning, and better able to do some fast recruiting.

After your attempt to discuss, and before you can decide what to do, take a moment to assess the situation. With which of two kinds of aides are you now involved?

- The PA still respects your concerns, is open to discussion, and will
  probably work with you in being replaced and moving out.

- The PA has become an irrational "Mr. Hyde" and seemed to be someone
  totally different from the reasonable PA whom you thought you hired. He
  now could care less about your concerns, is a probable threat to your
  possessions or personal safety, is cutting back on his help to you, and has
  no interest in moving out of your space.

In the first scenario, you should propose a game plan, discuss it with the live-in, and ask for his help with the transition. Set the stage for his working with you as a team during the upcoming transition. If this PA will cooperate, keep him in the loop and updated on your plans. Avoid turning him against you by having him read about your recruitment for his replacement in the classifieds before he hears about it from you.

Your game plan in this first case will often be the following:

- Decide how and where to advertise for new help, and get your ad posted.[7]
- Keep your current PA updated, and coordinate with him to get a smooth transition between his moving out and the new PA moving in.

If the live-in PA will discuss your concerns and work with you, follow the game plan outlined above for a cooperative person. The transition might go more smoothly than you expected, because the PA might have been hoping for a way to quit.

In contrast, if the live-in aide refuses to sit down with you and has become the enemy, then you should plan to move quietly and quickly. If this nasty PA is also your sole source of help, then it is best to start planning now for the worst possible outcome.

If you fear that the live-in aide might not help you into bed tonight, then start now—early this morning—to line up an alternative, on-call source. Typical sources for emergency help can include previous PAs, friends, PA friends (see preceding section), or even a local agency that provides professional aides. By lining up secondary help now, early in the first day after you get the PA's news, you do two things: you increase the chance that sudden replacement help will actually be available, and you reduce your growing emotional fear that it will not be.

Once you have a backup source for help, start advertising for the live-in's replacement. Yes, I have been exactly where you are now—and yes, you also can find and hire help perhaps within the same day.[8]

If you estimate that your personal recruiting will take too long, then consider getting temporary help from an agency.[9] If you fear that the live-in might become physically abusive, there are two strategies for you.

First, get the PA to move out. There is no simple, sure-shot formula for kicking out a live-in aide. Use whatever means will work. However, start by politely and assertively stating your need—and his—that he find another place promptly. You will be more convincing if you can point out advantages to him in moving out today. Please note the difference between stating, asking, and begging.

You should *never* beg. Second, until the PA does relocate, get some friends to hang out at your place. The PA will not harm you in front of your friends, and these buddies might make the PA sufficiently uncomfortable to speed up his departure. Before they arrive, brief them on the reason for your invitation. Ask that they be neutral in interactions with the PA—neither nasty nor friendly.

---

7. Strategies for creating PA ads are outlined in chapter 📖 8, **"Where and How to Advertise for Your Own PAs."**

8. Please see the section on same-day, power recruiting in that same chapter 📖 8, **"Where and How to Advertise for Your Own PAs."**

9. You might find it helpful to check out chapters 📖 1, **"Beyond Family Caregivers: Options and Settings for Finding Outside Assistance,"** 📖 4, **"Settings Where You Use Help,"** and 📖 6, **"Ten Steps to Getting All or Some of Your Help From Agency-Employed Aides."**

Chapter 4
Settings Where You Use Help

You probably do not spend your entire life at home. When the alarm rings each morning, you are ready to start your day and head into the mainstream.

If you are dependent on help from others, your aide arrives on time (or at least you hope she will) as you are shutting off the alarm. Your morning routine might take an hour or two, and then you are ready to hit the road.

There might be a variety of daily activities throughout the surrounding community and beyond. Your agenda might include a punctual, routine schedule of appointments and meetings, social and leisure activities, and educational or career responsibilities. There might be overnight stays during vacation or business trips. You will also occasionally stay in a hospital or rehab center to take care of a short-term ailment or new impairment.

Your own private (or family) housing

The most common setting for using caregiver or PA help is in your own private housing. That setting is usually a house or apartment.

The main advantages include the privacy felt within your own "castle," the comfort of surroundings that are familiar as well as those that can be ideally modified to any of your access needs. Additionally, you have a choice of live-in company that includes relatives, spouse, or friends. In short, your private home gives the greatest comfort because of your freedom to customize the environment.

If you need physical assistance, the typical contacts for finding help can include relatives, spouse, lover, aide (from either an agency or personal recruiting), or a friend.

Many people would be able to recruit, hire, train, and manage their own assistance from paid, outside providers, but well-meaning relatives and friends often interfere. It is additionally common for relatives and friends at home to insist on performing many duties for you that you could do for yourself. You might feel pressure from your family that prevents you from hiring outside PA help.

Caregiver assistance from relatives may be very comfortable initially, but eventually it may not be available to you, for any of several reasons. Relatives understandably become chronically tired of providing help day after day, or at least in being your only source of help, regardless of the sweet things they tell you to the contrary.

In addition, the situation cannot last forever, because young relatives grow up and move away to conduct their own private lives. Older relatives become older and can no longer meet the physical demands of assisting you. Other relatives, a spouse, and friends also need free time to pursue their own interests, education, or career desires, or simply to have private time to themselves.

Consequently, there are at least three cautions about living with, and accepting help from, family caregivers:

- insist that you be allowed to do all that you can for yourself
- view the unlimited and unconditional help that is stated by caregivers to be, instead, bounded by the limits and conditions of their unstated energy, stamina, and time
- insist that you be able to hire outside PA assistance for at least some of your needs, regardless of family caregiver protests.

Your insistence on doing all that you can for yourself, and hiring outside help for at least a portion of other needs, may be met with resistance or even resentment by parents, relatives, a spouse, and others around you. The common reasons for this are centered around assumptions that you are sick, and therefore unable to manage your needs, or that your polite decline of their help is actually a rejection of their love for you.

Your desire to manage your own needs might also be met with resistance by visiting aides or nurses. These people do not often encounter help recipients who are knowledgeable about their own care and want to manage it. They may also see you as sick and therefore incapable of making your own decisions. Furthermore, these health providers sometimes interpret your honest questions about their procedures as an evaluation of whether they are performing their procedures properly. By their own interpretation, they might believe you are questioning their expertise and authority—their problem, *not* yours.

Take the initiative to discuss these situations in an open manner. Explain why you want to do things for yourself and hire outside help for other needs. Talk to those who misunderstand your capabilities, and assertively state the reasons behind your desire to manage, while showing them your ability to do so. Explain that the physical impairment to part of your body does not affect your overall health or ability to think clearly, and therefore it does not affect your ability to manage your own needs.

Assure your relatives that you want their continued love and that there will still be many opportunities for them to do things for you. However, you wish to be self-sufficient—just as they are—in doing certain things for yourself.

Following this discussion, and when you see even a few signs of their willingness not to impede your hiring outsiders, patiently lay out your PA game plan. To increase the family's acceptance and decrease their objections, begin your employment with perhaps a one-month trial during which you:

- hire outside providers for a small total of weekly hours
- avoid parts of the family's weekly schedule that are already especially stressful (these will eventually be ideal times for liberating family members from caregiver duties, but not during this initial trial period)
- avoid parts of the schedule when the family traditionally enjoys private, family activities
- assemble the family each week or so to answer questions, to discuss what is working well and what is not, and to announce any changes
- all routinely consult this reference book, both to problem-solve and to plan innovations.

Day or evening meetings, appointments, and errands

As previously mentioned, few of us live our entire lives at home. There are medical appointments, many types of meetings, meals at restaurants, education and career responsibilities, church services, shopping and banking needs, romantic dates, and a huge variety of cultural, recreational, leisure, and social activities.

This is day and evening travel that does not require an overnight stay. It can be of any distance, whether a trip around the block to get a quart of milk or a day-long business meeting that requires a 400-mile round-trip flight on a commuter airline.

Assistance can come from a PA who travels with you the entire time, or—if your needs are minimal—from a stranger whom you briefly encounter. Many of us would find everyday independence considerably more difficult if friendly passers-by, or the staff in stores or on airlines, were not available to offer help with such quick, non-personal needs as:

- hard-to-open entrance doors
- hard-to-reach grocery items, cafeteria food, or shelved library books
- grocery sacks that are too heavy, numerous, or fragile to carry by wheelchair to one's car
- cafeteria or fast-food trays with hot and spillable coffee or tea
- heavy baggage to be carried through the miles of airport concourse.

Your title and role toward this assistance is clearly that of a manager. Only you know what you want from today's travel, and what help you need to accomplish those objectives. A few exceptions to the manager role might occur for very dependent people who travel on a specially planned private trip, or group tour with a close friend, relative, spouse, or medical personnel.[1]

---

1. For more detail about using the volunteer help of strangers and business staff, please see chapter ⌨ 2, "Volunteer Help: Don't Wear Out Your Friendships."

Overnight travel

When day outings just do not provide enough chill for your stress level, or when the business you own or work for demands your expertise at a week-long conference, it is time to hit the road or the skies with your aide.

Transportation might be provided by car, camper, van, bus, air, rail, or ship. And yes, folks in 'chairs—with and without their trusty PAs—do occasionally hitchhike across country! Lodging might be at any of a variety of settings: a $500-per-day luxury resort, small roadside motel, ski resort (in or out of season), campsite next to a fishing stream, Amtrak sleeper car, guest room on a cruise ship, RV or pop-up camper, or at a friend's house on the other coast.

> *Plan on a single PA traveling with you to need either relief or time off each three to four days. Travel on long trips either with two aides, or at a slower pace and with much patience!*

You are the direct manager of the PA assistance that you bring with you, and the PA will usually agree to travel without a salary, as long as you or your business covers all the expenses.

I have traveled from coast to coast many times and seldom paid an additional, hourly salary to the PA who traveled with me. If my travel is financially sponsored, I am very up-front with the financial source about my need to include the airfare, room, and board for my aide. If my travel is personal, I build the extra expense into my vacation budget, save receipts, and deduct my out-of-pocket PA expense on my taxes as a medical or business item.

Because my PAs are typically local college students, I have little trouble finding travel companions when I need them. I employ four to six part-timers, and within two or three phone calls I usually hear an enthusiastic "Yes!" in response to my request: "Hetty, I need to fly to San Francisco on the 11th, attend a three-day conference, and sample some great restaurants. I need someone to travel with me, do the PA stuff, and get all expenses paid except your personal spending money. Are you interested?"

Still, there are some cautions to being on the road, totally dependent on your companion, and a thousand miles from any of your backup aides. Here are some tips for making the most of your travel.[2]

- Select your travel PA carefully, screening for someone who is stable, mature, flexible, and drug-free. Remember also that an aide who is great at home is not always a great aide on the road. Some people simply do not travel well.

---

2. For additional notes about traveling with PAs, please see chapter 📖 **18, "Coping with and Reacting to PA Failures."**

- Regardless of how well you plan a trip, problems and crises are very common. Airlines routinely damage wheelchairs, hotel rooms are often not as accessible as they claim to be, and a sudden medical need will occasionally send you or your PA to the emergency room. Most of all, travel can make even the nicest people tired, cranky, and a little crazy. Select a companion who has the stability and "staying power" to be there, but also has the flexibility to deal with sudden problem situations.

- To test the stability and compatibility of an aide for several travel days, you might first want to enlist the aide's help for an especially active day trip. Hit the road early for a "shop-till-you-drop" day, or whatever turns you on. Observe how well the two or three of you get along, especially if your upcoming vacation will include a family caregiver and a hired aide.

- If you will be traveling extensively with a single PA or family caregiver, you can plan ahead on that provider needing time off each three to four days. Make long trips either with two aides, or at a slower pace and with lots of patience. Whether you are receiving help while at home or flying friendly skies, PA work is still work and not a vacation. It is a fact that X amount of help with your routine ADL needs at home will probably require at least 2X of help while traveling and camping out in hotel rooms. In addition to your usual ADL needs, your PA is packing, traveling, and unpacking—often performing all elements of this travel routine each day.

- If you are traveling several days with a one-and-only family caregiver or hired aide, you would be wise to routinely schedule "PA R&R" (rest and recuperation) time. You might be psyched for traveling eight successive destinations in eight days, but few single family caregivers or aides would survive. Ideally, plan for a half-day when a caregiver or aide has off-duty time to sleep, take a long walk, or spend down time—alone. If you can travel with a caregiver and an aide, or two aides, suggest that they alternate duty days or mornings and evenings. Let them negotiate their own scheduling between them, with you stepping in as an arbitrator only if needed.

- Before leaving home, discuss your PA's probable need for private time. At this early time, sketch out a tentative plan that sounds good. Then, as the trip progresses and changes occur, update the plan as needed. Some PAs depend on a daily fitness routine, and will need formal exercise during travel days. Once on the road, watch and listen for signs of chronic fatigue and respect them. Let your PA routinely recharge.

- If you are traveling with hired aides and are offering to pay travel expenses in lieu of salary, make sure that the financial terms are firmly understood in advance. Does there seems to be an expectation for cash spending money, or have you formally discussed all of the terms?

- Although assistance for very personal needs will come from your family caregiver or PA, be prepared to accept and manage supplemental help from strangers. Hotel staff, airline and cruise ship personnel, and passers-by often offer—or can be summoned to provide—valued help. Give your personal travel aide a welcomed break, and ask an airport skycap to carry the luggage!

- On a logistical note, folks with disabilities seldom travel lightly. Most of us use many items for our ADLs. You probably lay out these items all over your bed on the morning of departure, and wonder if there is a more organized alternative to shoveling it all into four duffel bags until each one bursts.

My suggestion is first to organize small piles of items by function or by work area. You might put your toothbrush, toothpaste, mouthwash, hairbrush, razor, and aftershave into one pile. All of your meds could go into another pile. Next, seal each pile in a gallon-size resealable bag, and then stuff the bags into your duffel.

Each time you pack and unpack, you will be sorting eight to 10 categorized resealable bags, instead of the 75 to 100 separate items within the bags. Also, be sure that each bag is zip-sealed tight, to minimize damages if a bottle of something leaks!

College residence hall or campus-area housing

Today's competitive career market usually requires a college education. College facilities include vocational-technical schools, community and junior colleges, and universities. Students often have an additional choice of attending classes while commuting from home or while living on or near the campus.

If you have a recent disability and are still learning to manage the disability and the required PA help, you might welcome the option of commuting from home to a nearby community or junior college program. Commuting for at least the first year of studies can enable you to get your personal concerns under control while learning to coordinate a bite-sized taste of academic life. You have the chance to prove your academic abilities to yourself, to your relatives, and perhaps to your state's office for vocational rehabilitation (an often-used educational funding source).

If you decide to begin as a community college commuter, you can even opt to complete a two-year associate degree before moving away from home for further studies at a four-year institution.

If you decide to live away from home, there are two main options: to live in commercial housing near the vocational-technical school or college campus, or to choose a campus that provides its own housing on or adjacent to its campus.

The primary source for PA help at a campus is fellow students, although a few students use commercial aides supplied by community agencies for at least some of their needs. The college campus is one of the all-time best PA recruiting markets, because college students are generally young and physically fit, flexible in their personal schedules, and looking for ways to earn money.

Often a college campus will feature a department or office with a title such as "disabled student services," "disability services," or "handicapped student center." You should feel free to ask these professional staffers, as well as other students with disabilities, for advice in recruiting PAs from students or the surrounding community.

You are the direct manager of the PA assistance that you require, unless you need a PA coordinator because of an inability to meet some of the physical, verbal, or visual requirements of direct management.[3]

Acute care hospital

It is as certain for those of us with disabilities as "death and taxes" are for everyone else: we become somewhat regulars at the local hospital. With our disabilities, we get a special menu that includes urinary tract infections (UTIs), upper respiratory infections (URIs), skin breakdowns (DUs, for decubitus ulcers), and sprinklings of other sporadic unknowns that often require MRIs just for the initial identification. Before you know what has hit you, you are an inpatient receiving IV treatments.

Sometimes the hospital objective is to cure a type of ailment. At other times, the best you can do is to reduce the ailment's negative effects when a complete cure is not possible. The end result of the hospital stay, when illness has been cured, can be to return home to life as usual. At other times, when you will have ongoing effects from the illness, you might be referred for further treatment or therapies to a rehab center, nursing home, or assistance while at home.

A hospital stay offers you a wide variety of help providers, including a nurse, medical technician, aide, and other health professionals. However, you have two kinds of relationships with these professionals, as a patient and a manager—and that is where their confusion starts.

Many of these health providers, especially nurses, med techs, and aides, have problems making the minute-by-minute transitions between when you follow their instructions and when they follow yours.

> *As a patient who receives care for a temporary, acute illness, you follow instructions from the hospital staff. However, as the manager of your routine ADL needs, you provide instructions to the staff.*

As a patient, you receive medical treatment and therapies for an ailment that is not part of your normal routine. You should feel free to ask questions, monitor, and participate in the treatment you receive. Here, you primarily entrust your illness and care to the wisdom of medical professionals and follow their suggestions and instructions. Your further responsibilities as a patient include learning about the procedures for your treatment after discharge, and remembering that you are welcome to call or consult with these professionals at any time in the future when you need medical advice.

---

3. For more detail about the advantages of using college-student PAs, and special strategies for recruiting them, please see chapters 📖 7, "Ten Steps to Getting All or Some of Your Help from Personally Employed Aides," and 📖 8, "Where and How to Advertise for Your Own PAs."

In contrast, for your routine ADL needs, you should change roles from being a hospital patient, who follows suggestions and instructions, to being a manager who provides instructions to the staff. As this manager, you politely and assertively make your needs known and provide instruction on how to assist those needs.

For these routine needs, the nurse, med tech, or aide will typically assure you, "If you would like any help with routine needs, please feel free to let me know what kind of help you need and how I can best provide it." Sometimes this is a valid, sincere offer, and at other times your requests will be met with reluctance, resistance, or even resentment.

As your own manager, you should make your needs known with regard to the equipment, procedures, and schedule or logical order that you usually follow. It is wise to discuss these factors early, perhaps at the admissions check-in when you first arrive in your room, with the primary nurse assigned to you. The primary nurse will ask you standard admission questions about your health, medical condition, usual diet, and the medications that you normally take.

This is an ideal time to discuss the types of physical assistance you will need, as well as how long you typically require assistance with each activity. If you require 45 minutes of help in the morning with a bed bath, your primary nurse should know this in advance to enable staff planning. Be prepared to make reasonable compromises about the types of equipment, procedures, and schedules around those that are available in this temporary hospital setting. Think of your stay as an adventure challenge or game of "camping out" for a few days where you will not have the schedule or many of the comforts of home.

> *You may have to compromise on the schedule of your daily routine, but never compromise on the quality of help you receive.*

You should not compromise, however, on the overall quality of treatment or assistance that you receive. Do not "do without" any truly essential needs just because the nurse seems too busy to help you, or the aide is in a bad mood.

If you encounter problems, try to explain the reasons why some part of your routine care is important to you and see if the reaction of the nurse or aide changes. If problems cannot be resolved in this way, ask to speak with your primary nurse or the nursing supervisor.

Explain the problem as objectively as you can, with a minimum of emotions or "bad attitude," and ask for the nurse's advice in resolving the matter. Regardless of how aggressively angry (or helplessly defeated) you feel, try to remember that your objective is to describe unfulfilled needs and not to evaluate the hospital or berate the uncooperative staff. Be cool in describing your unfulfilled needs, and let the supervisor draw his or her own conclusions about a solution. Again, further compromises in methods might be necessary, but never quality.

Feel free to refer to the "Patient's Bill of Rights" (*Figure 4-1*) that you probably received from the hospital at the admissions check-in. Almost every hospital issues such a listing to new patients. Refer to it if you wish specifics about your individual rights in the hospital, or if you simply wish some reassurance and confidence that the topic about which you are about to complain is justified.

Figure 4-1: **Sample Patient's Bill of Rights**

As a patient at Boston General Hospital (a fictitious example), you have the right to:

1. Receive emergency medical treatment as indicated by your medical condition upon arrival to the Emergency Department.

2. Considerate and respectful care.

3. The name of the physician responsible for coordinating your care.

4. The name and function of any person providing health care services to you.

5. Obtain from your physician complete current information concerning your diagnosis, treatment, and prognosis in terms you can reasonably be expected to understand. When it is not medically advisable to give you such information, this information shall be available to an appropriate person on your behalf.

6. Receive from your physician information necessary to give informed consent prior to the start of any procedure, treatment, or both. This information, except for emergency situations not requiring informed consent, shall include as a minimum the specific procedure or treatment or both, the medically significant risks involved, and the probable duration of incapacitation, if any. You will be advised of medically significant alternatives for care or treatment, if any.

7. Refuse treatment to the extent permitted by law and to be informed of the medical consequences of this action.

8. Privacy to the extent consistent with providing you adequate medical care. This shall not preclude discreet discussion of your case or examination of you by appropriate medical personnel.

9. Privacy and confidentiality of all records pertaining to your treatment, except as otherwise provided by law or third-party payment contract.

10. A response by the hospital to requests for usual services consistent with your treatment.

11. Be informed by your physician, or his or her designee, of your continuing health care requirements following discharge.

12. Receive information about the need to transfer you to another facility and any alternatives there might be to such a transfer.

13. The identity, upon request, of other health care and educational institutions that the hospital has authorized to participate in your treatment.

⑭ Refuse to participate in research and human experimentation affecting your care and treatment; such shall be performed only with your informed consent.

⑮ Examine and receive an explanation of your bill, regardless of source of payment.

⑯ Treatment without discrimination as to race, color, religion, sex, national origin, handicap, or source of payment.

⑰ Designate any accommodation to which you are admitted as a non-smoking area.

⑱ Without fear of reprisal, voice grievances and recommend changes in policies and services to our staff, the governing authority, and the Massachusetts Department of Health.

⑲ Submit complaints about the hospital care and services and to have the hospital investigate such complaints. The hospital is responsible for providing you, if requested, with a written response indicating the findings of the investigation. If you are dissatisfied, the hospital will then direct you to the appropriate office of the Massachusetts Department of Health.

⑳ Know the hospital rules and regulations that apply to your conduct as a patient.[4]

Rehabilitation hospital

If you are like many of us, you probably celebrated your original rehab hospital discharge several years ago as a one-shot deal. You had paid your dues of experiencing the onset of a disability, gritted your teeth to get through weeks of the daily therapies, and received your discharge handshake for surviving. You had been drafted into special service, paid your dues, and then put it all into the past so you could get on with life.

In the next few years, you realized that rehab graduates have an incredibly strong and active alumni association, and that the original rehab graduation (or tour of duty) was merely the first of a series.

Similar to acute care hospital stays, your rehabilitation is usually a lifelong process. Life with a disability is one of ongoing, in- and outpatient admissions. For a rehab center, common reasons for repeated readmissions include periodic re-evaluations (in-depth checkups) as well as the regrettable onset of new, secondary disabilities. The secondaries can be either brand new impairments to your body, or the development of new complications to the original impairment.

The typical contacts during the stay include the same kinds of medical professionals that were discussed for the acute care hospital. Your titles and roles toward these professionals include the same patient and manager functions as explained for a hospital stay, but in a rehabilitation hospital you have the additional title and role of *student*.

---

4. For more detail and examples about negotiating your ADL needs for help with hospital staff, please see chapter 📖 12, "Getting It Done—Your Way!"

As a student during your stay, you are wise to absorb all that you can of the information, strategies, and techniques offered by the various types of professionals around you. By learning and practicing these details, you will be maximizing your ability to live independently in the life ahead of you.

Some rehab patients are strongly tempted to discharge themselves early, in an attempt to escape their impairment as well as the therapies and other rehab responsibilities. Some others become angry and reject the suggestions of doctors, nurses, aides, physical therapists, occupational therapists, speech therapists, and counselors.

> *In receiving rehab services, you usually have just one chance at the medical pros giving you their best effort. Do you really want to go home early, or do you want to grit your teeth until you cross the natural finish line and get every inpatient advantage you can?*

This is another occasion when you are wise to react with a clear, rational head, instead of emotionally bursting forth from the gut. The bottom line is that the level of function and independence you have on leaving the rehab center will be the same level you will have for the rest of your life. When you leave the center, you will want to go home with an absolute minimum of the disability with which you were admitted. You usually have just one chance at the medical pros giving you their best effort. Don't go home early; stick it out until you cross the natural finish line.

Think of these folks as your "presidential cabinet of advisors" who will be suggesting shortcuts and inside tips on ways to make the most of your life despite your impairment. Stick with them and learn from them. This will be a temporary period of hard work—the most valuable investment chance you will ever be given toward making the rest of your life easier.

Be a willing, eager student in learning rehab techniques. Learn all that you can about your disability and ways to make the emotional adjustment as well as physical accommodations.

For independent activities, learn the shortcuts and tricks for doing all that you can for yourself. For dependent needs, learn from the pros around you about strategies for recruiting, interviewing, screening, hiring, training, managing, and parting ways with quality help providers. In turn, you will be able to get the help you need, when and where you need it. Upon rehab discharge, get into the swing of managing that help, and being overall independent, as soon as possible.

Transitional and residential independent living centers

Baseball legend Yogi Berra is credited with saying, "Nothing provides experience like experience." On being discharged from the rehab center, you will probably want to get out into the mainstream of life and fly as quickly as possible. The question is whether you want to fly with or without a safety net—whether you want to try out your wings with support from an independent living center (ILC) or do it on your own.

Before you attempt to take advantage of an independent living (IL) program, you would be wise to have learned all you can from your previous stay at the rehab hospital. The rehab hospital can provide basic IL skills, and then an IL center will offer you the chance to try out those skills in an actual living situation. If you want advice on increasing your skills beyond the resources of the rehab hospital, there are two primary types of IL programs or centers.

The most common IL programs are nonresidential programs that consist of a central office and a demonstration and classroom area. Counselors are available to individuals who are able to visit the area to receive counseling, or who ask that a counselor come to their home. In either case, the counselor can coach the individual on methods and strategies for increasing independence in performing specific types of daily living activities.

There is also an increasing number of transitional and residential IL centers. For admission to this type of program, you submit an application that details your specific personal goals. Residents live at the residential center for a temporary period in order to learn skills. A progressive program will be very clear in stating that it has no room or time for housing residents who desire simply to be dependent, passive patients and who are unwilling to work toward independent living.

If accepted, you live in a private apartment within or near the center for a period of time that typically ranges from 6 to 18 months. You are expected to participate routinely in two primary types of skills training activities: individual counseling sessions about personal concerns, and group classes and workshops that address common concerns shared by most of the residents.

Individual counseling might address ways of independently performing personal medical procedures and coping with specific problems of emotional adjustment. The group session topics might include PA management skills, managing personal finances, assertiveness training, and others aimed at preparing for educational and career opportunities.

The overall purpose of a transitional and residential program is to teach IL skills in a setting where residents can feel free to make mistakes while counseling support is available. The clear objective of the program is for residents to make steady progress toward independently managing their own living needs, and then to move into a more independent setting that is appropriate to their abilities. This is why such programs are termed "transitional and residential."

Because the setting is designed to simulate living on one's own while the program provides professional support, the professional contacts differ from the previously discussed hospitals. Aides are available for the residents to share and directly manage themselves. Skills instructors and counselors provide instruction and support for becoming as independent as possible. Nurses, therapists, and physicians are on call for approach by residents, just as they will be during a future life in the community.

The titles of your relationship to these professionals include "student," with the objective of learning independent living skills; and "manager," with the objective of learning and improving PA management skills. These titles and roles were discussed in detail for the two previous hospital settings.

Independent/assisted living facility or nursing home

There are three levels of group living facilities for persons with limitations due to disability or aging. The independent living center provides private apartments, group meals in a dining room, and accessible bus transportation. The assisted living facility provides more protective care, with on call aides, medication supervision, and special programs for clients who have attention and cognitive deficits. The nursing home, or health care center, emphasizes medical care with a nursing staff.

The most common professional contacts at a nursing home include social workers, nurses, aides, and therapists. Physicians and other health professionals are usually available on an on call basis.

The resident's relationship to these professionals is usually a mixture of manager and patient, in a proportion related to the number of daily needs that one is able and willing to coordinate for oneself. Residents usually become increasingly passive and dependent upon staff care and, as their stay continues, upon staff decisions. The price of being dependent on this care includes living by staff decisions as to the choice and schedule of daily activities.

For many residents who become truly passive and dependent, due to a cognitive inability to manage personal needs, this surrender of choices to staff decisions might not present significant problems. However, for those who are clear thinking and consequently have the ability to manage, but who choose not to do so, the surrender of choices can cause an emotionally devastating and progressive depression.[5]

---

5. For more detail about each level of residential care facility and typical program offerings, please see chapter 📖 1, "Beyond Family Caregivers: Options and Settings for Finding Outside Assistance."

Part II

Three Ten-Step Plans for Getting the Help You Need

Part II

Three Ten-Step Plans for Getting the Help You Need

The three ten-step plans of this part form the core of this book. Whether you are seeking help with a disability for the first time or you are a seasoned pro, you can refer to these plans again and again for useful information on defining your needs, developing a system to meet those needs, and ensuring that you get consistent, dedicated assistance.

The chapters are dedicated to three simple, ten-step programs for getting help from the three main types of help providers: family caregivers, agency-employed aides, and personally employed aides (or PAs). Each program begins with similar (although not identical) Planning Steps ❶ through ❸, which provide you with basic planning information and guide you through decisions that you have to make before pursuing any of the three sources of help providers. Each program then outlines Steps ❹ through ❿, which provide specific information for recruiting, training, managing, and parting ways with each type of help provider.

The ten-step program for family caregivers, chapter 📖 **5, "Ten Steps to Getting All or Some of Your Help from Family Caregivers,"** contains important information that will help your family, your caregivers, and you avoid the overwork, chronic fatigue, and depression that are typical of caregiver situations. As you will see, most of these problems can be avoided when the caregivers, family members, and help recipient do some advance research and planning as a team.

The key strategy is for this family team to prioritize family resources for preserving the strength of individual members and the family or marital unity. This priority also includes support to the help recipient for seven categories of special disability needs that can be uniquely addressed by the family. Ironically, the most obvious need of the help recipient which usually receives the most attention—help in the routine, physical ADLs (activities of daily living)—should be the family's lowest priority. These daily tasks can be addressed by family caregivers if any family resources remain. However, the majority, and often all, of physical ADL needs should be assigned to outside, paid providers.

The ten-step program for using agency-employed aides, chapter 📖 6, "Ten Steps to Getting Getting All or Some of Your Help from Agency-Employed Aides," outlines the procedure for selecting and working with an agency that will meet your needs. Included are guidelines for screening and selecting an agency that is right for you, and then strategies for training agency aides to accommodate your schedule. The chapter's emphasis is to empower you to maintain control over the quality of the agency, agency aides, and provided assistance so that you can also maintain control over your choice of lifestyle.

The ten-step program for using personally employed aides or PAs, chapter 📖 7, "Ten Steps to Getting All or Some of Your Help from Personally Employed Aides," addresses your recurring use of the RISHTMP cycle of recruiting, interviewing, screening, hiring, training, and parting ways with your PAs. The interviewing and screening phases include eight specially designed steps that enable you to identify and disqualify undesirable applicants *before* you would hire them. The entire chapter empowers you to find quality help providers, when and where you need them, and to keep them longer.

Following this three-chapter package of Part II, is Part III, "More Topics on Getting the Help You Need." These chapters provide supplemental, in-depth strategies for some of the management tasks introduced in this Part II.

Part III More Topics on Getting the Help You Need

📖   8 Where and How to Advertise for Your Own PAs

📖   9 Initial Training and Ongoing Management of Aides and PAs

📖   10 Recognizing and Resolving Your PA Problems, or Parting Ways

Chapter 5

Ten Steps to Getting All or Some of Your Help from Family Caregivers

If you receive help from family caregivers, you know it is usually the most compassionate, comprehensive, and dependable help available anywhere. You may also have seen your caregiver become chronically tired and perhaps depressed from all the tasks she or he does, morning and night, day after day. You might have felt a mixture of endless appreciation for the wonderful help you receive, sorrow for the fatigue and physical pain the caregiver tries to hide, and guilt for having your limitations be the reason for the caregiver's sacrifices.

If you are a family member who is not a caregiver, you might feel love and sympathy for the family's help recipient who is dependent on assistance. The caregiver concerns you, because she or he provides hour after hour of daily help and stops only when fatigue prevents working longer. However, you might also miss the time and events the family or marriage formerly shared before caregiving needs consumed them.

If you are the family caregiver, you take immense pride in providing the best help possible to your loved one. It seems unfair that the unconditional help you provide to another requires so many costs and sacrifices from you. Once, you had private time, personal space, and an identity that was unrelated to being a caregiver. Now, you may often feel tired, might increasingly feel depressed that those personal essentials are gone, and might occasionally feel a despair that they will never return.

According to the NFCA,[1] more than one-quarter of adults (more than 54 million Americans) provided help to a chronically ill, disabled, or aged family member or friend during the previous year (1999–2000). These unpaid family and friends typically provide 90 percent of all long-term services, worth an estimated $196 billion annually.

We can assume that some experienced "caregiver families" are successfully balancing the needs of all family members, while others are encountering problems. In addition, a group of inexperienced families want a quick course in how to balance everyone's needs, because a loved one is now expressing or demonstrating initial needs for family help.

---

1. National Family Caregivers Association, *Caregiver Survey-2000*, (Kensington, MD: Author, Oct. 2000).

123

Financial investors have an adage about managing money: "If you are not intentionally planning to succeed, then you are unintentionally planning to fail."

Without the benefit of a planning strategy like the one in this chapter, too many families have unfortunately experienced the truth of this adage. Too many family caregivers have attempted to provide physical help to loved ones without a game plan that equally safeguards—and balances—the needs of:

- the caregiver(s)
- the family and marital unity
- you, the help recipient.

Each family has different needs, and can sense the best planning schedule and style for addressing those needs. Some families will prefer advance or early planning, whereas others prefer to have some actual experience with concerns before addressing them. Another reason to delay planning is the overload of tasks and emotions that can accompany a loved one's sudden dysfunction due to a disability or illness. When a family begins accommodating the sudden paralysis resulting from a teen's car accident or an elder's stroke, a caregiver's depleted time and stamina can be valid reasons to delay planning for the future.

However, I maintain it is important that the family act at some point to establish a well-designed plan to balance everyone's needs and prevent family burnout. A plan, like the ten-step one proposed in this chapter, will enable the allocation or reallocation of family resources to benefit the family caregiver, family or marital structure, and the help recipient. By keeping the rest of the family strong, you are ensuring that assistance with your dependent needs will be uninterrupted. That may mean that assistance no longer comes entirely from the family.

To provide a quick illustration of how common problems can occur for a caregiver family when planning is not done, and to demonstrate the importance of this chapter's strategies, I offer these personal experiences.

Personal caregiver experiences with my mother and former wife

About 35 years ago, I was finally discharged to go home after 14 months of acute care and rehabilitation following my diving injury. Following what this chapter calls the "traditional, burnout approach to caregiving,"[2] my mother initially abandoned her personal needs to be my only source of help. We firmly believed that after the first three or four weeks, when my routine was established and the dust had settled, we would be able to reclaim her personal time.

---

2. Please see *Figures 5-2* and *5-3*, in **Step ❶** of this chapter, for outlines of a traditional, burnout approach to caregiving and a five-part strategy to preserving family strength.

By the way, the term *caregiver* is used throughout this book to refer to the volunteer, unpaid help provided by spouses, family members, relatives, and close friends. As noted earlier in the introductory chapter, 📖 **"Definitions of Titles and Terms Used in This Reference,"** the term has been used instead by society and the media to refer to almost any category of personal assistance provider. However, its use in this book is more precise, for the reasons discussed in that chapter.

As so commonly happens, our good intention never became reality. The ongoing days, weeks, and months never provided days with sufficient post-caregiving time or energy for planning her own concerns. After 18 months at home, I moved out to pursue studies and a new life at a college campus. I have often remembered seeing my mother wishing me well at the airport. I am convinced that my departure from home happened just in time to prevent her probable collapse from emotional and physical exhaustion.

I vowed to myself that I would take an initiative of responsibility to prevent that chronic fatigue, depression, and even anger from ever again happening to any unpaid family caregiver or paid outside provider who helped me.

Then, 15 years later, I met Peggy at Boston University, where we were both members of the administration. Each of us fell deeply into the euphoria of romance, casting aside most rational planning strategies so we could spend every possible moment with each other. Before we were aware of it, she had offered to assist most of my ADL daily needs. Again, we had firm intentions of easing her out of that role. We intended to create a healthy balance between her providing help during our private times, and hiring several part-time PAs to accommodate the other ordinary times.

Peggy and I, as much as we loved—and still love—each other, never found sufficient time to retool our priorities and schedule so that her needs were fulfilled as well as mine. Does that phrase sound familiar?

Even though I subsequently hired and managed a continuous aide staff of five or six part-timers for the next 14 years, and even though they accommodated 90 percent of my ordinary ADL needs, I failed to recognize in a timely manner the many other factors that eventually exhausted Peggy.

To cite a very abbreviated list, she became tired from being the only faithful backup to the hired help who often called in sick. She was also tired from setting her alarm to leave our bed a half-hour before my 6 A.M. aide arrived each morning, and from waiting until the late hours each night when my evening aide finally departed before she could join me in bed. In a third example, she was tired from being frequently interrupted by my help requests, and thus feeling that she was always on duty while at our house; I failed to limit most of my non-urgent help requests to the times when she was formally scheduled to help me.

After 15 years of marriage, I understandably lost Peggy to the divorce she needed—to get the rest that she had wanted and required for so long. (Today, we purposely live just three blocks from each other, and continue to be very supportive of each other. We just can't live together anymore.)

So, you can see my vested interest in urging you and your family to formally take the time to "intentionally plan to succeed," so you will not "unintentionally plan to fail."

If your disability is not congenital, you might begin this chapter's planning and ongoing series of routine family meetings very soon after the disability occurs and dependent needs become evident. If you have had your disability for a while, and perhaps the problems and fatigue have been piling up as high as the stressful emotions, then begin your family's balanced lifestyle as soon as any planning again seems to be possible.

At the least, please do not repeatedly postpone your planning until "tomorrow," because—as we saw for my mother and Peggy—tomorrow might never arrive!

This chapter has been carefully designed to help your family, your caregivers, and you (the help recipient) reduce stress, overwork, chronic fatigue, and depression. Each of the three family elements should be kept equally strong. Most of the traditional problems can be avoided by having the whole family join together in doing the research and planning that you are doing right now through this reference book. If, in contrast, these problems have become established, then the strategies of this chapter can be used as a remedy to return balance to the family's functions. Read on.

The remainder of this chapter has two main parts. A ten-step planning strategy is followed by explanatory narrative.

Figure 5-1: **A preview of planning Steps ❶ through ❿ for getting all or some of your help from family caregivers**

Step ❶ As the help recipient, you identify a planner and manager—ideally, yourself—to make decisions and provide ongoing monitoring of a variety of disability-related needs.

Step ❷ You or the planner-manager create your list and schedule of ADL help needs, be sure the needs are valid bases for requesting help, and then total the weekly and monthly hours on the list.

Step ❸ You, as the help recipient, and the family caregivers review each other's personal concerns; you or the planner-manager also review the qualities of being a first-class PA manager.

Step ❹ You and family members review a five-part strategy for preserving family strength and preventing family burnout, before deciding whether family caregivers should commit to providing routine physical help for all your ADL needs.

Step ❺ You help family caregivers decide if they still want to provide all or some of your physical ADL help. Additional decisions include how many hours of help they will provide, which tasks and schedule they prefer, and ways in which other family members will give them routine support.

Step ❻ If family caregivers will not initially be providing all or some of your physical ADL help (or decide later not to do so), identify the types of tasks and total hours to be assigned to outsiders. Decide the type(s) and source(s) of providers you will hire, and whether to use agency or personally employed providers.

Step ❼ You calculate the cost of hiring outside providers, and identify the source of funding.

Step ❽ You or the planner-manager hire outside providers, if and when your family needs help from them.

Step ❾ You or the planner-manager use family caregivers or other, current outside providers to train new providers with a three-step procedure.

Step ❿ You, family caregivers, and the rest of the family hold routine, state-of-the-family meetings to review what is working well and what needs improvement.

Although this ten-step planning strategy has been used successfully, some of its more innovative elements merit clarification. A discussion of several topics follows the ten-step presentation.

Planning steps ❶ through ❿

Step ❶   **As the help recipient, you identify a planner and manager— ideally, yourself—to make decisions and provide ongoing monitoring of a variety of disability-related needs.**

> • Decide who will perform the initial planning regarding your help needs and then the ongoing management of those needs and any outside help providers, far in advance of identifying the actual providers.
>
> **Step ❶** is not yet about who will provide the help, but instead first about who will be the planner-manager: the one who makes decisions and then provides ongoing, overall management. The planning decisions will begin with creating a list and schedule of help needs. The ongoing management functions are centered around the list of eight disability-related needs found later in **Step ❹** —the physical help with ADL needs is just one of them.
>
> Ideally, the help recipient is the best choice for making those decisions and is also the logical source for expressing them during the training and monitoring of providers, even when family caregivers are the providers. These decisions will determine the recipient's daily type and quality of lifestyle, so it is most appropriate for that person to form the decisions and then carry them out on a long-term basis. The upcoming plan gives the help recipient the first chance to consider the planner-manager role.
>
> Although the recipient is the ideal choice, that person is not always willing or able to assume those responsibilities. When the recipient has caring and competent family members or close friends, these people are the second choice. They would plan and manage during periodic meetings. When the recipient lacks family and friends who are willing to assume these roles, a health care agency or facility is the third choice for who must take over.
>
> ### *The Three Management Roles for Help Recipients to Consider*
>
> Because you, the recipient, would be the best planner and manager, you are first offered the position by reviewing a set of three possible management roles. There are such distinct advantages in your assuming this self-directive and empowering position! If it is at all possible for you to be the planner-manager, Roles One or Two will propose the way. If you are not able or willing to manage, Role Three will ask that family members be the next to consider this position.

You are encouraged to take as powerful a role as you are willing and able to assume. As you will find described for Role Two, you can maintain both an image and a fully active function of authority and control, despite having significant secondary limitations to doing some of the traditional management tasks.

So, to offer you the first choice as the planner and manager, decide which one of these three management roles applies to you.

> ‣ *Role One*—You can independently manage
> the people who help you.

You have the desire to manage help providers, as well as the cognitive ability to remember your needs, make routine decisions, and resolve problems. In addition, you have the functional abilities to manage and use your choice of providers.

Consequently, you can manage and use your choice of family caregivers, agency-employed aides, personally employed PAs, or any combination.

> ‣ *Role Two*—You can independently manage the people who help
> you, after you accommodate an impairment to your
> doing some of the management tasks.

You have the desire to manage help providers, as well as the cognitive ability to remember your needs, make routine decisions, and resolve problems. However, you have a learning disability, a limitation to physical writing or computer interfacing, or an impairment to speech, hearing, sight, or another function that limits your independently doing some of the functional management tasks.

You have already developed ways to accommodate this impairment in your daily lifestyle, and you do so again to fully manage the people who help you, by:
- ▾ doing the tasks in innovative ways
- ▾ using technology and adaptive equipment to do the tasks
- ▾ using extra help from your help providers.

Consequently, with the accommodation in place, you can manage and use your choice of family caregivers, agency-employed aides, personally employed PAs, or any combination.

> ‣ *Role Three*—You require someone else to remember your routine,
> make decisions, solve problems, and manage the people
> who help you.

You might have the functional abilities to be your own manager, but you lack one or both of the other two essentials:
- ▾ the desire to manage help providers

▼ the cognitive ability to remember your needs, make routine decisions, and resolve problems.

In Role Two, we saw that some functional limitations can be accommodated in ways that still enable you to manage independently. However, it is rare that help recipients who lack the desire to manage, or the cognitive abilities to do so, can create satisfactory accommodations.

Consequently, you will require a family caregiver, another type of personal representative, or an agency to make decisions, employ, and manage help providers for you.

The importance of reviewing management roles is to put you in as much power and control of your lifestyle and help providers as you want and are able to have.

The Three Management Roles for Family and Friends to Consider

When the help recipient is unable or unwilling to plan and manage, the family and close friends are offered this second set of considerations.

Next are three possible management roles for family and friends. The first, preferred role suggests that the recipient act as consultant to a group of family and friends who collectively do the planning and managing. Role Two applies when the group's interest is limited and seems to focus on just one or two members; it also assumes that these same people will later be likely to volunteer to take on the physical caregiver tasks. If neither Role One nor Two seems feasible, then the third proposes that a health care agency or facility must ultimately fill the position.

▸ *Role One*—The family or friends work as a team of advisors in planning and managing.

When there is a sufficient number of family and friends who agree to a long-term, active commitment, these people meet periodically to plan and manage collectively. They represent the help recipient in their decisions and actions.

▸ *Role Two*—One or two members of the family and friends agree to perform the planning and managing.

When the available and interested family and friends are limited to one or two members, these people do their best to represent the wishes of the help recipient.

When this considerable responsibility is assumed entirely by one or two persons, these persons should be especially guarded against acting on a common impulse to also provide the daily, physical ADL assistance. My heartfelt advice to families reviewing this **Step ❶** is to be careful to limit their current commitment to being *a planner and manager,* and to delay any additional impulse toward being *a help provider* until at least **Step ❹** (an essential discussion of cautions found later in this chapter).

▸ *Role Three*—In the absence of available family and friends,
a health care facility or agency is contracted to perform
the planning and managing.

When neither the help recipient nor his/her family and friends are available for these functions, a facility or agency is the final choice for these needs.[3]

Indeed, staffing this position of planning and managing the help needs is prerequisite to actually providing the help. It is common and acceptable for family and friends to volunteer their managing and planning, and then be unable to provide actual caregiver help. However, it is not logical that they would provide caregiver help after declaring themselves unable to plan and manage that help. If neither the help recipient nor the family and friends are willing or able to manage the needs, it is assumed that family and friends will also be unavailable for providing caregiver help.

When this situation is identified, there is no reason to further pursue this chapter on getting help from family caregivers. Instead, your resource for planning, managing, and providing help would seem to be entirely in health care facilities and agencies. The best introduction to these is in chapters 1 and 6.

Step ❷   You or the planner-manager create your list and schedule of ADL help needs, be sure the needs are valid bases for requesting help, and then total the weekly and monthly hours on the list.

The planner-manager from **Step ❶** begins to make some planning decisions. Please note that these steps continue to appropriately address the help recipient, regardless of who is actually acting as the planner-manager. If the recipient is unable or unwilling to be the planner-manager, his or her opinion should still be, as much as possible, the basis of the planning.

---

3. For considerations in selecting an outside facility or agency, please review chapter 📖 **1,** "Beyond Family Caregivers: Options and Settings for Finding Outside Assistance." For advice on selecting a full-service agency, please examine chapter 📖 **6,** "Ten Steps to Getting All or Some of Your Help from Agency-Employed Aides."

It might at first seem unnecessary to create a formal list and schedule of help needs if family caregivers are initially intended to be the sole source of help. However, the list and schedule will be a surprising asset to family planning. In addition, it will be an essential planning tool if the family eventually decides to assign some ADL tasks to outside providers.

- Create your list and schedule of needs.

  Identify what help you need and create a list that includes the "what, when, where, and how long" for your needs. This listing, according to your personal style, could be in the format of a carefully memorized outline, a handwritten listing, or a more detailed computer printout.[4]

- Be sure that all of your requests for help are valid.

  There is a fine line between respecting providers, by requesting help for valid needs, and abusing providers, by asking them either to provide unnecessary help or to become inappropriately responsible for you.[5]

- Total the weekly hours of help you will probably need, and assume that some of them will eventually be assigned to outside providers.
  - ▸ From your list of needs and schedule (above), add up the weekly and monthly hours for your routine needs.
  - ▸ Then add another 25 percent to the total hours for unforeseeable—but predictable and frequent—bowel and bladder accidents, illnesses, medical equipment repairs, and special needs.

Your total hours of need =
    Routine, predictable needs
+   25% allowance for sporadic, unpredictable needs

Example:
Your weekly total =
    32 hours of routine needs
+   8 hours of unpredictable needs
=   40 total weekly hours, or 160 monthly hours

---

4. For more detail about listing what help you need and when you need it, as well as confirming the importance of your preferences in how you want help provided, please see chapters 📖 12, "Getting It Done—Your Way!" and 📖 13, "Defining and Describing Your Help Needs."

5. Please see chapter 📖 11, "When It Is, and Is Not, Okay to Ask for Help."

Step ❸   You, as the help recipient, and the family caregivers review each other's personal concerns; you or the planner-manager also review the qualities of being a first-class PA manager.

This goal of this step is for family members to better hear and understand each other—as well as themselves. It is common that this understanding cannot be adequately achieved through routine family conversation, so you will be referred to two lists of concerns for caregivers and help recipients. In addition, another short chapter proposes a "bill of rights" common to all (Please see Part VII).

Attempts at face-to-face communication among family members are often not completely successful. When trying to convey your feelings and emotions, how many times have you just given up, in the belief that other family members have neither heard nor understood what you tried to tell them? Perhaps you feel they habitually do not listen to you, but that they might listen to someone else who understood your point of view. Well, today might be your lucky day!

In addition to better understanding others, reading your own concerns might give you a surprising new insight into yourself. While your lifestyle has its share of joys, it also has sad, painful, and depressing emotions. When these emotions become severe, you might want to deny or suppress what you don't want to think about. You have learned to get through some days by effectively using denial. However, denying a problem doesn't make it go away permanently; instead, ironically, denial empowers it. Reading through your own concerns can facilitate a re-identification of denied problems, so you can formally face and resolve them.

I have spent years compiling three lists of concerns, one each for help recipients, family caregivers, and outside, paid providers. Throughout the years, I repeatedly felt the "ah ha!" of epiphanies as I suddenly understood more about myself, my previously burned-out family caregivers, and paid providers who resigned before the end of their commitments.

Your family might be surrounded each day with real-life experiences of painfully active stress and burnout. The last thing you might think you want to do is read through two brief lists that simply seem to restate what you are now experiencing. However, make a deal with your family: tell them that you will read through their list of concerns if they agree to read through yours. Then, I suggest that each of you read through your own list to better understand your own feelings about certain topics.

- To facilitate communication and understanding, you and your family are encouraged to review the lists in these chapters:
  - ▸ Everyone is encouraged to review a proposal of personal rights in chapter 📖 **22, "A Bill of Rights for You as a Help Recipient, Family Caregiver, or Paid Provider."**
  - ▸ As a help recipient, you are encouraged to read chapter 📖 **24, "Your Personal Concerns as a Family Caregiver."**
  - ▸ In return, caregivers and other members are encouraged to read chapter 📖 **23, "Your Personal Concerns as a Help Recipient."**

> *While family caregivers provide support and help to your needs, you should be supporting and helping their needs.*

- Review the qualities for being a good PA manager. Throughout this book, a variety of special topics about being a respected and in-control PA manager are addressed. Use the index and table of contents to locate any topic of concern.

Step ❹ **You and family members review a five-part strategy for preserving family strength and preventing family burnout, before deciding whether family caregivers should commit to providing routine physical help for all your ADL needs.**

As an introduction, you can first review the outlines of the traditional, burnout approach to caregiving *(Figure 5-2)* and the five-part strategy to preserving family strength *(Figure 5-3)* before the latter is discussed in detail.

Figure 5-2: **The Traditional, Burnout Approach to Caregiving**

Traditionally, loving family caregivers have expressed their unconditional caring by placing the help recipient's needs ahead of their own. This generous gesture usually works well for short-term needs, but after a few weeks of their sacrificing so many personal essentials, many caregivers experience chronic fatigue and depression. The following steps additionally describe this problem situation; *Figure 5-3*, describes how to prevent it!

① A family member acquires (or is born with) significant functional limitations—a disability.
   • Causes include congenital conditions, an injury or illness, a stroke, or advancing age.

② Family members (often only the mother or significant other) become caregivers.
   • They drop everything to provide whatever help the recipient requires, whenever he requires it.

③ The family designs a system first to meet ongoing needs for the recipient, with caregiver and family needs being allocated any remaining time and stamina.
   • Initially, hiring outside help is not a consideration, as it might be interpreted as a lack of family caring or resources.
   • For the help recipient, it might also be interpreted as a sign of decreasing love and possible rejection by the family.
   • More and more recipient needs surface and are unquestioningly accommodated by family members, who usually feel too guilty to voice their increasing fatigue, depression, and need for relief.

④ Emotional and physical health crises begin to occur within the family.
   • First, the actual caregivers become overworked, chronically tired, and clinically depressed.
   • Second, other family members become angry at the caregiving priority, because the traditional needs of the family and marriage have gone unfulfilled.
   • Third, the help recipient feels these stresses and believes himself to be the shameful cause. He often feels shame, guilt, depression, and anger for what he and his disability seem to be doing to the family.
   • Fourth, the recipient begins to fear that the family will stop loving him and even abandon him by sending him to a nursing home.

⑤ Family members finally seek relief or replacement help. They then turn to volunteer or hired help from the outside, as they could—and should—have done initially to minimize the opportunity for this ultimate crisis.
   • Either help is brought into the home, or the beloved recipient moves out to a care facility.

Figure 5-3: **The Five-Part Strategy to Preserving Family Strength**

To reduce or avoid the risks that caregiver burnout will occur, you and your family should consider planning as a team to prioritize resources of time and energy, in the following order.

① First, maintain each member's individual personal needs—for keeping each person physically and emotionally rested and healthy.

② Next, maintain each member's roles, functions, and tasks within the family or marital structure—for keeping the family or marriage strong and unified.

③ Then, maintain the family's ability to share personal caring, love, and support—for continuing the times and activities that provide emotional and spiritual strength to the family and each member.

④ Next, allocate sufficient time and energy for the family to address these seven primary disability issues that the family—and not outside providers—can uniquely address:

- problem-solving help with sporadic, disability-related concerns of many kinds
- coordinating the scheduling of your daily, routine ADL needs between family and outside providers
- assisting in the training of newly hired, outside providers
- providing physical ADL help during private family events, romantic times, and family vacation travel
- providing physical ADL help for emergency and urgent needs that occur between the scheduled work shifts of hired, outside providers
- providing special physical help for temporary, especially complex medical needs, such as skin sores, fractures, or illnesses, as a supplement to the routine help from outsiders
- providing backup help for "no-shows" when scheduled, hired providers are unable, or fail, to appear for a shift.

⑤ Finally, use any remaining family resources—*if* any—to supplement the outside help that is hired for most, or all, of your routine physical ADL needs.

Here is a discussion of the five-part strategy outlined in *Figure 5-3*.

① First, maintain each member's individual, personal needs—for keeping each person physically and emotionally rested and healthy.

Before providing any help to someone else, caregivers and other family members should identify and maintain their own needs, especially the personal activities and private time that they currently enjoy and require.

Caregivers must maintain their own personal strength and health before they can help someone else. Therefore, they should plan ways for ensuring that they can continue to meet their own needs before considering new caregiver duties. You and caregivers should insist that most categories of a caregiver's current personal needs be maintained. If a daily walk in the park has been consistently important to this point, it will become even more important as a break in providing care.

If necessary, perhaps reduce the amount of time spent with some categories; however, think carefully about consequences before deleting any. If the caregiver's new daily schedule does not permit an hour-long walk, then reducing the time to a half-hour is preferable to completely abandoning the activity.

② Second, maintain each member's roles, functions, and tasks within the family or marital structure—for keeping the family or marriage strong and unified.

Caregivers should next maintain any essential roles and functions that contribute to the unity and strength of their family or marriage.

A unified and strong family can provide important support to both its caregivers and its help recipients. Therefore, after first maintaining their own personal needs, caregivers and other family members should next continue to meet needs of the family or marital structure before considering taking on new caregiver duties.

This family strength is often dependent on roles and functions that are already filled by each family member. Most caregivers will burn out if they try to maintain all their previous family duties while adding new, caregiver tasks. Some priorities should be established.

Caregivers should identify their family roles and functions, and might sort them into these three groups:

▸ Those family functions that the caregiver must maintain, as no other family member can perform them.

▸ Those family functions that the caregiver and family can suspend, because they are not essential to the family's strength.

▸ Those essential functions that the caregiver can transfer to other family members.

Other family members should begin to fill in some of the duties, caring, and support that the caregivers previously supplied to the family—and then grace the caregivers with a double dose!

③ Third, maintain the family's ability to share personal caring, love, and support—for continuing the times and activities that provide emotional and spiritual strength to the family and each member.

Family members should maintain the time required for continuing most of the traditional family events where they share their unique love, caring, and support.

The loving support that family members share will be especially important in the upcoming, trying times. If caregivers and other family members must ration their limited resources, it would be wise to continue this support and assign some of the disability-related physical needs to outside help.

④ Fourth, allocate sufficient time and energy for the family to address these seven primary disability needs that the family—and not outside providers—can uniquely address. This allocation is typically significant, and should not be squeezed as an afterthought into an otherwise busy schedule as another source of stress.

The seven disability-related needs that a family can best support are:

Disability need #1

▸ Problem-solving help with sporadic, disability-related concerns of many kinds.

A disability requires an ongoing process of resolving a wide range of concerns and problems. These routinely include diagnosing and treating periodic medical crises, devising strategies for performing activities of daily living (ADLs), maintaining inventories of medical supplies and prescriptions, and dedicating the double-planning time required in general for accommodating a disability. To avoid having these unforeseeable-but-predictable concerns create family stress, the family is wise to permanently reserve a few units of energy and time for them.

Disability need #2

▸ Coordinating the scheduling of your daily, routine ADL needs between family and outside providers.

Whether acquired through an agency or personal employment, outside help requires a significant amount of family time for the periodically necessary hiring of new help. To describe this process, I created the term *RISHTMP cycle* for recruiting, interviewing, screening, hiring, training, managing, and parting ways with providers. Sometimes the recipient of the help assumes most of this responsibility. However, family caregivers frequently find that if they want relief help from outsiders, it's up to them to recruit and coordinate it—in addition to the physical help they actually provide! When faced with this requirement to recruit their own relief help, caregivers unfortunately too often abandon their plans. They either don't know how to personally employ or don't believe they could do it while providing their own help. This book provides the "how-tos" for getting agency or personal aides, and it encourages family caregivers to consider assigning *all* of the ADL help they provide to outsiders, and using that freed-up time to manage outsiders instead of providing help.

Disability need #3

▸ Assisting in the training of newly hired, outside providers.

New help providers, whether from an agency or personal employment, require training. Part of training suggests using a family caregiver or currently hired aide to demonstrate the recipient's routine. Smart planning says that the family should permanently allocate time and energy for this task before agreeing to provide any help themselves.

Disability need #4

▸ Providing physical ADL help during private family events, romantic times, and family vacation travel.

Most families (and especially romantic couples) routinely schedule traditional activities, vacations, or simply quiet time "for family only." Regardless of extensive outside help for routine ADLs, families and couples usually want to isolate some routine times from the intrusions. A few more units of family time should be reserved for providing family help to disability needs during these private gatherings.

Disability need #5

▸ Providing physical ADL help for emergency and urgent needs that occur between the scheduled work shifts of hired, outside providers.

Regardless of how well outside help is scheduled and confirmed, there will be occasional needs for "crisis help." Bowel and bladder accidents, as well as the unpredictable need for an in-bed nap or out-of-refrigerator snack, are examples of needing help between the scheduled shifts of workers. More family time should be reserved.

Disability need #6

▸ Providing special physical help for temporary, especially complex medical needs, such as skin sores, fractures, or illnesses, as a supplement to the routine help from outsiders.

Life with a disability is full of routine, sporadic secondary disabilities. As unfair as it seems, the secondary challenges come in a variety of forms: bedsores, bone breaks, urinary tract infections, respiratory congestion, and even the common flu (that often brings special complications and the need for longer recovery to people who have disabilities). Each of these periodic bonuses requires extra, temporary care. If you live alone, you will be instructing your hired help in any special procedure of the day. However, it is common for a caring family member to supplement the hired help's usual duties by stepping in for a few minutes to provide a personal inspection or a hands-on special treatment.

Disability need #7

▸ Providing backup help for "no-shows" when scheduled, hired providers are unable, or fail, to appear for a shift.

It is not uncommon for scheduled outside providers to be suddenly unable to appear for a shift. Strategies are presented in this reference for having outside providers back up other outside providers; however, family caregivers often serve as the first line of backups. Once more, smart planning dictates saving some family resources for these sudden fill-in needs.

⑤ Fifth, use any remaining family resources—*if* any—to supplement the outside help that is hired for most, or all, of your routine physical ADL needs (disability need #8).

Finally, after first allocating time and stamina to the previous four parts, family caregivers should decide whether they have the remaining resources to actually provide the routine, daily help. If so, they should have first choice of your ADL duties and schedule. Outside help is then arranged for most (and sometimes all) of the remaining ADL tasks. This planning is outlined in the following steps.

Step ❺   **You help family caregivers decide if they still want to provide all or some of your physical ADL help. Additional decisions include how many hours of help they will provide, which tasks and schedule they prefer, and ways in which other family members will give them routine support.**

- Caregivers decide whether they have enough remaining time and energy to provide ADL help to you.

  Caregivers are cautioned against initially providing boundless help for whatever and whenever it is needed, while assuming that they will later be able to reclaim their personal time:

  ▶ from whatever time might be left over

  ▶ by working extra hours

  ▶ by working faster.

  Instead, caregivers are strongly advised to consider the priorities in the five-part strategy of **Step ❹**.

- Caregivers who do want to directly assist with ADL needs must decide how much help to provide.

  If the caregivers have remaining resources for providing your help, then coach them to conservatively decide how much.

- Encourage caregivers to take their first choice of specific ADL tasks and scheduling (ahead of outside providers).

  Family caregivers should consider at least these factors in making their selections:

  ▶ Type of task—Pleasant vs. unpleasant tasks; required lifting vs. none.

  ▶ Required effort—High effort and energy drain vs. light tasks.

  ▶ Complexity—Those tasks requiring frequent decisions, medical training, or experience vs. no-brainer tasks.

  ▶ Schedule—Morning vs. evening; avoiding schedule conflicts with their current commitments; their desire for a variety in schedule.

  ▶ Duration—Short vs. lengthy work shifts.

  ▶ Location—In-home vs. in-community or in-travel.

- After caregivers have a tentative list of the quantity and types of tasks, you might suggest that the whole family participate in a review exercise.

  Ask caregivers to reduce the chances for burnout by consulting with the whole family in an exercise for evaluating their ADL task selections.

Caregivers have some tough decisions coming up, and most will welcome advice from the help recipient and other family members. When faced with the difficult decisions about whether to directly help with ADL needs—and if so, how much—most caregivers have a heartfelt tendency simply to provide help for all the needs. However, these are decisions that should integrate both heart and head, and advice from other family members can be very valuable in keeping the process grounded.

The caregivers' provision of help unavoidably affects the entire family: the caregivers, the help recipient, and each other family member. In the Caregiver-Workload Advisory Exercise (*Figure 5-4*), I suggest that all family members examine the caregiver's proposed list and schedule of ADL tasks. The resulting balanced decisions will better safeguard the concerns of each part of the family.

While this whole-family approach to planning increases the chances of having everyone's concerns represented, it also makes communication, support, and the sharing of tasks whole-family responsibilities.

Figure 5-4: **The Caregiver-Workload Advisory Exercise**

Your family caregiver(s) have given other family members a tentative list and schedule of your ADL tasks with which they are considering assisting. Their list is usually a discrete part of all your needs, unless they have selected all of them. This simple caregiver advisory exercise is a very effective way for the entire family to communicate their predictions about the effects of the proposed list, schedule, and workload on caregivers and other family members. It is also effective in achieving family-wide empathy and support for the caregivers.

This exercise is fully effective only when the whole family participates: the caregiver(s), recipient of help, and the other members. This full-family feedback is very helpful to the caregivers who are making decisions about their selection of tasks and schedule. Caregivers usually welcome this family participation, because each family member will be directly or indirectly affected by the caregiving situation. They prefer not to make the decisions alone and solely bear the responsibility for outcomes. If the decisions later adversely affect family members, the family's full involvement now in making those decisions will increase the probability of their constructive suggestions for improvement, and decrease the probability of poor and passive communication that often airs only unproductive complaints.

After family caregivers have presented the tentative list, they request each family member to provide opinions about the following questions and topics.

Figure 5-4: **The Caregiver-Workload Advisory Exercise (continued)**

"After examining the tentative list and schedule of ADL tasks that our family caregiver(s) are considering, what effect do I foresee that each of these bulleted topics will have for me and each other family member during these next six months? Also, where I foresee problems, what modifications do I suggest the caregivers consider?"

- The types of tasks listed for family caregivers
- The amount of daily, weekly, and monthly work listed for family caregivers
- The schedule of each day's work for family caregivers
- The amount and schedule of time off that is free from scheduled work for family caregivers
- The types of tasks, and amount and schedule of work, that are alternately listed for assignment to volunteer or hired, outside help providers

As each family member considers the effect of each bulleted topic on each family member, some of these questions might help in formulating answers. Please note that "unrelated" means "not related to the caregiver tasks done for the help recipient."

What is my relationship to the caregiver(s) and the help recipient?

- Am I dependent on either of them for the unrelated functions they already do for the family, and could their continued ability to perform these family functions be affected by any of the bulleted items?
- Am I dependent on either of them for my unrelated physical needs or emotional support, and could their continued ability to accommodate my needs be affected by any of the bulleted items?
- Are they dependent on me for the unrelated functions I already do for the family, and could my continued ability to supply this help to the family be affected by any of the bulleted items?
- Are they dependent on me for their unrelated physical needs or emotional support, and could my continued ability to supply this help to their needs be affected by any of the bulleted items?
- If I will not be one of the caregivers, are there ways I could assist the caregivers with their own personal needs, or assume (and relieve them of) some of their unrelated family functions?

- Ask the family to plan for supporting itself and the caregivers.

  After caregivers and other family members have consulted in finalizing the caregiver list and schedule of ADL tasks, the entire family can additionally help with the following planning:

▸ ways that the help recipient and non-caregiver family members can assume some of the *family functions and support* that the caregivers can no longer supply because of their new disability-related tasks

▸ ways that non-caregiver family members can further reduce chances for caregiver overload by assuming some of the caregivers' *personal needs.* According to NFCA member surveys, 65 percent of caregivers do not receive consistent help from other family members.

When family caregivers generously provide unconditional help to a loved one, they are often caught in a double bind. In some families, they are additionally expected to maintain all of their previous family functions as well as their own personal needs. In each 24 hours, a caregiver often provides early-morning, mid-day, late-night, and even middle-of-the-night ADL assistance. In addition, some families expect a housewife and mother (or househusband and father) to maintain meal preparation, laundry, housecleaning, and other typical family functions. In a third category, caregivers have personal needs such as educational, career, and leisure interests—or just getting the car washed.

By now, it is easy to see that by keeping the caregivers strong, the whole family can stay strong. It is wise for the whole family to contribute extra help wherever necessary, to keep each part of the family or marriage strong. It is unfair to expect caregivers to do it all: their new caregiver tasks, their traditional functions within the family, and their own personal needs.

Each non-caregiver family member can plan ahead and be proactive in volunteering—and not just passively waiting to be asked—to fill in family functions and personal needs. Proactive means that members take responsibility both for identifying extra chores they can do and performing them. Too often, members merely offer to respond to caregiver requests. This approach does not reduce the caregiver workload, but adds to it.

Step ❻   If family caregivers will not initially be providing all or some of your physical ADL help (or decide later not to do so), identify the types of tasks and total hours to be assigned to outsiders. Decide the type(s) and source(s) of providers you will hire, and whether to use agency or personally employed providers.

Many families decide to be the sole source of help with ADL needs. For some families, this plan works well for many years. Others find it necessary to assign some or all of the needs to outside providers after family caregivers become chronically tired and require relief or replacement help.

• Identify the types of help providers you will probably use. There are several factors to consider.

   ▸ Identify the type(s) of help provider you need by examining:

- ▼ the kinds of help you need
- ▼ the type(s) of providers available to you
- ▼ the type(s) of provider that you require to accommodate your variety of help needs
- ▼ the type(s) that your funding source stipulates or that you can afford.

▶ Provider types include the following. Some types are restricted, when employed by agencies, in the kinds of help they are allowed to provide:
- ▼ nurse
- ▼ certified nursing assistant (CNA)
- ▼ personal care provider (PCP)
- ▼ personally employed aide or personal assistant (PA)
- ▼ homemaker
- ▼ transportation driver
- ▼ companion.

▶ Identify the source(s) of help providers that you will pursue:
- ▼ at-home assistance: volunteers, agency-employed aides, or personally employed PAs
- ▼ community assistance: respite or day care, independent living center, assisted living center, or a skilled nursing home.

- Research the pros and cons of the main two sources of outside help providers.

▶ Become familiar with these ten-step chapters to choose the source of provider that works better for you:
- ▼ For agency-employed aides, please see chapter
  📖 6, **"Ten Steps to Getting All or Some of Your Help from Agency-Employed Aides."**
- ▼ For personally employing PAs, please see chapter
  📖 7, **"Ten Steps to Getting All or Some of Your Help from Personally Employed Aides."**

Step ❼ You calculate the cost of hiring outside providers, and identify the source of funding.

- Calculate the cost of your help.[6]
  ▶ If you are using personal funds and personally employing PAs, research the hourly salary rate that others are paying their PAs in your community.
  ▶ If you are using agency aides, ask the agencies for their hourly rates.
  ▶ Multiply the total hours of your needs by one of these rates.[7]

---

6. For points to remember in estimating costs, please see chapter 📖 19, **"Your Costs of Recruiting, Training, and Keeping PAs Happy."**

7. For more detail about calculating the total hours of your help needs, as well as the total salaried cost (including taxes and other extras), please see chapter 📖 20, **"Paying Salaries: Cash, Non-cash, or Both."**

> Your total cost of aides or PAs =
>   Total hours of help needed
> x   Hourly salary or agency rate
>
> Example:
> Your weekly cost =
>   40 total hours
> x $8.50 (personal salary) or $20.00 (agency rate) per hour
> = $340.00 weekly ($1,360.00 monthly) or
> = $800.00 weekly ($3,200.00 monthly)

- Decide how to pay for this outside help.
  - ▶ Decide whether to use personal funds or outside funding for your help:
    - ▼ personal, out-of-pocket funds
    - ▼ federal or state agency or assistance program
    - ▼ accident or insurance settlement
    - ▼ health or long-term care insurance
    - ▼ other.
  - ▶ If using personal funds and personally employing PAs, use your cost estimate to plan your personal budget. If the cost exceeds your personal funds, then you will need to research sources of some outside money.
  - ▶ If using outside funding, identify the source(s), research the eligibility criteria, and apply for the funding. Be sure to note if the funding source places any restrictions on the type or source of help you can hire. Some funding sources will limit you to using only a specific agency with which the funding source has a contract. With this stipulation, you will not be permitted to personally employ your own PAs if you want the source to pay for your providers.

Step ❽   You or the planner-manager hire outside providers, if and when your family needs help from them.

If—and when—the family decides to hire outsiders, the planner-manager prepares to recruit either an agency or personally employed aides.

- Get ready to describe your routine.
  - ▶ Create and rehearse both a brief, 30-second and a detailed, 5-minute description of your needs and schedule, plus some basic notes about how you employ PAs.
  - ▶ Give the appropriate description to applicants when answering initial phone inquiries, during face-to-face interviews, and when training new PAs.

Each time you or your representative describes your routine, you will want to impress your own PA applicants, or the supervisor and aide from the agency, that you are someone who is organized, sharp, and worthy of their help. This first impression is important to your authority, power, and control of the work relationship. Each description should be well organized, concise, and to the point.[8]

As mentioned earlier, it might initially seem inappropriate to discuss costs and funding in a chapter about using unpaid family caregivers. However, a primary strategy to preventing caregiver chronic fatigue and stress is eventually to assign many needs to outside providers. It is wise at least to introduce these topics at this early time. In calculating these cost estimates, you can decide to use your total hours of current needs or just a portion. The important objective at this planning stage is to be aware of the process so it can be readily and intelligently used later.

- Use these chapters to pursue your choice of outside help providers.

  ▸ For using agency-employed aides, please see chapter
    📖 6, "Ten Steps to Getting All or Some of Your Help from Agency-Employed Aides."

  ▸ For using personally employed PAs, please see chapter
    📖 7, "Ten Steps to Getting All or Some of Your Help from Personally Employed Aides."

It is ideal for the help recipient to assume responsibilities of recruiting and coordinating outside help. However, when this is not possible, this is a function with which other family members—and not only caregivers—can assist. The caregiver's role is most difficult when she or he becomes overtired, realizes the urgent need for outside relief help, and then must single-handedly recruit and manage it.

Step ❾ You or the planner-manager use family caregivers or other, current outside providers to train new providers with a three-step procedure.

- Train each new aide in what needs you have, as well as how and when you prefer to receive that help. Use family caregivers or current outside help to train new help in three steps:[9]

  ▸ Have the new aide watch a family caregiver or current aide perform each part of your routine.

  ▸ Have the new aide do the routine once or twice while a current provider stands by.

  ▸ Finish her training by having her work directly with you, while receiving your occasional reminders and lots of patience.

---

8. For more detail about what goes into each of the two descriptions, and when to use each one, please see chapter 📖 13, "Defining and Describing Your Help Needs."

9. For more details on using family caregivers or outside providers in this three-step method for training new help, please see chapter 📖 9, "Initial Training and Ongoing Management of Aides and PAs."

Step ❿ **You, family caregivers, and the rest of the family hold routine, state-of-the-family meetings to review what is working well and what needs improvement.**

- Encourage your entire family to hold routine review meetings.

  It is wise to schedule family review meetings routinely, in advance of any identified concerns or problems:

  ▸ to facilitate communication when family members need it most, and often find it increasingly difficult to achieve

  ▸ to identify and discuss both obvious and hidden concerns and problems before they grow into crises.

  Get the whole family together at least once each week or each month (Sunday nights after dinner?) for a "state-of-the-family" meeting." To encourage members to state their individual opinions, you could consider starting each meeting by answering these rank-ordered questions, and then having an open discussion about both individual and family (or marital) concerns.

  ▸ At each family meeting, each caregiver might answer these questions—to most closely express her/his personal feelings—by providing a number, from one to five (1 to 5), where
  1 = Strongly agree, 2 = Agree, 3 = Somewhat agree,
  4 = Somewhat disagree, and 5 = Strongly disagree
  - ▾ "In reviewing this week's events, I feel the assistance I provided to the recipient was appreciated."
  - ▾ "In reviewing this week, I feel that the personal energy level available for my caregiving duties exceeded my available energy on at least three days this week."
  - ▾ "I would like to transfer some of my caregiving duties to outside help providers."

  ▸ At each family meeting, the caregiver, the help recipient, and each non-caregiver family member could answer these questions—to most closely express personal feelings—by providing a number, from one to five:
  - ▾ "In reviewing this week, I was not able to spend as much time as I wanted with the whole family."
  - ▾ "In reviewing this week, I feel I did have enough time each day (yes, "each day" and not merely "each week"!) for my own, private needs."
  - ▾ "In my opinion, in comparing this last week to the week before, the stress level within the family was higher."
  - ▾ "Overall, I am getting sufficient rest each night."
  - ▾ "I think it would be a good idea to transfer some of the family's caregiving duties to outside help providers."

▸ You, as the recipient of help, should answer these questions—to most closely express your personal feelings—by providing a number, from one to five:

  ▾ "In reviewing this week, all of my personal ADL needs for help were satisfactorily fulfilled."

  ▾ "All of my personal non-ADL needs for help were satisfactorily fulfilled."

  ▾ "I felt comfortable—and not uneasy—whenever I requested help this week."

  ▾ "There were things that I could not do this week because I did not have help when I needed it."

  ▾ "I would like to bring in some additional, outside help."

A balanced strategy

At the core of this chapter's preventative approach is a balanced strategy that attempts to safeguard the personal needs of your caregiver(s) and other family members, the structural needs of your family or marriage, and your personal and disability-related help needs, as the help recipient.

As we showed at the beginning of the chapter with the personal caregiver experiences of my mother and former wife, the traditional approach to caregiving usually lacks adequate advance planning.

The key to the five-part family preservation strategy is in wisely planning to use caregiver and family resources of time and stamina first to maintain the strength of individual caregivers and the family or marital structure. With this two-fold foundation solidified, caregivers and family next can decide which of your needs to address with their remaining resources. Your needs are divided between those that only the family can address and those that could be assigned to outside help providers.

As someone with a disability, you have both emotional and physical needs, and they are both personal and disability related. As a person, you need the same emotional caring, love, and support from your family or marriage that you needed before (or outside of) the disability. In fact, you and other family members now require more support than ever.

As shown in *Figure 5-3,* the five-part strategy for preserving family strength, you have at least these eight types of disability-related needs. Your family can be especially helpful with the first seven of them, listed below in **Step ❹** .

It is wise to address the seven personal and disability-related needs (of **Step ❹**) by combining the family's support with their collective problem solving and planning. If you live alone, do not despair. Strategies throughout this book will show you how to use outside providers and health care professionals for these seven needs. However, if you have willing family, prioritizing their help around these needs makes your life considerably easier.

In contrast to the first seven needs which are best addressed by the family, your eighth, most obvious help need is the mostly physical, no-brainer type. By no-brainer, I am not implying that these needs can be assigned to stupid people, but that they are highly repetitive and tend not to require many complex decisions. ADL needs are cognitively easier, but physically more demanding—and therefore ideal candidates to reserve *from* family and *for* outsiders. This routine, repetitive, daily help with your ADLs consists of physical help with some or all of the following:

- urinary collection
- bowel program
- bathing or showering
- getting dressed
- transfers among bed, commode chair, wheelchair, and car
- food preparation and eating
- taking medication
- wound care.

These are the hard-core needs for which you require rock-solid, dependable, and continuous help providers. Although ADL help is essential to your lifestyle, it can be provided by both family members and outsiders.

Because ADL help can be assigned to outside providers, it should be the lowest priority for using family resources. It is such an irony that families mistakenly give it the highest priority. Instead, some help recipients insist that their ADL help needs be assigned to outside providers from Day One. It is wise not to wait until family caregivers first show signs of burnout to consider outside help.

Why must you prioritize family resources? Simply stated, few families have sufficient resources to do it all—to meet all of their own needs, as well as yours—without some supplemental, outside help. Planning is essential to deciding how much help the family can realistically provide, and to which kinds of needs it is best allocated.

Experience has proven that family members have a finite amount of time and energy. Few family members have the resources both to continue meeting personal and family needs and to provide help for all the new, disability-related needs. Too many families make the mistake of simply trying to "do it all" by working extra hours or working faster. The result of burning the family candle at both ends is, predictably, family burnout.

If asked to make a choice between having a family provide either emotional support or physical caregiver help, most people with disabilities would reserve the family's finite time and energy for providing its unique, loving support. They would wisely decide to hire outsiders for most of the physical assistance. Families and caregivers should make the same decision.

Compassionate caregivers often view providing physical help with the needs of a loved one much as they would providing immediate attention to the sudden flare-up of a stove-top grease fire. In either case, their own personal needs are quickly abandoned and all of their available resources (time and energy) are nobly allocated to the urgent need. This all-out reaction is appropriate and physically possible for a short-term emergency, but not for long-term disability needs. Disability needs merit a careful planning of resources before action is undertaken.

Traditionally, physical help in your routine ADLs is the most obvious need seen by family caregivers. Ironically, as you can now see, it should be the last priority for the caregivers and family to consider. As a result of identifying the needs to which the family should give priority before considering ADL help, the ultimate family decision might be that it does not have sufficient remaining energy for all—or even some—of the ADLs. The caregiver and family should guard against abandoning their own needs in order to provide caregiver help for whatever (and whenever it) is needed.

Do these priorities imply that physical help for your disability-related needs is not important, or that family needs are more important than yours? Not at all. Your life depends on getting routinely dependable physical help. The importance of the help you need is not being questioned, only the source.

Too many families assume that family caregivers, because they have unlimited love for the help recipient, will also have unlimited time and energy for disability-related, ADL needs. They would like this to be true, but it is not. Within a brief period, the overworked caregiver becomes fatigued and unable to continue without relief or replacement help. In addition to the caregiver's problems, you, the help recipient, become concerned that your needs will not be met.

Therefore, to reduce the chances for these crises, it is important to carefully select the source(s) for your ADL help. Careful planning should be performed in advance to find help providers who satisfy these objectives. The source of your help:

- should be dependable and continuous
- should not jeopardize the well-being and strength of either the individual caregiver/family members or the unity of your family or marriage
- should not be jeopardized by the status of your personal relationship with either the individual caregivers or your family or marriage
- should not jeopardize your family's ability to continue its love, caring, and support among all of its members
- should not jeopardize your ability to have urgent or emergency help between scheduled shifts of outside providers when they are not available
- should provide you with readily available backup help when an outside provider is unable to, or fails to appear for, work
- should assist you in coordinating and scheduling your help
- should provide a variety of people to meet your variety of needs, schedules, and locations of help.

Carefully planning the source of your help ensures that your essential needs are assigned and scheduled to providers who have adequate time, energy, and availability. Experience has shown that few families can fulfill this wide, exhaustive variety of your needs. The resources of both family and outsiders should be carefully balanced and coordinated.

If this means that your family, mother, father, or spouse decides that physical help with your daily, routine needs cannot come from your family, you should not feel rejected or no longer loved. Instead, feel so loved that your family believes that your physical needs should not be forced to compete with their own needs, and for their finite supply of time and energy. Instead, they believe that many, or perhaps all, of your help needs should be entrusted to outside providers who are paid specifically to provide that help. Consequently, you will also be able to better trust that your family will remain strong, and continue to provide the love and support that are available from no other source.

In short, your family will have wisely reserved its resources for being there when you need them most.

Different needs, different help

You might wonder, "My mother, father, spouse, and family have always been there when I needed them. Now I have additional disability needs. Why can't my family keep things simple and provide this help as well? What makes these needs so different?"

There are big differences between the traditional help that family members routinely provide to each other and the unique ADL help that you now need for your disability. In short, your disability needs are of a different type, frequency, and extent.

First, your needs are personal and medical, and of a special type that not everyone is comfortable in satisfying. When one family member needs, and another member provides, this very intimate and personal help, the family relationship often changes. Yesterday, the relative roles and functions of family members were well established between husband and wife, independent senior and dependent children, and strong and stronger family members. Today, any of those roles might be completely reversed. These realities can be quite upsetting for them and for you.

Second, the need for this help occurs every day of the week, month, and year. There are usually no holidays or vacations, as there are for other household duties of meal preparation, laundry, or career demands. In addition, one usually cannot expect that these needs will lessen with time; indeed, these needs usually become more complex and time-consuming. This day-after-day, month-after-month grind can become very tiring. From your viewpoint, you might want to believe that you need just a little help; however, from a provider's viewpoint of stark reality, what you routinely require is hard work.

Third, few family needs are as extensive as disability needs. Unlike other types of help that are exchanged among family members, few experienced help providers or recipients would tend to trivialize disability needs as favors. In addition, the tradition of family members sharing help usually means an actual, physical exchange. Joyce provides five units of help to Judy, and it is expected that Judy will later return five units to Joyce. These routine exchanges among family members result in a desired balance of both granted favors and energy. However, when a family caregiver provides you with five units of personal help, time, and energy for a disability need, your physical limitations mean that you probably will not be able to fulfill your part of the exchange or "reimbursement." For each family member, this is one-way expenditure with little expectation of an actual payback outside of your return of love.

In summary, disability help is not ordinary family help—it is extraordinary family help. It is routine, never-ending, extensive, and tiring. It is usually beyond the reasonable capabilities of family members alone. Family members will unavoidably be providing some of the help, but they are best reserved for providing their unique brand of love, caring, and support.

Family caregivers cannot do it all. Please do not ask them to do so, or make them feel guilty if they try to set limits on what they can do. Their love for you is not being questioned; the issue is their human energy, stamina, and well-being.

Caregivers and family members have personal needs that can be provided only from within themselves. The number one priority must always be to meet their own, basic needs before they can meet those of someone else. All people require an certain amount of routine food, sleep, self-esteem, joy, spirituality, and private time. All people must provide these things for themselves. No one else can provide them, or should be expected to provide them.

In addition to member needs, the family's needs and strength must also be addressed. Once more, the family's needs must come from within itself; no outsider can provide them. The primary cause of failure in family caregiver systems is caregivers' and family's lovingly giving more than they actually have to give.

Out of pure love, and some guilt, these selfless people give so much to a recipient that they themselves start operating from a personal deficit. When they expend all their available energy for others, and their bodies and spirits painfully tell them to stop and rest, their love prompts them to deny the symptoms and continue their help. They routinely "run out of gas" and then attempt to continue running on mere fumes.

When a person continues to drive that personal engine on only fumes, the engine soon fails. The symptoms frequently include chronic fatigue, spiritual sacrifice, insufficient self-esteem, and depression. The caregiver collapses, the family structure or marriage often collapses, and you, the help recipient, are suddenly in a crisis without help (or with unreliable help).

The exhausted and depressed caregivers lose; the weakened family or marriage loses; and now, having neither physical help nor a strong family, you twice lose!

To turn most of these potential losses into wins, share this chapter's planning strategies with your family. You might ask each family member to review this chapter before you all gather to discuss its points. Assure them that it is okay with you that they reserve their limited resources primarily for maintaining their own personal strength (strength that you require them to have), and that they hire outsiders for most of your daily, routine needs. You might be relieving them of guilt they would otherwise be experiencing.

These are hard-core decisions to be made carefully in advance with a rational head, and not to be made hastily in crisis with an emotional heart.

For the physical help with your routine ADLs, the family can combine any of its remaining resources with outside help—or, indeed, use only outside help. A small percentage of outside help might come from volunteers, but most will be hired from agencies or personal employment.

Chapter 6

Ten Steps to Getting All or Some of Your Help from Agency-Employed Aides

Perhaps you read the previous chapter, 📖 5, "Ten Steps to Getting All or Some of Your Help from Family Caregivers." Consequently, you have decided to reserve family help for its special uses and times, and arrange for outside help for some—or even all—of your routine, activities of daily living (ADL) needs. Perhaps the family caregiver alternative is not available to you, and you have decided to use agency aides as your sole source of assistance. As a third possibility dictated by financial stipulations, you might be pursuing agency aides because your funding source requires them.

You might also be attracted to having an agency supply your aides because it seems much simpler than personally employing your own. However, you may be curious about using a combination of both, and having the agency help as a back-up to personal recruiting. There are pros and cons to using each source.[1]

In any case, an agency's role is to recruit, interview, train, schedule, pay, and otherwise manage aides on behalf of the actual recipient of services. Agencies perform an essential set of services for people who:

- are unwilling or unable to manage their own care
- prefer agency help because their needs are temporary, and therefore they have no desire to take the time to learn management skills
- receive funding for services and are required by the funding source to use assistance only from certain approved agencies
- are new to a community, have an immediate need for help, and are as yet unaware of where to personally recruit PAs within their new locale
- have a personally employed PA who suddenly quits, and consequently require immediate fill-in help until personal recruiting is again successful
- intend to personally employ PAs, and need agency assistance while they ready themselves to begin the process of personal recruiting.

---

1. For a comprehensive comparison of these options, please see chapter 📖 1, "Beyond Family Caregivers: Options and Settings for Finding Outside Assistance."

Agencies can supply several categories of staff. The titles for these staffers may vary among agencies, but the three primary types are:

- companions (or personal care providers, PCPs) who have minimal, non-medical training
- home health aides (or certified nursing assistants, CNAs) who have usually completed at least one, six-week training course on basic medical details
- registered nurses (RN) or licensed practical nurses (LPN) who have completed several years of formal medical training and licensure.

A ten-step process will guide you through selecting and contracting an appropriate agency, while including strategies for maintaining quality control over the aides assigned to you and the help you receive. *Figure 6-1* is a preview of the later, more detailed version.

Figure 6-1: **A preview of planning steps ❶ through ❿ for getting all or some of your help from agency-employed aides**

Step ❶ As the help recipient, you identify a planner and manager—ideally, yourself—to make decisions and provide ongoing monitoring of a variety of disability-related needs.

Step ❷ You or the planner-manager create your list and schedule of help needs, and then total the weekly and monthly hours on the list. Next, calculate the cost and identify the source of funding for hiring agency services.

Step ❸ You, as the help recipient, review the personal concerns of paid help providers (as well as your own); you or the planner-manager also review the qualities of being a first-class aide manager.

Step ❹ You check local resources for the names of agencies that might fit your specific needs.

Step ❺ You call these agencies for preliminary details by phone.

Step ❻ You meet at your residence with each agency representative to discuss details in depth.

Step ❼ You check other agencies, if the first agency is not satisfactory.

Step ❽ For a seemingly satisfactory agency, you check the agency's references, its Better Business Bureau status and rating, and its service contract. Know the agency's reputation as well as your rights.

Step ❾ You ask to meet the aides who have been assigned to you.

Step ❿ You or the planner-manager use family caregivers or other current aides to train new agency aides with a three-step procedure.

By definition, you would have fewer personal tasks to perform when using an agency, and many more tasks and concerns when using family caregivers or personally employed PAs. Consequently, you will find fewer details in this chapter's ten steps than you do in the ten steps for the other two sources. Our lighter treatment of agency aides here is not symptomatic of omissions, but simply a realistic reflection of the fewer tasks and concerns you have when using agency aides.

Planning steps ❶ through ❿

Step ❶   **As the help recipient, you identify a planner and manager— ideally, yourself—to make decisions and provide ongoing monitoring of a variety of disability-related needs.**

- Decide who will perform the initial planning regarding your help needs and then the ongoing management of the providers, far in advance of identifying the actual providers.

Step ❶ is not yet about who will provide the help, but instead about who will make the initial planning decisions and then provide ongoing management.

First, the planning decisions include creating a list and schedule of what needs require help, as well as exploring the cost of agency help and how to fund those costs. When using an agency, the ongoing management applies to approving of the assigned aides, coordinating their training, and monitoring the quality of help they provide. However, some families have no choice but to entrust all these responsibilities to the agency.

Ideally, the help recipient is the best choice for making those decisions, and is also the logical source for expressing them during the training and monitoring of providers. These decisions will determine the recipient's daily type and quality of lifestyle, so it is most appropriate for that person to form the decisions and then carry them out on a long-term basis. The upcoming plan gives the help recipient the first chance to consider the planner-manager role.

Although the recipient is the ideal choice, that person is not always willing or able to assume those responsibilities. When the recipient has caring and competent family members or close friends, these people are the second choice. They would plan and manage during periodic meetings. As mentioned, when the recipient lacks family and friends who are willing to assume these roles, the health care agency or facility is the third choice for who must take over.

The Three Management Roles for Help Recipients to Consider

Because you, the recipient, would be the best planner and manager, you are first offered the position by reviewing a set of three possible management roles. There are such distinct advantages in your assuming this self-directive and empowering position! If it is at all possible for you to be the planner-manager, Roles One or Two will propose the way. If you are not able or willing to manage, Role Three will ask that family members be the next to consider this position.

You are encouraged to take as powerful a role as you are willing and able to assume. As you will find described for Role Two, you can maintain both an image and a fully active function of authority and control, despite having significant secondary limitations to doing some of the traditional management tasks.

So, to offer you the first choice as the planner and manager, decide which one of these three management roles applies to you.

> ▸ *Role One*—You can independently manage
> the people who help you.

You have the desire to manage help providers, as well as the cognitive ability to remember your needs, make routine decisions, and resolve problems. In addition, you have the functional abilities to manage and use your choice of providers.

Consequently, you can manage and use your choice of family caregivers, agency-employed aides, personally employed PAs, or any combination.

> ▸ *Role Two*—You can independently manage the people who help
> you, after you accommodate an impairment to your
> doing some of the management tasks.

You have the desire to manage help providers, as well as the cognitive ability to remember your needs, make routine decisions, and resolve problems. However, you have a learning disability, a limitation to physical writing or computer interfacing, or an impairment to speech, hearing, sight, or another function that limits your independently doing some of the functional management tasks.

You have already developed ways to accommodate this impairment in your daily lifestyle, and you do so again to fully manage the people who help you, by:
- ▾ doing the tasks in innovative ways
- ▾ using technology and adaptive equipment to do the tasks
- ▾ using extra help from your help providers.

Consequently, with the accommodation in place, you can manage and use your choice of family caregivers, agency-employed aides, personally employed PAs, or any combination.

> ▸ *Role Three*—You require someone else to remember your routine, make decisions, solve problems, and manage the people who help you.

You might have the functional abilities to be your own manager, but you lack one or both of the other two essentials:

- ▼ the desire to manage help providers
- ▼ the cognitive ability to remember your needs, make routine decisions, and resolve problems.

In Role Two, we saw that some functional limitations can be accommodated in ways that still enable you to manage independently. However, it is rare that help recipients who lack the desire to manage, or the cognitive abilities to do so, can create satisfactory accommodations.

Consequently, you will require a family caregiver, another type of personal representative, or an agency to make decisions, employ, and manage help providers for you.

The importance of reviewing management roles is to put you in as much power and control of your lifestyle and help providers as you want and are able to have.

The Three Management Roles for Family and Friends to Consider

When the help recipient is unable or unwilling to plan and manage, the family and close friends are offered this second set of considerations.

Next are three possible management roles for family and friends. The first, preferred role suggests that the recipient act as consultant to a group of family and friends who collectively do the planning and managing. Role Two applies when the group's interest is limited and seems to focus on just one or two members; it also assumes that these same people will later be likely to volunteer to assume some caregiver tasks. If neither Role One nor Two seems feasible, then the third proposes that a health care agency or facility must ultimately fill the position.

> ▸ *Role One*—The family or friends work as a team of advisors in planning and managing.

When there is a sufficient number of family and friends who agree to a long-term, active commitment, these people meet periodically to plan and manage collectively. They represent the help recipient in their decisions and actions.

▶ *Role Two*—One or two members of the family and friends
        agree to perform the planning and managing.

When the available and interested family and friends are limited to one or two members, these people do their best to represent the wishes of the help recipient.

When this considerable responsibility is assumed entirely by one or two persons, these persons should be especially guarded against acting on a common impulse to also provide the daily, physical ADL assistance. My heartfelt advice to families reviewing this **Step ❶** is to be careful to limit their current commitment to being *a planner and manager,* and to delay any additional impulse toward being *a help provider* until at least Step ❸ , (an essential discussion of cautions found later in this chapter).

▶ *Role Three*—In the absence of available family and friends,
        a health care facility or agency is contracted to perform
        the planning and managing.

When neither the help recipient nor his/her family and friends are available for these functions, a facility or agency is the final choice for these needs.[2]

Indeed, staffing this position of planning and managing the help needs is prerequisite to actually providing the help. It is common for family and friends to volunteer their managing and planning, and then be additionally unable to provide actual caregiver help. However, it is not logical that they would provide caregiver help after declaring themselves unable to plan and manage that help. If neither the help recipient nor the family and friends are willing or able to manage the needs, it is assumed that family and friends will also be unavailable for providing caregiver help. When this situation is identified, your resource for planning, managing, and providing help would seem to be entirely in health care facilities and agencies.

---

2. For considerations in selecting an outside facility or agency, please review chapter 📖 **1,** "Beyond Family Caregivers: Options and Settings for Finding Outside Assistance."

Step ❷   You or the planner-manager create your list and schedule of help needs, and then total the weekly and monthly hours on the list. Next, calculate the cost and identify the source of funding for hiring agency services.

The planner and manager from **Step ❶** begins to make some planning decisions. Please note that these steps continue to appropriately address the help recipient, regardless of who is actually acting as the planner-manager. If the recipient is unable or unwilling to be the planner-manager, his or her opinion should still be, as much as possible, the basis of the planning.

• Create your list and schedule of needs.

    ▸ Identify what help you need and create a list that includes the "what, when, where, and how long" for your needs. This listing, according to your personal style, could be in the format of a carefully memorized outline, a handwritten listing, or a more detailed computer printout.[3]

    ▸ Be sure that all of your requests for help are valid.

There is a fine line between respecting providers, by requesting help for valid needs, and abusing providers, by asking them either to provide unnecessary help or to become inappropriately responsible for you.[4]

• Get ready to describe your routine.

    ▸ Create and rehearse both a brief, 30-second and a detailed, 5-minute description of your needs and schedule, plus some basic notes about how you employ PAs.

    ▸ Give the appropriate description to applicants when answering initial phone inquiries, during face-to-face interviews, and when training new PAs.

Each time you or your representative describe your routine, you will want to impress the supervisor and aide from the agency, that you are someone who is organized, sharp, and worthy of their help. This first impression is important to your authority, power, and control of the work relationship. Each description should be well organized, concise, and to the point.[5]

• Total the weekly hours of help you will probably need.

---

3. For more detail about listing what help you need and when you need it, as well as confirming the importance of your preferences in how you want help provided, please see chapters 📖 **12, "Getting It Done—Your Way!"** and 📖 **13, "Defining and Describing Your Help Needs."**

4. Please see chapter 📖 **11, "When It Is, and Is Not, Okay to Ask for Help."**

5. For more detail about what goes into each of the two descriptions, and when to use each one, please see chapter 📖 **13, "Defining and Describing Your Help Needs."**

‣ Total up the weekly hours of help that you need, for both routine and unforeseeable needs:

▾ Use this total when calculating a budget for personal or outside funding.

▾ From your list of needs and schedule (above), add up the weekly and monthly hours for your routine needs.

▾ Then add another 25 percent to the total hours for unforeseeable—but predictable and frequent—bowel and bladder accidents, illnesses, medical equipment repairs, and special needs.

Your total hours of need =
    Routine, predictable needs
+   25% allowance for sporadic, unpredictable needs

Example:
Your weekly total =
    32 hours of routine needs
+   8 hours of unpredictable needs
=   40 total weekly hours, or 160 monthly hours

• Calculate the cost of your help.

‣ Estimate the salary cost for your help.[6]

▾ Multiply the total hours of your needs by the agency's hourly rate.

Your total cost of aides or PAs =
    Total hours of help needed
x   Hourly salary or agency rate

Example:
Your weekly cost =
    40 total hours
x $20.00 (agency rate) per hour
= $800.00 weekly, or ($3,200.00 monthly)

• Decide how to pay for this outside help.

‣ Decide whether to use personal funds
or outside funding for your help:

---

6. For points to remember in estimating costs, please see chapter 📖 **19, "Your Costs of Recruiting, Training, and Keeping PAs Happy."**

▼ personal, out-of-pocket funds

▼ federal or state agency or assistance program

▼ accident or insurance settlement

▼ health or long-term care insurance

▼ other.

▸ If using personal funds and the cost exceeds your budget, then you will need to research some sources of outside money.

▸ If using outside funding, identify the source(s), research the eligibility criteria, and apply for the funding. Be sure to note if the funding source places any restrictions on the type or source of help you can hire. Some funding sources will limit you to using only a specific agency with which the funding source has a contract.

Step ❸ **You, as the help recipient, review the personal concerns of paid help providers (as well as your own); you or the planner-manager also review the qualities of being a first-class aide manager.**

The goal of this step is for you to better understand the personal concerns of a typical, paid help provider. By better understanding these concerns, you will be a better manager. Ideally, each agency aide would also review your list of concerns; however, few will probably be interested in taking the time. In addition to reviewing the provider's list, you might find advantages in reviewing your own.

• To facilitate communication and understanding, check the lists in these chapters:

▸ Everyone is encouraged to review a proposal of personal rights in chapter 📖 **22, "A Bill of Rights for You as a Help Recipient, Family Caregiver, or Paid Provider."**

▸ As a help recipient, you are encouraged to read chapter 📖 **25, "Your Personal Concerns as a Paid Help Provider, plus Ten Reasons Why PAs Quit and Are Fired."**

▸ In return, caregivers and other members are encouraged to read chapter 📖 **23, "Your Personal Concerns as a Help Recipient."**

• Review the qualities for being a good PA manager. Throughout this book, is a variety of special topics about being a respected and in control PA manager are addressed. Use the index and table of contents to locate any topic of concern.

Step ❹ **You check local resources for the names of agencies that might fit your specific needs.**

• Start with a phone book Yellow Pages. Some communities have at least three sources of agencies, commercial, government, and nonprofit. Try these common headings: nurses, home care, health care, employment services, or temporary employment services.

- Referral from a physician, hospital, or friend. Some hospital departments that might be helpful include social welfare, discharge planning, outpatient nursing services, or case management.

- Referral from your outside funding source. If you will be receiving funding for your aides, check first with that funding source. Some funding sources will stipulate which agency you must use.

These are the three most common sources for finding an agency that employs and coordinates nurses, aides, and housekeepers. If you will be using the phone book Yellow Pages, you should note the difference between two of the sources. Employment services (termed temporary employment services or temp agencies in some locales) usually employ a variety of workers, including secretaries, gardeners, computer programmers, and other people who want part-time or entry-level jobs. These temp agencies often directly employ health-care providers and have a separate internal branch that specializes in these providers, or they may refer you to another outside agency that does so.

Step ❺   You call these agencies for preliminary details by phone.

- Use the short or long description of your needs (from **Step ❷**), as appropriate. Find an agency that can provide the types and schedule of help that you need.

- Ask about the agency's fees.

- Schedule a face-to-face meeting at your residence with an agency rep.

When you have identified some favorable-looking agencies, your next step is to call these prospects with some preliminary questions. Your first impressions, from both factual and intuitive information, are important. Can an agency provide the services and schedule that you need, and is your conversation with the staffers comfortable?

You are interviewing these agencies, and you should have the right to select an agency that seems to be efficient as well as easy to work with. Remember, when calling these prospects, that you are in the driver's seat and in control. Directly or indirectly, the agency will be working for you.

If possible, try to find at least two agencies that are worthy of a meeting at your residence. The more choices you line up, the more selective you can be in finding the best available services, and the more empowered and in control you will feel. You will always be somewhat dependent on the daily services you receive from the aides of any source. Consequently, it is especially important that you balance this feeling of dependence with a feeling of control in selecting the best source of aides, and aides who will listen to you.

Step ❻   You meet at your residence with each agency representative to discuss details in depth.

- Provide an outline of basic personal data:
  ▸ Your medical history

▶ The tasks and schedule of help that your lifestyle requires.

▶ Your funding source—outside funding or personal budget.

- Get details about the agency's operating policies and compare them with your needs.

  ▶ Ask for a list of duties that the aides are permitted to do or restricted from providing. If the restricted list includes tasks that you require, ask for advice on how to get that help.

  ▶ Ask whether you will be routinely working with a common core of aides, or frequently working with new and different aides. A reasonably common core of the same aides will mean less training for you. Less frequent changes also mean longer-term working relationships with established trusts and less stress.

  ▶ Check the availability of extra help, between scheduled shifts, for bowel accidents and other urgent needs. Even if it seems that your family can provide this non-routine help, you should first try to get it from outsiders.

  ▶ Ask what to do if you have a sudden change of personal schedule, whether same-day scheduling changes can usually be made, and how to request them.

  ▶ Ask about the supply of substitutes and backups when a regular aide is sick, regardless of whether subs might be available from your family:

    ▾ Will the agency call you before sending a sub?

    ▾ Will the sub aides usually be able to maintain your regular schedule?

    ▾ Is the agency willing to assign you two or three aides, on a rotating basis, so that more than one aide will know your routine and make subs easier to work with?

  ▶ Ask whether you can meet with the proposed aides before they are assigned and scheduled to work with you, and whether you have the right to decline an aide and request another.

- Get general details about the agency's aides.

  ▶ You ask about the level of training and experience for a typical aide, and how much training you must typically provide for your specific needs.

- Get details about the agency's fees and billing.

  ▶ You might want to ask for a listing (itemization) of each type of cost that makes up their overall charges.

  ▶ If you use outside funding, ask whether the agency will bill the funding source, or whether you must pay the agency and then be reimbursed by your funding source.

  ▶ If you use outside funding, will the funding ultimately cover all agency charges, or will you be responsible for some?

  ▶ If you will use personal funding, is a personal (non-funding source) fee discount available to you? How often will you be billed?

- Ask the agency rep for a business card and post it on your refrigerator for fast reference when problems or questions arise.
  - ‣ The card should include an after-hours and weekend contact. Ask whether your after-hours call will reach a staffer or a commercial answering service.
  - ‣ If the agency uses an answering service, will your call merely be recorded and stacked until Monday morning, or will the service immediately contact an on-call staffer who will promptly return your call?

Step ❼ **You check other agencies, if the first agency is not satisfactory.**

- Be sure that your funding source does not limit you to a specific agency—you might not have another choice.

- Tell the first (unsatisfactory) agency's rep that you need some time before signing their contract. Get back to your agency list and call another.

- Shop other agencies for the best policies, customer rep, and aides.

Step ❽ **For a seemingly satisfactory agency, you check the agency's references, its Better Business Bureau status and rating, and its service contract. Know the agency's reputation as well as your rights.**

- Before signing, ask the agency for a list of client references and call them to ask whether the clients are satisfied with agency services. Ask for at least one or two improvements the agency should make (there are always at least one or two). If the cited problems concern you, call the agency and ask what it is doing to improve those service areas.

- Call the local chapter of the Better Business Bureau and identify the agency you are considering. Ask if the agency is a BBB member and if the Bureau knows of any pending consumer complaints. This is a free service and the primary reason the BBB exists.

- Call the discharge planning office or case management office at your local hospital, and ask the BBB questions.

- Before signing a contract, ask about any restrictions about changing your preference to another agency. Know your rights. Ask whether the contract commits you to use the agency for at least a minimum period of time.

- Many agencies will provide you with a "Patient's Bill of Rights." If you are interested, ask for this listing from each agency that you interview.

Step ❾ **You ask to meet the aides who have been assigned to you.**

Ask to meet with your proposed aides before they are assigned and scheduled.

- Greet the aide and ask about her or his training and experience.

- Ask about her experience with people who have your type of disability and needs.

- Ask how long she has worked with this agency and whether she likes working there.

- Provide her with an outline of your needs and schedule, and ask about any concerns.

- Ask each aide how she would prefer that you train her. Outline the three-step procedure (please see **Step ⑩**).

- Ask how to make last-minute, small schedule changes. Can you simply call her directly, or must you contact the agency and seek permission through its formal channels?

- Ask that she call you directly whenever she will be delayed for a work shift.

- If your initial meeting with any aide leaves you feeling uncomfortable, feel free to call the agency representative to discuss your concerns.

Step ⑩ **You or the planner-manager use family caregivers or other current aides to train new agency aides with a three-step procedure.**

The agency supervisor who met with you undoubtedly took some detailed notes about your needs for help, or she was delighted when you handed her your printed list. She will use this list in selecting which of the agency's aides to assign to you, and for briefing those providers about the general types of needs that you have. It would be impossible for her to actually train anyone from this list; that will be your job, or that of your representative.

You will have to train each new agency aide in what needs you have, as well as how and when you prefer to receive that help. Remember that regardless of an aide's extensive training and experience (or lack of them), each new aide from any source will greet you on the first day and say, "Please tell me what help you need, and how and when you prefer that I provide that help. Also be sure to let me know each day how well I am doing."

Use family caregivers or current outside help to train new help in three steps:[7]

- Have the new aide watch a family caregiver or current aide perform each part of your routine.

- Have the new aide do the routine at least twice while a current provider stands by.

- Finish the aide's training by having her work directly with you, while receiving your occasional reminders and lots of patience.

---

7. For more details on using family caregivers or outside providers in this three-step method for training new help, please see chapter 📖 **9, "Initial Training and Ongoing Management of Aides and PAs."**

Chapter 7

Ten Steps to Getting All or Some of Your Help from Personally Employed Aides

Employing your own aides (also known as personal assistants or PAs) can dramatically improve the quality of your lifestyle. It's as simple as that.

I know, because I have exclusively used personally employed PAs to assist my needs for decades, while listening to the unfortunate experiences of some of my peers who use agency help. I estimate that I am able to avoid 90 percent of the problems that they routinely encounter by being in direct control over both who supplies me with help and the quality of help they provide.

Hiring your own PAs—or, as a family caregiver, hiring them for a loved one—can be a reliable, effective, and even empowering way of getting the help you need. Once you enjoy the control and freedom of personally employing your own PAs, you will probably not want to consider trying, or going back to, agency help.

If you use family caregivers to supply all or part of your care, PAs can be a welcome (and life-saving) supplement. If you are on your own, PAs can provide you with the independence you need to maintain an active, involved lifestyle. Your own PAs can be asked to accommodate a wide variety of medical and non-medical activities, ranging from transfer help during a physician's appointment, to help with changing into swim trunks for a SCUBA lesson, to traveling during a two-week vacation. If you need to move across the country or across town, your own PAs can again be tapped for help that is not available from agency aides.

The ten-step hiring plan presented here has been designed from years of collecting comments and suggestions from hundreds of help recipients like you, as well as from help providers. I have directly hired aides through this procedure for more than 30 years. Though no procedure is infallible, this one works better than any other I have encountered. Most importantly, it should work for you!

Just who is out there?

PA applicants come in all shapes and sizes, and with good and bad reasons for wanting to work for you. Whether this is your first hiring ever, you have been screening and hiring for 30 years, or you are a professional home health agency, you will go through the same process. You will hear from diamond-quality applicants as well as barely sober ones, just as the pros do.

It is a fact that the majority of people who inquire about your job are undesirable as PAs. Consequently, your goals are:

- to attract several potentially good people to apply for your job

- to screen out the candidates who cannot or should not be your next PA, before they are hired

- to hire and train the desirable candidates

- to keep your PAs as long as possible by being a good manager.

> *The majority of people who inquire about your PA job should not be hired.*

By using a good interviewing and screening process, you will be able to identify undesirable applicants and disqualify them. In addition to your efforts, at least one-quarter—and occasionally all—of the applicants will disqualify themselves. They will fail to show up for interviews or to call you back with their job decision. These are failures of the applicant, not of you or this procedure. This procedure is designed to expose weaknesses in applicants who are undependable or irresponsible. If an applicant is undependable, it is far better that he or she fails now to show up for the interview or demonstration that you require, rather than failing to show up on one of the first mornings to get you out of bed.

This procedure has been specially structured to accomplish the two primary objectives of any well-designed job interview:

- to provide you with the information you need about each applicant so you can screen out people who make you uncomfortable, are not responsible, and cannot meet scheduled commitments

- to provide applicants with the information they need to decide about committing to your job, by meeting you and another aide and by actually observing your routine.

Figure 7-1 is a quick preview of the ten-step process; you will find a more detailed version in the following pages.

Figure 7-1: **A preview of planning steps ❶ through ❿ for getting all or some of your help from personally employed aides**

Step ❶   As the help recipient, you identify a planner and manager—ideally, yourself—to make decisions and provide ongoing monitoring of a variety of disability-related needs.

Step ❷   You or the planner-manager create your list and schedule of ADL (activities of daily living) help needs, be sure the needs are valid bases for requesting help, and then total the weekly and monthly hours. Next, calculate the cost and identify the source of funding.

Step ❸   You first identify the type and source of providers you might need. Next, you, as the help recipient, review the personal concerns of paid help providers (as well as your own); you or the planner-manager also review the qualities of being a first-class PA manager.

Step ❹   You advertise for your own PAs.

Step ❺   You receive responses to your PA ad, and identify who to call back (Screening 1).

Step ❻   You call back the selected ad applicants, and identify who to interview (Screening 2).

Step ❼   You and a current PA host an interview and demonstration of your routine, and ask interested candidates to call you back the next day (Screenings 3 and 4).

Step ❽   You receive next-day callbacks from still-interested candidates, check their references, and identify who to hire (Screenings 5 and 6).

Step ❾   You hire the finalists, schedule training sessions, and then decline the others (Screening 7).

Step ❿   You or the planner-manager use family caregivers or other, current outside providers to train new PAs with a three-step procedure. Occasionally, a new PA will fail to appear for the first or second scheduled shift (Screening 8).

As you scan the ten steps of *Figure 7-1,* you will notice brief references to eight screening opportunities. These eight screenings have been designed around standards that identify the responsible and dependable type of PA that you require. In addition to the four times you screen applicants, they screen themselves four times. Each screening provides you with more information about each applicant, and provides the applicants with more information about you and the PA position. Throughout the process, your privacy and security are protected. These eight screenings are summarized at the end of this chapter in *Figure 7-2.*

There will be occasions when all of your callers and candidates will be eliminated, leaving you with no one to consider from this group of inquiries. This occurrence is:

- rare

- not the sign of a weakness in this ten-step procedure, but a strength that is purposely built in

- not a sign that you are being rejected, that no one wants to work with you, or that you are doing anything wrong

- simply a sign that this was a crummy group of applicants who were either not interested in your type of job, or not qualified to do it.

When this occasionally happens, you simply call the newspaper and tell them to "play it again, Sam."

So how long does all this take? The steps of this procedure—from receiving phone inquiries to beginning the training of one or more new PAs—can be completed in less than 24 hours. However, the average time is three to five days. You will find an important benefit in each step. Try to avoid the temptation to abbreviate or simplify the strategies.

Following this plan will not guarantee that you will hire only quality aides, but it will significantly increase your chances of doing so. You will succeed in routinely (though not continually) hiring high-quality PAs, and you will be in control of who helps you as well as how that help is provided.

After you have hired a new PA, the training begins. If you are not entirely at ease with the thought of being an instructor, you may take comfort in knowing that PA training has been summarized into just three basic steps.[1]

This upcoming ten-step procedure has been carefully designed and tested over the years with one goal in mind: getting you the reliable help you need, when and where you need it, and advising you about how to keep it longer. Although you may find it tempting to eliminate some of the screenings and keep more people in the hiring pool, that would be a mistake. By doing so, you could be bringing into your home (and working with) the wrong people. Even if these people were hired, they would usually not last very long. Soon after you finish their training and begin to trust them, they typically fail to be dependable, unexpectedly quit, or even steal from you before quitting.

The objective of a well-designed interview and screening process is to weed out people who should not be your PAs *before* you unknowingly hire them. By following all ten steps, you too can hire—and be in full control of—reliable help that allows you to live an active, independent lifestyle.

---

1. These steps are neatly contained in **Step ❿** and discussed in chapter 📖 **9, "Initial Training and Ongoing Management of Aides and PAs."**

The decision made in **Step ❶** is basic to the planning to be done in the other **Steps ❷** through ❿ . **Step ❶** calls for establishing a planner and manager, purposely much in advance of deciding who will provide the actual help. The function of planner and manager is first offered to you, the help recipient, and then to family and friends. If neither group can fill the function, it is wise to realize at this early stage that the planning, managing, and eventual provision of help must be usually contracted to an outside health care facility or agency.

Although this ten-step planning strategy has been used successfully, some of its more innovative elements merit clarification. Therefore, a discussion of several topics follows the ten-step presentation.

Planning steps ❶ through ❿

Step ❶   **As the help recipient, you identify a planner and manager— ideally, yourself—to make decisions and provide ongoing monitoring of a variety of disability-related needs.**

- Decide who will perform the initial planning regarding your help needs and then the ongoing management of the providers, far in advance of identifying the actual providers.

Step ❶ is not yet about who will provide the help, but instead about who will make the initial planning decisions and then provide ongoing management.

First, the planning decisions include creating a list and schedule of what needs require help, as well as exploring some introductory financial concerns about the cost of outside help and how to fund those costs. When needed, the ongoing management begins with selecting one or more sources for outside help providers and hiring them. If, however, the family is firm about currently using only family caregivers, the management functions can be set aside for possible later use.

Ideally, the help recipient is the best choice for making those decisions, and is also the logical source for expressing them during the training and monitoring of providers—even when family caregivers are the providers. These decisions will determine the recipient's daily type and quality of lifestyle, so it is most appropriate for that person to form the decisions and then carry them out on a long-term basis. The upcoming plan gives the help recipient the first chance to consider the planner-manager role.

Although the recipient is the ideal choice, that person is not always willing or able to assume those responsibilities. When the recipient has caring and competent family members or close friends, these people are the second choice. They would plan and manage during periodic meetings. When the recipient lacks family and friends who are willing to assume these roles, a health care agency or facility is the third choice for who must take over.

The Three Management Roles for Help Recipients to Consider

Because you, the recipient, would be the best planner and manager, you are first offered the position by reviewing a set of three possible management roles. There are such distinct advantages in your assuming this self-directive and empowering position! If it is at all possible for you to be the planner-manager, Roles One or Two will propose the way. If you are not able or willing to manage, Role Three will ask that family members be the next to consider this position.

You are encouraged to take as powerful a role as you are willing and able to assume. As you will find described for Role Two, you can maintain both an image and a fully active function of authority and being in control, despite having significant secondary limitations to doing some of the traditional management tasks.

So, to offer you the first choice as the planner and manager, decide which one of these three management roles applies to you.

▸ *Role One*—You can independently manage
  the people who help you.

You have the desire to manage help providers, as well as the cognitive ability to remember your needs, make routine decisions, and resolve problems. In addition, you have the functional abilities to manage and use your choice of providers.

Consequently, you can manage and use your choice of family caregivers, agency-employed aides, personally employed PAs, or any combination.

▸ *Role Two*—You can independently manage the people who help
  you, after you accommodate an impairment to your
  doing some of the management tasks.

You have the desire to manage help providers, as well as the cognitive ability to remember your needs, make routine decisions, and resolve problems. However, you have a learning disability, a limitation to physical writing or computer interfacing, or an impairment to speech, hearing, sight, or another function that limits your independently doing some of the functional management tasks.

You have already developed ways to accommodate this impairment in your daily lifestyle, and you do so again to fully manage the people who help you, by:
  ▼ doing the tasks in innovative ways
  ▼ using technology and adaptive equipment to do the tasks
  ▼ using extra help from your help providers.

Consequently, with the accommodation in place, you can manage and use your choice of family caregivers, agency-employed aides, personally employed PAs, or any combination.

> ▸ *Role Three*—You require someone else to remember your routine, make decisions, solve problems, and manage the people who help you.

You might have the functional abilities to be your own manager, but you lack one or both of the other two essentials:

- ▾ the desire to manage help providers
- ▾ the cognitive ability to remember your needs, make routine decisions, and resolve problems.

In Role Two, we saw that some functional limitations can be accommodated in ways that still enable you to manage independently. However, it is rare that help recipients who lack the desire to manage, or the cognitive abilities to do so, can create satisfactory accommodations.

Consequently, you will require a family caregiver, another type of personal representative, or an agency to make decisions, employ, and manage help providers for you.

The importance of reviewing management roles is to put you in as much power and control of your lifestyle and help providers as you want and are able to have.

The Three Management Roles for Family and Friends to Consider

When the help recipient is unable or unwilling to plan and manage, the family and close friends are offered this second set of considerations.

Next are three possible management roles for family and friends. The first, preferred role suggests that the recipient acts as consultant to a group of family and friends who collectively do the planning and managing. Role Two applies when the group's interest is limited and seems to focus on just one or two members; it also assumes these same people will later be likely to volunteer to assume the physical caregiver tasks. If neither Role One nor Two seems feasible, then the third proposes that a health care agency or facility must ultimately fill the position.

▸ *Role One*—The family or friends work as a team of advisors
in planning and managing.

When there is a sufficient number of family and friends who agree to a
long-term, active commitment, these people meet periodically to plan
and manage collectively. They represent the help recipient in their decisions and actions.

▸ *Role Two*—One or two members of the family and friends
agree to perform the planning and managing.

When the available and interested family and friends are limited to one
or two members, these people do their best to represent the wishes of
the help recipient.

When this considerable responsibility is assumed entirely by one or two
persons, these persons should be especially guarded against acting on a
common impulse to also provide the daily, physical ADL assistance. My
heartfelt advice to families reviewing this **Step ❶** is to be careful to limit
their current commitment to being *a planner and manager,* and to
delay any additional impulse toward being *a help provider* until at least
Step ❸ (an essential discussion of cautions found later in this chapter).

▸ *Role Three*—In the absence of available family and friends,
a health care facility or agency is contracted to perform
the planning and managing.

When neither the help recipient nor his/her family and friends are
available for these functions, a facility or agency is the final choice for
these needs.[2]

Indeed, staffing this position of planning and managing the help needs
is prerequisite to actually providing the help. It is common and acceptable for family and friends to volunteer their managing and planning,
and then be unable to provide actual caregiver help. However, it is not
logical that they would provide caregiver help after declaring themselves unable to plan and manage that help. If neither the help recipient nor the family and friends are willing or able to manage the needs,
it is assumed that family and friends will also be unavailable for providing caregiver help. When this situation is identified, there is no reason
to further pursue help from family caregivers. Instead, your resource for
planning, managing, and providing help would seem to be entirely in
health care facilities and agencies. The best introduction to these is in
the two most recently footnoted chapters.

---

2. For considerations in selecting an outside facility or agency, please review chapter 📖 **1,**
"Beyond Family Caregivers: Options and Settings for Finding Outside Assistance." For advice on selecting a full-
service agency, please examine chapter 📖 **6, "Ten Steps to Getting All or Some of Your Help from Agency-**
Employed Aides."

Step ❷ You or the planner-manager create your list and schedule of ADL (activities of daily living) help needs, be sure the needs are valid bases for requesting help, and then total the weekly and monthly hours. Next, calculate the cost and identify the source of funding.

The planner and manager from **Step ❶**, begins to make some planning decisions. Some of this planning applies to using both family caregivers and outside providers, while other points apply mostly to outsiders. I am purposely presenting a comprehensive planning approach for the best preparation. If the current intention is to use only family caregivers, you should still be aware of the additional steps for obtaining outsiders—if or when they are needed—for relief or replacement help. These steps continue to appropriately address the help recipient, regardless of who is actually acting as the planner-manager.

- Create your list and schedule of needs.
  - ▸ Identify what help you need and create a list that includes the "what, when, where, and how long" for your needs. This listing, according to your personal style, could be in the format of a carefully memorized outline, a handwritten listing, or a more detailed computer printout.[3]
  - ▸ Be sure that all of your requests for help are valid.

  There is a fine line between respecting providers, by requesting help for valid needs, and abusing providers, by asking them either to provide unnecessary help or to become inappropriately responsible for you.[4]

- Get ready to describe your routine.
  - ▸ Create and rehearse both a brief, 30-second and a detailed, 5-minute description of your needs and schedule, plus some basic notes about how you employ PAs.
  - ▸ Give the appropriate description to applicants when answering initial phone inquiries, during face-to-face interviews, and when training new PAs.

  Each time you or your representative describe your routine, you will want to impress the PA applicants, or the supervisor and aide from the agency, that you are someone who is organized, sharp, and worthy of their help. This first impression is important to your authority, power, and control of the work relationship. Each description should be well organized, concise, and to the point.

---

3. For more detail about listing what help you need and when you need it, as well as confirming the importance of your preferences in how you want help provided, please see chapters 📖 **12, "Getting It Done—Your Way!"** and 📖 **13, "Defining and Describing Your Help Needs."**

4. Please see chapter 📖 **11, "When It Is, and Is Not, Okay to Ask for Help."**

- Total the weekly hours of help you will probably need.
  - ▶ Total up the weekly hours of help that you need, for both routine and unforeseeable needs:
    - ▼ Use this total when calculating a budget for personal or outside funding.
    - ▼ From your list of needs and schedule (above), add up the weekly and monthly hours for your routine needs.
    - ▼ Then add another 25 percent to the total hours for unforeseeable—but predictable and frequent—bowel and bladder accidents, illnesses, medical equipment repairs, and special needs.

Your total hours of need =
    Routine, predictable needs
+   25% allowance for sporadic, unpredictable needs

Example:
Your weekly total =
    32 hours of routine needs
+   8 hours of unpredictable needs
= 40 total weekly hours, or 160 monthly hours

- Calculate the cost of your help.
  - ▶ Estimate the salary cost for your help.[5]
    - ▼ If using personal funds and personally employing PAs, research the hourly salary rate that others are paying their PAs in your community.
    - ▼ Multiply the total hours of your needs by this going salary rate.[6]

---

5. For points to remember in estimating costs, please see chapter 📖 **19, "Your Costs of Recruiting, Training, and Keeping PAs Happy."**

6. For more detail about calculating both the total hours of your help needs, as well as the total salaried cost (including taxes and other extras), please see chapter 📖 **20, "Paying Salaries: Cash, Non-cash, or Both."**

- Decide how to pay for this outside help.
  - ▶ Decide whether to use personal funds or outside funding for your help:
    - ▼ personal, out-of-pocket funds
    - ▼ federal or state agency or assistance program
    - ▼ accident or insurance settlement
    - ▼ health or long-term care insurance
    - ▼ other.
  - ▶ If using personal funds and personally employing PAs, use your cost estimate to plan your personal budget. If the cost exceeds your personal funds, then you will need to research some sources of outside money.
  - ▶ If using outside funding, identify the source(s), research the eligibility criteria, and apply for the funding. Be sure to note if the funding source places any restrictions on the type or source of help you can hire. Some funding sources will limit you to using only a specific agency with which the funding source has a contract. With this stipulation, you will not be permitted to personally employ your own PAs if you want the source to pay for your providers.[7]

Step ❸ **You first identify the type and source of providers you might need. Next, you, as the help recipient, review the personal concerns of paid help providers (as well as your own); you or the planner-manager also review the qualities of being a first-class PA manager.**

- Identify the types and sources of help providers you will probably use.
  - ▶ Identify the type(s) of help provider that you need by examining:
    - ▼ the kinds of help you need
    - ▼ the type(s) of providers available to you
    - ▼ the type(s) of provider that you require to accommodate your variety of help needs
    - ▼ the type(s) that your funding source stipulates or that you can afford.
  - ▶ Provider types include the following. Some types are restricted, when employed by agencies, in the kinds of help they are allowed to provide:
    - ▼ nurse
    - ▼ certified nursing assistant (CNA)
    - ▼ personal care provider (PCP)
    - ▼ personally employed aide or personal assistant (PA)

---

7. For definitions and details about each type of provider, as well as typical restrictions on the kinds of help they can provide, please see the introductory chapters 📖 **"Definitions of Titles and Terms Used in This Reference"** and 📖 **"Two Types of Assistance Providers: Unpaid and Paid."**

   ▾ homemaker

   ▾ transportation driver

   ▾ companion

   ▸ Identify the source(s) of help providers that you will pursue:

   ▾ at-home assistance: volunteers, agency-employed aides, or personally employed PAs;

   ▾ community assistance: respite or day care, independent living
   center, assisted living center, or a skilled nursing home.

• Another goal of this step is for you to better understand the personal
concerns of a typical, paid help provider. By better understanding
these concerns, you will be a better manager. Ideally, each PA would
also review your list of concerns; however, few will probably be interested in taking the time. In addition to reviewing the provider's list,
you might find advantages in reviewing your own.

To facilitate communication and understanding, check the lists in these
chapters:

▸ Everyone is encouraged to review a proposal of personal rights in
chapter 📖 22, **"A Bill of Rights for You as a Help Recipient, Family
Caregiver, or Paid Provider."**

▸ As a help recipient, you are encouraged to read chapter
📖 25, **"Your Personal Concerns as a Paid Help Provider, plus Ten Reasons
Why PAs Quit and Are Fired."**

▸ In return, caregivers and other members are encouraged to read chapter 📖 23, **"Your Personal Concerns as a Help Recipient."**

• Review the qualities for being a good PA manager. Throughout this
book, a variety of special topics about being a respected and in-control
PA manager are addressed. Use the index and table of contents to
locate any topic of concern.

Next, **Steps ❹** through **❿** outline a specialized plan for recruiting, interviewing,
screening, hiring, and training your personally employed aides.

Each of these steps is quite detailed. In answer to your probable need for periodic explanations, most of these numbered steps are followed by a section called
"Strategies to make step x work for you." So, if an outlined step needs clarification, flip
forward a page or two for the discussion. If you still have questions about a topic,
check the footnotes, table of contents, or index for the locations of more details.

It is first obvious that by increasing the number of people who apply for
your position, you can be more selective in whom you hire. Conversely, if you
need one new aide and get only one applicant, you cannot be as selective as you
might want to be.

Step ❹ is about advertising for your own PAs. With these ad strategies, you will be able to write ads in special ways that will attract more PA prospects to call you about your job offer.

So your well-designed ads succeed in getting several inquiries. Next, you respond to the phone inquiries and decide which callers to screen out as undesirable, and which others to invite into your home for an interview.

Does your desire to hire someone new, and get it done as soon as possible, tempt you to talk someone into working for you? When you describe your routine, do you sometimes "sugarcoat" it by mumbling through or leaving out the less attractive duties? These are common mistakes we have all made, and they are discussed in this chapter.

The more you know about the applicants, the more educated a decision you can make about whether you should hire any of them. The next **Steps ❺** through ❾ enable you to research the applicants, screen out undesirables, interview some who deserve your consideration, and then hire a select few. These steps will also enable applicants to become fully acquainted with you and your job, so they can make educated decisions about whether they want to commit to performing this type of work. Why is that important? A PA who knowledgeably makes a commitment to want to work with you will tend to keep the job longer. Near the end of the chapter, **Step ❿** introduces you to training.

Step ❹ You advertise for your own PAs.[8]

- Create and post the newspaper or Internet ad, bulletin board notice, or poster that you will use to advertise your PA job:
  ▸ Identify the type of people in your community who would be good aides.
  ▸ Determine which benefits they want that you can offer, and include those benefits in your ad.
  ▸ Decide how and where you will advertise to reach the target people.
  ▸ Create your ad, review its content and layout, and have some friends review it.
  ▸ Place your newspaper or Internet ad, bulletin board notice, or poster.

Step ❺ You receive responses to your PA ad, and identify who to call back (Screening 1).

- Record a special outgoing message on your phone's voice mail (or answering machine).

---

8. For more detail about advertising to employ your own aides, please see chapter ▢ 8, **"Where and How to Advertise for Your Own PAs."**

▸ Use your phone's voice mail (or answering machine) to record an outgoing message that both encourages applicants to leave a message and to tell you a little about themselves and their reason for wanting your job.

▸ Using your phone's voice mail, where you listen to the callers, is preferred by many to reading a written, e-mail reply. A compromise, when advertising with an Internet ad, is to ask people to reply by phone and not by e-mail.

▸ Callers inquire about your ad, and record their name and inquiry on your phone's voice mail.

• Listen to the responses and screen out any undesirable callers.

▸ Within a few hours of callers recording their responses, you listen to each caller's factual information and personal attitude. This step's screening opportunity does not require you to make any calls or speak with anyone unless you want to. You can do the screening completely alone or with a friend or current aide. Your listening can be done at any hour and at your convenience. Play back the inquiries as often as needed without the pressure of listening to a live call.

▸ Screen out and erase a first group of obviously undesirable callers.

• Identify those desirable callers whom you want to call back.

▸ Write down their names, phone numbers, and details.

• During this first screening, you can expect to screen out as many as half of the callers as being undesirable.

Strategies that make Step ❺ work for you

Shortly after your PA advertising appears, you will start receiving phone inquiries. Rather than answer the phone directly, many people prefer to record the inquiries on an answering machine.

First, your machine's outgoing message can be tailored to ask callers for the kinds of information that are helpful to your decisions:

> *Hi there. Thank you for calling 555-7033. If you are calling about the home health aide ads, both the salaried and live-in jobs are still available. Please leave your name, phone number, and tell me a little bit about yourself. Please do leave me a message.*

Second, recording the inquiries gives you several advantages. If you are away, you will not lose inquiries; if you are at home, you aren't forced to personally answer each call, but instead can monitor the incoming calls (if you use an answering machine instead of a phone company voice-mail service). Either way, you will be able to take your time and critically listen to each applicant one or more times. Try to get interested inquirers to record a voice reply on your phone's system, instead of replying by e-mail. A voice reply will tell you much more about their personality, attitude, and even lifestyle.

You will also be able to compare a recorded collection of several callers against each other, and not have to rely on your memory's playback. In listening to recorded inquiries, you never feel the on-the-spot pressure of speaking with live callers, who often try high-pressure sales tactics to convince you to give them an interview.

Finally, your voice mail will accurately record each name, number, and set of comments, instead of your fumbling with a pen and paper during each call. If it is useful, one of your current PAs can later write down the data from each desirable caller.

This recruiting step provides much more than just the chance to record phone numbers. In this step you can screen out up to half of the callers as undesirable applicants. How? Simply by listening carefully.

Your decisions about selecting callers should be based on two factors: the factual information of *what* each tells you and the personal attitude behind *how* it is said. Factually, is this caller's experience, desired type of work, and reason for wanting to work with you appropriate for being a PA? In addition, what is her attitude? Ask yourself, "Does this sound like an angry or fog-headed person to stay away from, or does it seem to be a warm, clear-headed person I feel comfortable inviting into my home?"

A word about theoretical employment discrimination

If you are a professional who is accustomed to working within strict corporate personnel policies, you will notice that one or two of the proposed strategies of this chapter differ from the norm. Everyone who interviews, hires, and employs help providers should be as concerned as corporations in avoiding discriminatory practices. However, we help recipients often find it necessary to modify corporate-style employment policies with those that give us extra safety and security.

What I loosely refer to as corporate is any employment policy mandated by federal, state, and occasionally municipal laws that specify the dos and don'ts of how small and large businesses can employ people. These laws very specifically attempt to assure employees that they will be treated objectively and fairly, without discrimination. One way corporations avoid accusations of discrimination is by basing their employment decisions on objective facts that can be documented. Most businesses could be accused of potential discrimination if they made decisions on subjective intuition and assumptions—sometimes without even meeting candidates.

In contrast to hiring employees who work in a corporate office or hospital room, you hire PAs who work with you while you are alone. In addition, they work in your residence with access to your possessions and medications. Your cautious strategies safeguard you while interviewing and screening complete strangers, whether done in a public place or in your home, and with or without the company of a current PA. They protect you during the training of still unknown, new PAs that is done partly with a current PA and partly alone. You must also be especially cautious while initially working alone with new PAs, until you believe you can trust them.

Consequently, you are far more vulnerable than corporations to bodily harm and theft of possessions during both initial hiring and subsequent employment. You will find it essential for your own personnel strategies to provide you with more caution and protection than most of the traditional corporate policies with which you might be familiar.

In the screening, interviewing, and hiring steps that follow, you will be advised to avoid meeting with—and interviewing—initial phone applicants who make you feel uncomfortable for reasons that will be illustrated and discussed. You will be repeatedly advised to trust your subjective intuition, often giving it more importance and weight than objective, factual information. It is often more important to evaluate *how* applicants say something than *what* they say. The former can tip you off to a candidate's unfavorable attitude toward people with disabilities or inappropriate reasons for wanting your job, while the latter can falsely try to assure you that the person will be the best PA you could possibly hire!

Of course, you should attempt to base your employment decisions on factual evidence whenever possible. However, there will be occasions when you will be wise to refuse to consider applicants because of assumptions you must make when evidence is not available, or when acquiring it might place you in harm's way. Be sure your assumption that an applicant should not be interviewed or would not be a quality PA is based on an obviously dangerous situation or the apparent lack of an essential qualification, and not merely a difference in personal style, clothing, taste, or music preferences.

In reviewing the advisories of the following steps, remember that *you* are ultimately responsible for formulating the policies and strategies that you use in employing your help providers. The purpose of this book is to provide you with advice from actual experiences gathered from many of us help recipients. We continually try to be as fair as possible in employing providers. However, given a circumstance of possibly jeopardizing our personal safety to interview a stranger who genuinely makes us uncomfortable on the phone, most of us will refuse to interview—and theoretically risk an accusation of discrimination.

Which callers would you call back?

Here are ten examples of actual inquiries that your author has received on his answering machine from running the following ad in the local college newspaper.

$9 for Help to Man with Disability
Get experience working with a disability. Cool, active guy who uses wheelchair needs help with living activities, 6-8 hrs weekly. Just 10 min from campus (car required), routine easy to learn. Needed now. Call Skip today & lv message, 555-3721.

Which of these callers would you call back? In deciding, use both the factual information and your intuition before checking my evaluations in parentheses.

1) I'm calling about the ad for your live-in position. My name is Jennifer, but I'm really calling for a good friend of mine. He's really a nice, gentle guy who's interested in this job. Please call me back at xxx-xxxx and I'll be glad to tell you more about him." (I won't consider "hand-me-down" applicants. If her friend is really interested, he must take the initiative of calling directly. I erased this one.)

2) [Happy, bubbling, warm voice] "Hi, Skip. My name is Christy, and I saw your ad. I'm 28 years old and a first-year grad student in Occupational Therapy at SIU. I would like the experience of working with a person with a disability who has the positive attitude you seem to have from the ad you placed. I think I could learn a lot from working with you. Could you please call me at xxx-xxxx. Again, my name is Christy, and I hope to hear from you." (Yes! Christy's tone of voice and message content tell you that she is cheerful, warm, and well organized. She is an OT student, so she wants experience for fattening her resume in addition to the salary. I hired Christy, and had dependable help from her for two years. She is now a full-time OT, and we still exchange holiday cards.)

3) "Ah, yeah (sniff), I'm callin' 'bout the disabled who wants someone (cough, cough) to care for him. My uncle was on crutches for awhile, so working with them doesn't bother me none. Call me and we can talk 'bout what he needs. Thanks." [No name or phone number] (Chances are that this guy didn't call early in the morning, but in the late afternoon when addicts typically "get it together" each day. Whatever the reason, his head is not organized, he forgot to leave any contact details, and he is obviously not comfortable with people who have disabilities. Bye, bye, Sniffles.)

4) [Clear, pleasant voice] "Hello, I'm calling for Skip. I'm Sarah, a 38-year-old massage therapist here in town. I would like to supplement my income and would be glad to provide you with references. Please call me at xxx-xxxx so I can learn more about your needs and the hours you require. Thank you very much." (Like Christy, this woman is clear thinking and has taken time to consider why she really wants this job. Be sure to call back anyone like this.)

5) "My name is Heidi and I'd like to know more about the disabled gentleman who needs help. I think these people are so brave and inspiring. I've helped out several of them before. Yes, I have access to a real good car; my current boyfriend says I can use his. Please call me at xxx-xxxx, suite 110." (Out of curiosity—however, with no desire to reach her—I called the phone number and reached the main desk of a local cockroach motel that rents rooms by the week for $100. "Suite 110" was their room number. Again, a poor attitude. She is probably sincere in viewing "these people" as "brave and inspiring"; however, these terms within this context indicate her lack of comfort with people who have disabilities. That lack of comfort is not optimum for a PA. Also, she and her boyfriend are probably desperate for money, and consequently a poor security risk. Small, valuable items would start disappearing from your home and reappearing in pawn shops. Sorry, Heidi.)

6) [Quiet, pleasant voice] "Hello, Skip, my name is Lea. I'm a 42-year-old single mom with two daughters. I've done some home health aide work before. If you would please return my call, I would like to discuss what needs you have. Please call me at xxx-xxxx. I'll look forward to hearing from you." (She sounds pleasant, and has a sincere reason for wanting part-time work. You can invite her for an interview and demo of your routine, but insist that she bring employment references. She could be very stable and dependable, or there may be a reason why—at the age of 42—she is still going from one part-time job to another and willing to work for just $9.00 an hour. I have encountered two women with Lea's background, and honored my intuition that advised me to check references. Lea's previous employers loved her, and there was an honorable reason for her leaving each job. Another woman, with a similar background, did not sail through my reference calls. Her most recent employer, at a drive-through gas station, said that she worked well for the first two weeks. Then, one morning, she suddenly became angry with a customer, threw a Coke bottle at him, hopped over the counter, and tried to punch him out. In "iffy" situations like this, trust your gut and check references—or, indeed, you might decide always to check references.)

7) [Rushed, very fast, mumbled message] "This is Erin, saw your ad, 'm interested, xxx-xxxx." (From students at a college campus, calls like Erin's are common. Erin is "job fishing." She is taking ten minutes to rip through the ads in today's newspaper or Internet. She is not paying much attention to any specific ad, and is leaving the same, generic message for your job and the ones at the pizza parlor and the liquor store. She will go to class and come back to check for any "nibbles" left on her voice mail. So why not hire her? You could, if you were in desperate need and you realized that she would not last very long. She would typically promise you a six-month commitment, and then resign three weeks later when a more attractive job came her way—or she simply tired of yours.)

8) [Nervous, respectful voice] "My name is Jenny. I'm a 19-year-old sophomore, pre-veterinary student at BU. I would like to speak with Skip about the help he needs. I grew up on a ranch in Wyoming. I'm used to getting up early, and I'm a hard worker. Please call me at xxx-xxxx." (If you conclude that she sounds like a sincere, warm, and hard-working young woman with probably very down-to-earth values, you are right. Jenny provided me with very reliable help. When she saw my bowel routine for the first time, she remarked, "Hey, I've delivered calves on our ranch—your routine is easy." Be sure to call back any "Jennys" that come your way.)

9) "Hi, my name is Todd and I'm calling about your ad. I currently work at XYZ fast food restaurant. I just got into town and I don't have a phone, so you'll have to call me here between the hours of 7:00 A.M. and 3:30 P.M. The phone number is xxx-xxxx. Hope to hear from you." (I insist that all my PAs have a phone that can be heard from where they sleep. I would put Todd in a low priority.)

10) "Hi, Skip, my name is Scott. I'm a CNA (certified nursing assistant) who works for the GSU home care agency. I would like to work some extra hours directly with you. Please call me at xxx-xxxx any weekday after 4 P.M. I've worked for the agency for four years, and I'll be happy to supply you with references." (He sounds great, but you should call his references to be sure he is not making up his CNA certification or job history.)

A corporate personnel office is not required to grant each applicant an interview, and you are not required to call back each applicant. The understanding with most callers is that you will return their call if you are interested in them and the position is still open. Simply erase those respondents who are clearly undesirable. For the worthy candidates, write down the name, phone number, any of their important personal details and experience, and perhaps your 1-to-10 ranking that compares them to other callers.

Step ❻   You call back the selected ad applicants, and identify who to interview (Screening 2).

- Call back the initially desirable applicants, briefly describe your routine, and listen to their responses and attitude.
   ▸ Call back within 24 hours of their recorded inquiry to your newspaper or Internet ad.
   ▸ Become acquainted with candidates, ask about their backgrounds and reasons for wanting the job, and do a few minutes of "small talk." Listen both to what they say and how they say it.
   ▸ Describe your routine, using the shorter description of your routine that you created.[9]

- During this conversation, you screen out a second group of any undesirable applicants.
   ▸ Thank them for their inquiry and tell them you are now speaking with several people who inquired about the PA ad, and you might call them back again. Scratch those names from your list and make your next call.

- For worthy candidates, you continue your conversation with your more detailed description of the routine, and then schedule an interview.

---

9. For a discussion about your creating and rehearsing short and long descriptions of your routine, please see chapter 📖 13, "Defining and Describing Your Help Needs."

▶ Schedule them to meet with you and a current PA for an at-home interview and demonstration of your routine. As many as three candidates can be scheduled for the same time.

• Request that each candidate bring employment references, if you wish.

▶ Ask candidates to bring to the meeting a resume and/or a list of three references from previous employers.

▶ Both the interview and demonstration of major parts of your routine are usually held in the same place—at your residence. However, if you are uncomfortable about inviting total strangers into your home, you can schedule the interview for a public place, such as the food court of a shopping mall. You would interview the applicants and collect their employment references. After you return home, you would check their references and decide whether to invite them to your residence for the demonstration of your routine.

• During this conversation and second screening, you can expect to screen out up to 10 percent of callers.

Strategies that make Step ❻ work for you

As soon as you identify desirable phone responses to your PA ad, call them back within 24 hours of their leaving the recorded message. Hot interest in your job gets significantly colder with each 12 hours that you delay. By waiting 48 hours before you begin callbacks, you can often lose 25 to 50 percent of the candidates. They will find another job or simply lose interest in yours.

The second screening opportunity happens while you talk to candidates who initially sounded good on your answering machine. You can say good-bye either when you dislike an applicant (for valid reasons related to essential qualifications), or when an applicant disqualifies herself by not being able to handle the type of work, schedule, or some other aspect of the job. After five or ten minutes of dialogue you can usually decide whether to drop a candidate or invite her for an interview.

If it becomes evident from whatever carefully selected criteria you have decided to use, that someone is not appropriate, then thank her for calling, hang up, and scratch her name from the list. For desirable callers, schedule interviews during the same phone call. They could be held later that same day, or certainly within 24 hours.

The interview and the demonstration of your routine are usually combined into one meeting. You can even schedule two or three applicants for the same time, even though you might have only one position to fill. Because the demonstration must be held in your residence, combining the two steps means that both are held where you live. The only reason for separately scheduling the two meetings would be for your comfort, security, and peace of mind during the interviews.

Some interviewers feel better when they interview candidates and check their references before inviting them into the interviewer's residence for the demonstration. If security is a concern, the interview can be held in a public place such as a coffee shop or the food area of a shopping mall. If the candidate sounds and feels good during the interview, schedule the at-home demonstration right away.

Is it important to check each applicant's references? Some of us cannot be bothered to take the time, whereas others consider a careful scrutiny of references to be essential before hosting the at-home demonstration. If you would rather not routinely check references, but you will do so in special circumstances, then read through the ten sample phone calls (above) for two examples where reference checks were warranted.

In checking employment references, a few folks call an agency and pay for an employee-background security check. This information can include previous employers, a financial credit history, marital status, and any criminal record. I have also spoken with one PA employer who requires each PA applicant to complete a personality-profile survey. This survey form is sent for processing to a company that provides a psychological profile with their best guess about the applicant's tendency toward committing crime.

Companies that specialize in running background security checks, including drug testing, are increasingly in demand. Charges can range from $25 and up, per person.

My advice is to consider your neighborhood as well as the type of people applying. Are your neighborhood and its residents (the job applicants) known for a high or low crime rate? If robberies and house break-ins are frequent because people need money, then your job advertisement will probably attract some applicants who are more interested in your possessions than in helping you. In high-crime areas, objective checking of references or running formal background checks is a must. In contrast, are college students applying for your job? Although they are certainly not without tendencies toward crime or abuse, students do provide, on the average, high-quality, responsible, and dependable PA applicants.

If you are ethically uncomfortable with this selective style of deciding when to check references, you should perform such checks on all candidates. That is also the safest approach.

Step ❼ You and a current PA host an interview and demonstration of your routine, and ask interested candidates to call you back the next day (Screenings 3 and 4).

- As a third screening, as many as 25 percent of the candidates will either call to cancel their interview, or simply decide not to show up.

- You and a current PA welcome the applicants who appear for the meeting, and ask about their background and reasons for wanting the job.

  ‣ Make them feel comfortable by engaging in some small talk.

▸ You might begin the interview by outlining the two primary parts of the evening's agenda. Ask the applicants (1) to observe the routine while asking all the questions they wish of you and your PA, and then (2) to go home, think about the job, and call you back the next day with their decision about whether they are still interested in being considered for the job.

• During the interview, briefly describe your disability, the schedule and outline of duties, the essential qualities of a PA, and operational policies.

▸ During the interview (usually held in your living room) you describe the duties, schedule, and nature of the PA job. In addition, discuss the qualities that you require of each PA, the procedure for scheduling work shifts, the one-month minimum notice that you need for resignations, the hourly salary rate and schedule for issuing paychecks, and any other policies.

▸ You outline your staff size and structure, how the monthly scheduling meetings work, and how PAs are responsible for finding their own replacements if unable to work.

▸ Once more, invite applicants to ask questions of you and your current PA. Assure them that no question is too personal to ask.

▸ Ask for any comments from your current PA, and then ask him to give the candidates a tour of the work area, to set up any equipment for the upcoming routine, and to narrate to the candidates what he is doing. Leave them alone for a few minutes to get acquainted.

• During the demonstration, the applicants observe you and a current PA performing an important part of your routine, while you both observe the applicants.

▸ During the demonstration (usually held between your bathroom and bedroom) have the applicants observe you and the PA actually doing major parts of your routine. Be sure to explain the other parts that the applicants will not see.

▸ While the applicants watch you and your PA, you both should observe them for indications of whether each is comfortable with each of you as well as the nature of the work.

• At the end of the meeting, you ask applicants to call you back the next day with their decision about whether they still want to be considered for the job.

▸ At the end of the routine, thank the candidates for coming. Ask that they go home, carefully consider the position with their other commitments, sleep on their decision, and then call you back the next day to let you know if they still want to be considered for the job. If you intend not to be directly available, ask that candidates leave a detailed and complete message.

> ▸ Ask your PA to show the candidates out, and tell them that they are welcome to ask the PA any additional questions after they are outside. This step is pretty important, and will enable your PA to get an overall impression to share with you.

- After the applicants leave, you and the current PA compare notes. In a fourth screening, you decide which candidates you are willing and not willing to consider further, regardless of their next-day reply.

  > ▸ After the meeting, compare observations and impressions with your current PA. Tell her that her opinion of each candidate is important to you, and indeed it is. Thank her for doing a good demonstration. Ask her for any suggestions for you to improve your interviewing style.

  > ▸ In this fourth screening, combine your PA's impressions with your own and identify which applicants you would and would not be willing to hire, regardless of their next-day response.

- Expect that you will approve of most candidates from this meeting, but up to 30 percent of them will either call back the next day to decline the job, or simply decide not to call back. This is the fifth screening.

Strategies that make Step ❼ work for you

Whether the meeting is held in your residence or a public place, it is usually a good idea to include one of your current PAs. The PA provides you with a sense of security, provides a current member of your PA team for the applicants to meet, and enables you to demonstrate part of your routine. In addition, if you are older than the college age or younger bracket of your PAs, your greeting applicants with a current PA who is their age will help the applicants picture themselves as your next aide.

These PA applicants are often nervous—this is, after all, a job interview. How you set up the interview will either add to their stress or help to reduce it and make them feel comfortable. Throw out any books on conducting power interviews where you do things like position chairs to make people feel inferior while enhancing your authority, power, and control.

Instead, arrange the interview to make candidates feel comfortable. Eliminate or minimize sources of stress, anger, whining, and depression such as a blaring TV, loud stereo, barking dogs, street noise, and screaming kids. I put some soft-but-upbeat jazz on the stereo and slightly dim some of the brighter room lights. (Don't confuse this with a romantic "date." It is all carefully designed—and experience-proven—business marketing. I want the candidates to go home feeling, "Wow, that would be a nice place to work!")

This meeting usually involves three people: the applicant, one of your current PAs, and you. If you have more than one interested applicant, feel free to schedule up to three for the same meeting, especially since one of the three might drop out by not showing up. By no means should you ever limit the number of candidates you interview to the number of job positions you need to fill. If I have just one or two posts, I will still spend two or three consecutive "bowel-shower nights" interviewing every desirable candidate I have. I often interview seven, eight, or more candidates for one or two slots.

If your routine has more than one "part" (perhaps a morning "get dressed and out-of-bed" and an evening "bowel and shower"), then this demonstration should show the more involved and less attractive one.

The primary objective for showing your routine to applicants is for them to actually see—and sometimes get their hands into—the nature of the work. Otherwise, they would be making a commitment based on what they imagine you, your current PAs, and the work to be like. This kind of work is not meant for everyone. This is full disclosure time.

Additionally, they are watching one of your current PAs very informally zip through the routine. The candidates get the impression that this "medical procedure" is doable, not a big deal, and easy to learn.

Consequently, your selection of a current PA to perform the demonstration should be made carefully. Select a PA who remembers details well and zaps through them in a way that makes them look easy. This current aide should be pleasant and able to carry on a good conversation.

The current aide has three selling jobs to do:

- to make the tasks of your routine look reasonably easy

- to help you appear to be someone who is nice to work with

- to make himself appear to be someone who will be nice to work with as one of the PA team members.

After I have selected a current PA who meets these objectives, I never tell the PA about them. I simply select a PA who will naturally accomplish them without obviously attempting to act that way.

Also, while the applicants watch you and a current PA go through the routine, both of you should be observing them. Do their reactions tell you they would be comfortable doing what the current aide is doing? In contrast, are they so uncomfortable that they often look away from the activity, stand back from the activity, and otherwise show that they can't wait for the demo to end?

It is a good idea to wear clean clothes and have your living area reasonably neat and clean before the candidates arrive. The kitchen, bathroom, and bedroom need not be sterile clean, but should be reasonably picked up. This is the first time they meet you, so first impressions of several types are again important. What they see of you and your surroundings will be considered to be the standard of your expectations. Have this initial appearance set a good example.

So, with everything ready for a first-class interview and demonstration, welcome the applicants and make them comfortable in a living room area with you and the current PA. For security reasons, interview applicants should never be left alone within your residence. Keep a casual eye on them, especially if they "wander" into another room on their own—if they do, call them back.

Provide a brief, layman's description about how you acquired your disability, and your functional abilities and disabilities. Take five minutes, max. Do not put anyone to sleep with too much detail. Invite them to ask additional questions at any time. Assure them that they cannot embarrass you. If medical, physical therapy, or occupational therapy majors have applied for your job, a major incentive is being able to learn first-hand the non-textbook, nitty-gritty details of your life with a disability.

Discuss your staff size, the advance scheduling of shifts, and the responsibility for finding one's own work-shift replacement. Explain the advantages of dividing your needs among two, three, or more part-timers.[10]

Explain that you hold an hour-long staff meeting each four or five weeks. PAs bring their calendars or appointment books and decide among themselves who wants to commit to each shift for the next few weeks.

Once a PA has committed to a shift, and then decides that he cannot or does not want to work it, that PA has a choice. He either calls the other aides, finds his own replacement, and then calls you to inform you of the exchange; or he must work the originally scheduled shift. In short, people who want to make changes are responsible for finding their own replacement, or working the shift. They *are not permitted* to call you to tell you simply that they will not be coming to work. For your interests, this is a golden policy—and yes, it works smoothly as long as you are firm about it from the beginning.

Discuss your expectations of the PAs who help you: complete and utter dependability, punctuality, confidentiality, and honesty. There simply is no such thing as a no-show.

With regard to punctuality, explain that if aides expect to be more than five minutes late, they must call you with an estimated time of arrival. For example, if their car won't start, they should call and say, "Skip, my car is not starting. If I will be more than 20 minutes late, I will call again." Explain that even though you might not be able to physically answer the phone, you always keep the volume turned up on the speaker-monitor of your answering machine and you can always hear it.[11]

Discuss your expectations about the minimum period of the job commitment, your need for at least one month's advance notice of resignation, and concerns about scheduling assistance during holidays. State the hourly salary rate, whether the funding comes from you or another source, how often checks are issued (I suggest each two weeks), and that you must deduct FICA contributions (social security) but not income taxes.

Ask the applicant for any questions. Additionally, ask your current PA if you have left out any important points. This gesture makes your PA feel part of the process and indicates to the applicant that you and your PAs work as a comfortable team. In addition, your current aide might indeed bring up some things that you forgot.

---

10. For more detail about the advantages and how to do this, please see chapter 📖 **16, "Dividing Your Needs, and Assigning Work Shifts, Among Several PAs."**

11. For more detail about what to do if a PA fails to appear on time for a shift, please see chapter 📖 **18, "Coping with and Reacting to PA Failures."**

If you asked the applicant for employment references, collect the list, regardless of whether you intend to use it. Each reference should list:

- an employer's name and phone
- the type of job
- the approximate dates of employment
- any comments.

At the conclusion of this interview part of the meeting, ask your current aide to show the applicant the bedroom-bathroom area (or wherever the demonstration will take place). He can provide a "tour" of the work area and set up everything for the routine, while explaining to the applicant what he is doing. Leave them alone for a few minutes, so they can talk aide-to-aide if they wish. After all, the newcomer should also become acquainted and feel comfortable with her future teammates.

While you and the current PA demonstrate the routine, narrate the main activities. To break up the process, ask the applicant some fun questions, to show that a work shift is not all work. Some of the standard conversation questions, especially for college students, include:

- "What movies have you seen lately?"
- "What do you like to read?"
- "What TV programs do you watch?"
- "Where is the best pizza (or ice cream) in town?"

If the applicant is really interested in the routine, and occasionally offers to lend a hand, let her. She is probably very interested in the job, and wants to help with one or two tasks to see if she is "hands-on comfortable" with the personal nature of the work.

At the conclusion of the session, ask the candidate to carefully consider— overnight—the responsibilities and commitment of the job. Ask that she call you sometime the next day to leave a phone message to indicate whether she wishes to be further considered for the job. At this stage, keep your options open by not stating or implying that if she calls back she will automatically be hired.

It is also wise, throughout the session, to guard against statements like, "After you are hired," "After the first few days of doing the routine, you will find," or "You won't have any problem learning this routine." Each of these statements implies that you have already decided to hire the candidate. From years of experience, I have learned not to express or even imply a hiring commitment unless I am making a formal job offer as part of the later **Step ❾**. Between now and that more appropriate time, you might learn something about this candidate that confirms him to be a bad choice, or a better candidate might appear. For now, preface statements like these with, "If you are hired for this job," or "If we decide to work together in this job." Be noncommittal and preface statements with "If."

Leave yourself an escape route in case you decide not to hire one or more of them. Make your position very clear by stating that you are considering other candidates (regardless of whether you really are) and that you will be making a hiring decision within a couple of days. Since you hope they will delay considering other jobs until they hear from you, assure them that you will call each of them with your final decision—and be sure that you do so.

At the moment the candidates are about to leave, you might choose to perform a small gesture that has proven to be remarkably powerful in encouraging desirable candidates to want the job. If you tentatively believe certain candidates to be especially desirable, as they are about to leave provide them with encouragement by making good eye contact, giving them a sincere smile, and telling them that you both enjoyed meeting them and think you would really enjoy working with them. If they are genuinely interested in the job, they will often be personally flattered by your comment and unconsciously break into a big smile. For some reason, this simple gesture has a surprisingly positive effect on their calling back the next day to still want the job. Your gesture often gives a shot of confidence to conscientious and nervous candidates who might otherwise feel unworthy of being seriously considered.

At the end of the session, openly ask your current PA to walk to the door with the applicant. Invite the applicant to confidentially ask any last-minute questions of your PA while outside. When your current aide returns, thank her for doing a great demonstration. Ask her for any suggestions for improving your interviewing or demonstration style

After the candidates leave, perform your fourth screening by deciding whether you are still willing to consider all of them, regardless of whether they call back the next day. While they are still fresh in your mind, consider your conversations with each candidate and your observations of them while they watched the demonstration. Ask your current PA for his evaluation. You will be screening out very few candidates at this fourth stage.

However, you can expect that up to 30 percent of today's candidates, regardless of how eager and committed they seemed, will either call back tomorrow to decline the position or decide not to call back.

Step ❽ You receive next-day callbacks from still-interested candidates, check their references, and identify who to hire (Screenings 5 and 6).

- As a fifth screening, some candidates will either call to cancel their interest in the job, or simply decide not to call you back.

- Still-interested applicants will call you back the next day and ask to be further considered for the job.

- You check their references, if you wish.

- In a sixth screening, from everything you know about each candidate, screen out undesirables and decide whom you will finally offer to hire.

Strategies that make Step ❽ work for you

In receiving callbacks the next day, it is again a good idea to record the responses on a phone answering machine. Once more, recorded messages enable you to take your time making final decisions. You are protected from the on-the-spot pressure of a live person anxiously asking, "Well, do I get the job? When will you know?!"

If you will be checking references, wait until after you have received positive responses from candidates before doing so. If you decided in a previous step that someone is not desirable, or someone does not call back the next day, or she declines the position, then you will have wasted time (and sometimes the cost of fees from a company that provides background checks) on the advance checking.

For each reference you are calling:

- Introduce yourself and state that you are calling because (applicant's name) has offered them as an employment reference. State that you have a disability and are considering this person as a home health aide. Ask if you may ask a few confidential questions.

- Verify the type of job and dates of employment that the candidate claims to have worked for this employer.

- Identify in advance what traits you would like each PA to have, and ask the reference if the applicant proved to have them. For example, "How would you rate this person from one-to-five, with five as "excellent," for her:

  ‣ responsibility
  ‣ dependability
  ‣ punctuality
  ‣ honesty in communicating
  ‣ security toward your possessions
  ‣ ability to follow instructions
  ‣ other traits you may desire.

- A strategy is often used to evaluate a candidate's true former responsibilities, and to evaluate whether he or she was exaggerating or lying to you about them. Try to restate what the candidate told you about his or her position and responsibilities, and ask the reference merely if the accounting is accurate. "Kim informed me that she was the sole night cashier and was completely responsible for all sales, store security, recordkeeping for her shift, five nights each week, from May 11 to November 13 of last year. Are these facts accurate?"

- Ask the reference if they would rehire the applicant. This is perhaps the most important question. The answer best sums up both the reference's experience and evaluation of the candidate. A negative reply to this summation question will tell you what the former employer might be otherwise unable to say openly. If you receive a firmly negative answer, then you can safely assume that there is a serious reason why you should come to the same conclusion.

- Ask if there is anything else you should know with regard to hiring the applicant as a home health aide in your home.

- Thank the reference.

If you have not heard back from all the desirable candidates on the next day, give them one extra day. It is not advisable to call and "track down" a missing candidate. If applicants really want the job, they will be sure to call you on schedule. You can expect that up to one-third of applicants will never call back.

Remember, these people have not forgotten to call you back. Instead, they have intentionally made the decision not to call. In their set of personal values, not calling is their way of telling you they are not interested. Yet another screening opportunity in this ten-step procedure has done its job. Accept—and don't reject—its advice.

If you run out of applicants to consider (all of the original inquirers have been disqualified), then put your ad back into the newspaper. Occasionally, this will happen.

For those applicants who called you back, perform this sixth screening by deciding on the candidate(s) you want to hire. As mentioned, consider both the accumulated factual data as well as your intuition.

Your intuition about whether a final-stage candidate "feels comfortable" is very important. A successful businessman was once asked for his advice on hiring employees. He replied quite simply, "Never hire anyone whom you don't trust and with whom you feel uncomfortable. If you suspect that somehow someone might screw you, they probably will."

Step ❾ You hire the finalists, schedule training sessions, and then decline the others (Screening 7).

- Call the finalist(s), in your order of preference, and offer them the job(s).

- In a seventh screening, some candidates to whom you offer the job will have found a reason why they should not take it, and will decline your offer.
  - ▶ In this screening, a few candidates to whom you finally offer the job will decline. Consequently, to minimize the chance of their finding another job and declining yours, call the desirable candidates within 24 hours of their calling you back the day after the interview.

- If your favorite candidate declines your offer, call and make the job offer to the next in line, until the jobs are filled or you run out of desirable people.

- For candidates who accept your job offer, use this same phone call to schedule them for the first training sessions.

- Call and decline any remaining candidates, but keep them on file for future job openings.
  - ▶ After your favorite candidate(s) accepts the job, you should have the integrity to call any other final-stage candidates to tell them that you regret you will not be hiring them at this time. However, keep handy the phone numbers of any well-qualified "runners-up" in case a new PA does not work out or you need a PA backup.
  - ▶ Here is one more item that merits your cautious optimism. Expect that 25 to 75 percent of hired, quality PAs will resign before completing the full duration of their original employment commitment. Consequently, keep handy your file of desirable-but-not-hired candidates.

Strategies that make Step ❾ work for you

When everything seems to check out for your finalist candidates, you might finally have a done deal. Cautious optimism is still warranted. Call back the desirable finalists as soon as possible to offer to hire them, and to schedule the first training sessions with a current PA.

Notice the use of the phrase "offer to hire." Indeed, the candidates occasionally decline. Your role is simply to offer to hire; the candidate has the final decision of accepting or not. To increase your chance for success, do not delay calling with your offer. You could still lose them to another job.

If you have a greater number of desirable candidates than you do PA positions, be sure to hire the desirables before rejecting the others. For obvious reasons, be sure your desired people actually accept and commit to the position before you decline anyone. It is rare that a candidate would decline at this stage, but it can happen, especially if you delay more than 24 hours.

You should speak directly with the people being hired. This is not a time for merely leaving a phone message of, "Hi, Stacie, this is Jerry. Congratulations, you are hired. If I do not hear from you, I will see you this Tuesday night at 7:30 for training. Bye."

Make no assumptions. Do not consider finalists to be hired until you speak directly with them, and hear them say "yes!" In a similar vein, also insist on speaking to candidates when you are unable to hire them.

It is easier to hire someone than to be unable to do so. Indeed, if you think in terms of being unable to hire some candidates, instead of rejecting them, you might feel less guilty when delivering the bad news. The dictionary defines *to reject* in terms of "to refuse, rebuff, discard, (or) deny ... as imperfect, unwanted, unsatisfactory, unfit, unqualified." This is all quite negative stuff, and it is clear why many personnel people would rather have a root canal than make such phone calls. Instead, the task is much easier if you are calling a candidate whom you would like to employ, but are unable to hire.

If you are faced with telling people that you will not be hiring them, do have the courage to make the phone call. Avoid the temptation to just drop applicants and assume that if they do not hear from you they will get the message. We have discussed how disappointing it is for you not to receive an applicant's callback. Do not perpetuate the discourtesy.

There are two situations that should prompt you to decide not to hire some candidates who want to work with you:

- a candidate is undesirable, and you do not want to hire
- a candidate is desirable, but you do not have an available position.

In the second case, you are wise not to burn the bridge to the possibility of hiring this desirable candidate if an opening occurs in the future. In perhaps 1 of every 25 hires, new PAs will resign during the first few days or month of work. The most common reasons include their sudden realization that taking on your job overloads them, their family or significant other forbids them to continue the new job, they discover they do not want this kind of work, or they don't get along with you. When this happens, you can simply offer the job opening to a candidate who was recently interviewed but not hired.

In either event, consider this overall formula for making these difficult phone calls to break the news that you are unable to hire a candidate:

1) Greet the candidate and identify yourself and the reason for calling. Use a reasonably friendly tone, and identify yourself and the topic of your call. "Hello, Nicole, this is Joel. I am calling about the home health aide position that you interviewed for on Thursday."

2) Compliment the person. State two or three positive impressions from your having met with the candidate. You might have to be creative. There are always two or three positive things you can say. Don't lie, or you will probably contradict yourself in step (3) when you state your inability to hire them. (For example, avoid stating, "I think you would be a terrific PA...however, I am unable to hire you.") Keep the compliments simple and quick. "I would like to thank you for interviewing the other night. I really enjoyed meeting you and hearing your opinion on the movies we both like."

3) Provide an introduction and a logical transition to your main message. Change your tone of voice to be just a bit more serious, so the candidate will sense that something different is about to happen. Consider using the past tense for this decision that has been firmly made. "Nicole, as I may have mentioned at the interview, I had just two openings this time."

4) Deliver your main message. Make it clear and concise. Also remember that if you have not been looking forward to making this phone call, this is the part during which you might have a tendency to mumble. If you do, the candidate will be asking you to repeat the message. "I regret that I was not able to offer you one of these current openings." If this candidate was desirable, but you had more desirable candidates than you did job openings, say so. "Nicole, you are well qualified for this job and I would hire you if I had an additional job. May I keep your name and number handy, and call you when my next opening occurs to see if you are available? In return, would you please let me know if your phone number changes?"

5) Promptly wrap up the phone call, perhaps by offering a polite consolation. Again, this should be a clear and concise statement. Avoid a long (or short) rambling of reasons or excuses; there is no need to provide any at all. If you are asked for a reason, be vague; the candidate is usually only trying to open up an argument. Different from an excuse is a consolation, technically "something that alleviates grief or sorrow." Consolations have become a traditional way of coming down from the delivery of bad news. If the candidate is truly desirable, and she has agreed to let you call her with future openings, then this isn't merely a consolation, but a confirmation of your intention. "However, may I call you the next time I hire to see if you are available? Again, I would like to thank you for applying and interviewing with me. Good-bye."

Step ⑩   **You or the planner-manager use family caregivers or other, current outside providers to train new PAs with a three-step procedure. Occasionally, a new PA will fail to appear for the first or second scheduled shift (Screening 8).**

• Use the three-step procedure to train new PAs.

▸ Have new PAs watch a current PA perform each part of your routine.

▸ Have new PAs do the routine at least once for simpler groups of tasks, or twice for more complex groups, while a current PA stands by.

▸ Finish their training by having them work with you, while they receive occasional reminders and lots of patience from you.

The new aides will learn more quickly and better remember the details if these three steps for each part of your routine take place within a seven- to ten-day period.

• In a rare eighth screening, new PAs might drop out during the first one or two training sessions. If you follow our three-step process, a current aide will be assisting these two initial sessions. Consequently, if the new PA fails to show up, you are protected by your current aide.

Strategies that make Step ⑩ work for you

Now that you have hired the new PAs, it is time to get ready for training sessions. There are two primary ways to train new PAs: You do it alone, or you do it with a current PA.

If you perform the training by yourself, it will be up to you to describe each step of your routine clearly enough that a trainee can picture the action and follow the instructions. With a current PA, the PA is providing both the demonstrations and the standby help to accompany your instructions.

If you try to go it alone, you will quickly gain an appreciation for the adage, "A picture is worth a thousand words." Training with a current PA is much easier.

First, have the new PA watch a current PA perform each part of your routine. This observation provides the new person with a clear visualization of the routine's objectives. If new PAs saw a part of your routine demonstrated a few days ago when they interviewed as candidates, then you can skip this step for the parts that they saw.

Second, have the new PA complete the routine once (for a simple routine) or twice (for a longer, more detailed one). The current PA should "shadow" the new aide in case there is a need to jump in and demonstrate, or to fill in during a task. In addition, most new aides are nervous about doing something wrong, and the presence of the current PA provides a comforting confidence that help will be available if needed. The new provider does not worry as much about making mistakes.

Third, you and the new PA begin working one on one. All that is now required is your patience and doses of appreciation as reinforcement.

With a rare, one-in-fifty or so new PAs, an eighth screening takes place during the first or second training session. Here, your current PA will appear on schedule, but the new aide fails to appear. There are equal chances that the newbie has not yet adjusted to the new schedule, or has suddenly decided to quit when faced with the cold reality of the first actual work shift. If you follow our three-step training process, you are protected by having also scheduled a current aide for these initial shifts.

The Eight Screening Opportunities

Here is a summary of the eight opportunities that have been discussed in **Steps ❶** through **❿** of this chapter.

Figure 7-2: **The Eight Screening Opportunities**

Screening Number	Who Actually Screens?	Description	Effect— Screens Out
One	You	After your newspaper or Internet ad appears, your phone will start ringing. You listen to the ad inquiries that are recorded. You screen out (and simply erase) the obviously undesirable callers. See **Step ❺**	Up to 50% of callers
Two	You	You call back the desirable inquirers, provide a short description of your routine, and engage in a conversation with applicants. Based on this conversation, you screen out some and invite the remaining candidates to an interview and demonstration of your routine. See **Step ❻**	Up to 10% of inquiries
Three	The candidate	Some candidates will disqualify themselves by deciding not to come. Some will either call to cancel or simply decide not to show up. See **Step ❼**	Up to 25% of candidates
Four	You and your PA	Once you and a current PA have completed the interview and demonstration of your routine, you ask all the candidates to carefully consider the position and call you back the next day. They will indicate whether they are still interested in being considered for the job. After they leave, you and your current PA identify those whom you will not consider further, regardless of whether they call you back the next day. See **Step ❼**	Very few

Figure 7-2: **The Eight Screening Opportunities** *(continued)*

Screening Number	Who Actually Screens?	Description	Effect— Screens Out
Five	The candidate	Some candidates will disqualify themselves either by calling to cancel their interest in the job, or simply not calling you back. However, the majority will call to express their continued interest. See **Step ❽**	Up to 30% of candidates
Six	You	For those finalists who do call back and express their continued interest, you might decide to check their employment references. You finally gather all of your experiences, facts, and impressions about the candidates, and decide who you are willing to hire. See **Step ❽**	Very few candidates
Seven	The candidate	You call the finalist(s), in your order of preference, and offer them the job. Some candidates to whom you offer the job will have found a reason why they do not want it or should not take it. They will disqualify themselves by declining your offer. You then continue calling the desirable candidates until your positions are filled. See **Step ❾**	Very few candidates

Figure 7-2: **The Eight Screening Opportunities** *(continued)*

Screening Number	Who Actually Screens?	Description	Effect— Screens Out
Eight	**The candidate**	After you hire new PAs, you will be training them using a three-step process. In step one, each new PA watches a current PA perform part of your routine. In step two, the new PA performs the routine while the current one shadows. In step three, you begin working alone with the new PA. Besides being an effective training process, this strategy protects you in the rare instance when a new PA fails to show up for the first or second training session— your current aide will still be there. The new aide might have temporary trouble adjusting to the new schedule, or might suddenly quit when faced with the first actual work shift. This rare screening (when a new PA actually quits at this stage) happens with only 1 or 2 percent of newbies; however, your three-step training protects you when it does occur.	**Very few new PAs**

Part III

More Topics on Getting the Help You Need

203

Part III

More Topics on Getting the Help You Need

In Part II, you found three ten-step chapters for getting the help you need from family caregivers, agency-employed aides, and personally employed aides or PAs. The chapters in this Part III supplement the previous ones by providing in-depth discussions of selected, specialized topics.

In chapter 7, on getting your help from personally employed aides, you saw the logical importance of attracting a maximum number of quality applicants to inquire about your PA job. The greater the number of applicants who inquire about your newspaper or Internet ad, the more selective you can be in hiring the highest quality PAs. Part III's chapter 📖 **8, "Where and How to Advertise for Your Own PAs,"** includes many of the valuable principles used by professional ad agencies—all of them specially tailored to attracting your next help providers.

The first section of the chapter addresses where to advertise specifically for aides and PAs. It lists the places and types of publications typically found in most communities. The second section provides experience-proven strategies for writing effective ad copy. Topics include the five essential parts of any powerful ad, illustrations of the three types of newspaper ads, tips on how to quickly produce recruiting posters and bulletin board notices that will attract the eyes of PA applicants from ten feet away, and many examples of actual ads that have been very successful.

Chapter 📖 **9, "Initial Training and Ongoing Management of Aides and PAs,"** applies to all three types of help providers. Whether your paid providers come from agencies or personal employment, they will all need training directly from you (or your personal representative) in the specific help tasks that you need, as well as when, where, and how you prefer that help to be provided. First, you will find a three-step training procedure accompanied by helpful hints that shorten the learning curve for your PAs. Once new PAs have been trained, they require ongoing management—feedback that addresses what they could be doing better as well as routinely expressed appreciation about what they are doing correctly. The strategies for ongoing management ensure that you receive a consistently high quality of help, and that your aides will want to stay with you longer because they feel appreciated.

Chapter 📖 10, "Recognizing and Resolving Your PA Problems, or Parting Ways," is packed with checklists and strategies that discuss recognizing, analyzing, and resolving performance problems, ill feelings, and worker job dissatisfaction. The goal is to resolve uneasy feelings to keep both you and your PAs happy, and to avoid needless PA resignations and firings. You will find a list of PA habits and mannerisms that will often enable you to realize that PAs are planning to resign even before they realize it. You will know how, why, and when resignations typically occur, as well as how to react to your PA's resignation announcement so that most PAs will loyally stay with you until their replacement is up and running. If you carefully interview and screen PA applicants, and then provide them with appreciative ongoing management, your need to fire a provider will be a rare occasion. However, when a firing does become necessary, this chapter provides effective ways of getting the job done while protecting you from any negative repercussions.

Following the topics of this Part III are the four chapters of Part IV, "Taking Control of Your Help Needs." These next chapters provide tactics on identifying your help needs, ensuring that all items on your list are appropriate for help requests, and assuring you of the importance of your preferences about how you want to receive help—even though these preferences draw frequent criticism from your PAs. How often have you heard additional critiques about your making too many demands, being too demanding, or making other mistakes both in what help you request and in how you request it? In answer, two more chapters will coach you in how to be clear and direct with assertive communication, as well as how much control and supervision are warranted—and how much can suddenly be too much.

Part IV Taking Control of Your Help Needs

📖 11 When It Is, and Is Not, Okay to Ask for Help

📖 12 Getting It Done—Your Way!

📖 13 Defining and Describing Your Help Needs

📖 14 Say It, Ask for It, and Act—Assertively!

Chapter 8
Where and How to Advertise for Your Own PAs

For many of us, this is the most important chapter of this book. It attempts to answer our most basic, recurring question: "Where can you find a new PA when you need one?"

The answer to the question begins with deciding whether you will be using aides employed by an agency or directly employed by yourself. If you are using an agency, the task already is done; the agency will recruit, employ, and (partially) train the aides. But if you are not using an agency, you will need to learn how best to find competent, reliable assistance in your community. The first section of this chapter discusses *where* to recruit PAs in a typical community.

The second section provides strategies for *how* to write newspaper and Internet ads, bulletin board notices, and eye-catching posters. You need to know how to catch the eye of good applicants. It's a lot like fishing. Once you know where there are good fishing spots, the next step is knowing what bait to use and how to cast to make the bait look most attractive. That's what this chapter's all about: where and how to fly-cast for PAs and then reel them in!

Where to Advertise for Your Own PAs

If you want to directly employ your own PAs, there are usually several sources in a typical community for finding people who are willing to provide assistance. Some of these people will have considerable experience, but most will have none. The latter must first be oriented to the personal nature of the work, so they feel comfortable, and then trained so they perform duties in the ways you prefer. By combining the guidelines in this book with a little practice, you will soon be able to briefly introduce your help needs to job applicants during interviews, and then provide in-depth details during the training of newly hired PAs.

The rest of this section is a listing of the most common sources for recruiting any PAs whom you will directly employ. It should not be viewed as an exhaustive list, as you will probably develop additional sources particular to your locale. This sample listing is ranked in descending order of typical success, beginning with the most fruitful sources.

Previous PA applicants or employees

Before spending effort, time, and money on recruiting new PAs from scratch, be sure that all currently known resources have been used.

When you last recruited PAs, you might have kept a listing of the applicants who were fully qualified and desirable, but who were not hired. I hope you asked these second-stringers if you could call them later for future needs. Now is the time to make those calls to ask if they are still interested in working for you.

Referrals from current PAs

When a current PA announces to you that she wants to take vacation time or resign, she and other current PAs can sometimes assist in finding either temporary fill-in help or a longer-term replacement. If you recruit with newspaper ads or bulletin board posters, and need physical help doing so, also feel free to enlist her nimble fingers.

Your request of your current aide is simple, to ask whether:

- she has any advice about new ways or places where you can recruit aides

- she knows of any friends or PA colleagues who might be looking for work

- if she is a college student, whether she would make a brief announcement at the beginning of each of her appropriate classes about your job opening. She would briefly cite your need for help, and then invite anyone to see her after class for details. If you are unwilling to have her give out your name and phone number, you might ask her to take down the names and numbers of people interested in the position so that she can pass them on to you.

Peers who have disabilities

Although peers will seldom be able to provide you with physical help, they are usually your top source of advice. No one understands your disability concerns as well as someone who has a similar disability.

Peers who have been hiring and managing help for their own needs know from experience where to find help in their locales. When your efforts are just not paying off, do some networking with peers.

Disability organizations in a campus or community

Disability organizations can include independent living programs, state or city offices for those with disabilities, the administrative office or student organization at a college campus, and local citizen groups.

Any of these groups might be handy in your personal recruiting efforts for at least two categories of information. First, they might be able to advise you about the PA market in your living area, including where and how to recruit. This advice might also include the current range of hourly salary rates being paid to PAs. The organization might even have established a roster of folks who have registered with the organization because of their interest in being employed as PAs. However, as mentioned in the college campus section, "attendant rosters" have several limitations and are becoming outdated.

Second, the group might publish a periodic newsletter and be willing to include your PA notice. The trick in using newsletters is to hope that a monthly or bimonthly newsletter will be printed and promptly distributed within the time that you are recruiting a PA. That schedule match-up is often very difficult to accomplish.

Recruiting from a nearby college campus

If you live near a campus, you are lucky: college students have several qualities that make them excellent PA prospects. From a physical standpoint, they have youth, strength, and health. Their personal schedules are flexible because of a lack of local family life, and they have few time commitments beyond classes, meals, studying, extracurricular activities and sports, and romantic pursuits. Perhaps most importantly, most college students either need money or think they do.

On the downside, some students tend to be immature. Some are poor planners, become overextended with too many responsibilities, and are forced to drop some commitments—including your PA job—after just two or three weeks. Some occasionally dismiss outside commitments in favor of upcoming exams and papers, higher-paying and easier jobs, or satisfying their libidos.[1]

If you have never used college students as PAs, and you are beyond college age, you might initially be concerned about using a 22-year-old person (usually female) for personal help. As someone who is 30, 40, 50, 60 years old or older, your success at using twenty-somethings as PAs will depend primarily upon how young you feel. If you enjoy mixing with younger folks, respect them, and find their young pursuits interesting, then you will probably relate well to younger PAs. In contrast, if you look at the campus population as loud, always immature, untrustworthy, and having intolerable habits that sharply contrast with your own, then you would be better off employing PAs who are within your own age bracket.

Overall, students usually provide excellent PA help. I have passed the 50-year mark and have been directly employing my own PAs for more than 30 years, with 95 percent of them college students.

I also prefer college students because their population tends to present me with fewer problems directly related to PA performance than non-college applicants. I rarely check employment or character references for full-time students. Very few successful college students are able to maintain good grades while also maintaining a serious substance addiction or a lifestyle that is not conducive to the sharp mental acuity required by rigorous academics. Stated another way, successful college students don't have time for significantly bad habits. In contrast, I am more defensive and cautious when interviewing part-time working people who are not students.

---

1. However, the interviewing and screening procedure outlined in chapter 📖 7, **"Ten Steps to Getting All or Some of Your Help from Personally Employed Aides,"** was designed to build in factors that reduce the chances of hiring job applicants who are already overextended with other commitments.

As disabled people who are dependent on help from others, we want to avoid hiring people who:

- are unable to keep jobs, because they lack the responsibility required to routinely meet commitments

- are substance abusers, and demonstrate unpredictable behavior and schedules

- are in financial trouble, and thus may end up stealing our possessions

- have other hidden, undesirable traits and potentially are undependable, not trustworthy, or prone to take some sort of advantage of us.

Consequently, I feel comfortable placing ads in the student newspaper of the nearby college campus. The applicants will usually be academically successful, hard-working students. I become more careful and defensive when I occasionally must advertise in our community-wide newspaper. Although my particular community is generally a low-crime, God-fearing, respectful population, my community ads for aides often attract people who have more undesirable personal baggage than do full-time students. I am wary of 40-year-old people who have worked a short time for a part-time minimum wage at a gas station, and are additionally willing to work a few weekly hours for me at $9 an hour. I have found that the reason why they are not well established in a long-term, full-time job is often also a reason why I should not hire them.

In stating my additional concerns about non-college aides, I am not implying that I avoid hiring from the general community. Indeed, I routinely hire non-students, because they add a stabilizing diversity to my eclectic team of providers.

I usually divide my help needs among five or six part-time aides, for the several reasons discussed in chapter 16. I have found additional advantages in employing a PA mix of both college students and non-students. The advantages are most evident when it comes to scheduling issues. If I employ only college people, my availability of PA help is sharply influenced by student vacation periods and campus-wide exam schedules that all students have in common. When employing at least 20 percent— one in five—non-college people in my mix, I encounter few completely dry periods when an adequate number of providers is not available to me.

However, my own 30-plus years of hiring experience have shown me that the non-college population tends to have a greater number of undesirable traits—of the type that directly affect work performance as a PA—than do successful, full-time college students. I have consistently found the need to screen a greater number of non-college applicants—and to screen them more carefully—than college students, to find enough desirable applicants for my PA positions.

For these reasons, I enjoy hiring and working with college student PAs![2]

2. For further details on PA applicant traits to prefer and avoid, see chapter 📖 25, "Your Personal Concerns as a Paid Help Provider, plus Ten Reasons Why PAs Quit and Are Fired."

In screening students, it is wise to favor upperclassmen (juniors and seniors) and graduate students over freshmen and sophomores. The eager first- and second-year students are often the first respondents to PA ads, and they will also often require a bit more screening—or at least coaching. The eager freshman often does not yet have a realistic sense of the time demands of college life, whereas the upper-classman often has worked out a study routine and can make commitments with more reliability. Use of high school students is rarely recommended.

Although college students can be recruited at almost any time, there are some notably good and bad recruiting times at any typical college campus. Especially fruitful times include:

- The last three or four weeks of a semester, so they can commit themselves to a job that starts with the end of this semester or the beginning of the next.

- The first two weeks of any semester, before academic responsibilities start to pile up and while students are still rested from vacations.

- Right after Thanksgiving break through the beginning of December final exams, for positions beginning in January.

- For either salaried or live-in positions, right after spring break in March until the end of April, for positions beginning in summer or fall.

Logically then, bad times to recruit are most likely to be when exams, term papers, vacation weeks, and other sources of fatigue are overwhelming student desires for taking on new responsibilities. These poor times to recruit include:

- The week before and during midterm exams
  (at the midpoint of any semester).

- The week before and during final exams
  (the last two weeks of any semester).

- Vacation periods—
  - The week of Thanksgiving break
  - The six weeks between the December holidays and the January date when students return for spring semester
  - The week of spring break in mid-March
  - The week of May or June graduation.

The schedule of when semesters, spring breaks, and vacation times begin and end varies among colleges, but the details are readily available by calling the campus information desk, by speaking with the campus newspaper staff, or by checking the campus calendar at the campus Web site.

If you live on or nearby a college campus, there are several routes for finding interested and capable students to supply different categories of PA help. If you are currently employing student PAs from the local campus, these folks can be a big help in advising you on finding and using the following resources.

Many colleges have established a professional administrative office for the special needs of campus members with various disabilities. Popular titles for these offices include Disabled Student Services, Disability Services, Rehabilitation Services, or the Disabled Resource Office. Of all campus resources, this department should be the most helpful in answering your questions about where, when, and how either to advertise for PAs or to provide services as a PA. They should also be able to tell you about the current salary rate; some departments even attempt to sponsor a list of willing PAs, sometimes referred to as an "attendant roster." The help-provider registrants in attendant rosters tend to become unavailable within a few weeks, and in general, these lists are becoming nice ideas of the past.

The student newspaper at the campus is often the best way of advertising a PA job with students. Most campus papers welcome paid classified and display ads of any kind, regardless of whether you are a campus member. A phone call or Web visit to the paper's office can get prices, and ads can often be placed over the phone or the Web when payment is made by credit card. Salaried jobs are often best placed in the "Help Wanted" or "Employment" section, whereas ads for live-ins go under "Roommates," "For Rent," or "Housing."

Bulletin and notice boards on a campus are usually spread throughout residence halls (dormitories), dining halls (cafeterias), student lounges (such as that in the campus student center), academic buildings, and administrative buildings. Many of these cork boards have clearly printed limitations regarding the subject matter and size of notices that can be posted; violating notices are often torn down.

Campus buildings are often open to the public. You may wish to take a tour through some of the primary campus buildings to "case" the locations of bulletin boards and the type of notices displayed. With this advance information, make up your posters or notice cards of an appropriate type and size, and then return to the campus to put them in strategic places for maximum visibility. More detail on composing and strategically posting notices is found later in this chapter.

The student employment office of most campuses assists students in finding part-time jobs while they are students. This office is different from the career planning/placement office, which helps students with post-college careers, or the personnel office, which helps the college in recruiting faculty and staff for its own professional employment needs. The student employment office will often accept job announcements from both on- and off-campus employers. These announcements are usually posted on notice boards, filed in job notebooks, or posted on the Web that job-seeking students browse through each day. You should feel free to call a campus student employment office to inquire about their announcing your PA job.

There are usually many student clubs and organizations at any campus. It may take some inquiry from insiders, but locating certain types of clubs can be very useful in spreading the word about your PA needs. Groups with a medical concentration are often centered around academic majors in physical therapy, occupational therapy, rehabilitation counseling, nursing, or pre-med. These students can be especially good candidates for PA jobs, because they value the career-related experience.

You can often locate these groups by calling the student program office that coordinates and supervises all student clubs, by calling the academic department for a medical field and asking about its student club, or by directly contacting an actual club. Inquire about posting your job notice in that office, in the club's newsletter, and/or at the club's Web site, or having a member read your notice aloud at the club's next meeting.

Recruiting in the surrounding community

The community around you contains several categories of people who will probably be interested in PA work:

- Aides who are already employed in a local hospital or by home health aide agencies, and who would like extra money from a "moonlighting" job like yours

- Aides who are not employed by institutions or agencies because they prefer the self-employment freedom of directly contracting their services to private individuals like you

- Anyone else looking for a part-time job who is dependable, responsible, and inclined to do this kind of work.

Some such people will have medical training or considerable experience in performing PA duties, but most will have no experience. The vast majority of PAs you will hire will be inexperienced, although you will find them interested in learning while earning. There is a slight advantage to those with any degree of experience. The advantage is not in their actual training in medical procedures, but in their basic awareness of and comfort with the personal nature of the work. Remember that all PAs, experienced or not, will still depend on your instructions for providing the help you require.

A moonlighting aide is a nice find, but a rare one. It is probably a good idea not to advertise exclusively for them, but to have them among the people who answer your general "aide wanted" ad.

Initially, an inquiry from an experienced aide might seem to be a slam-dunk, done deal, to be accepted without question. However, take advice from those of us with hiring experience. Maintain your usual caution and follow the routine steps for screening. Regardless of the impressive employment references they spout out or impressive promises they make, there are both reputable aides and some very slick con artists. These applicants especially merit checking employment references. Always call two or three previous recipients of their help.

An ad in the local newspaper is usually the most effective way to reach the greatest number of community people. Posters in supermarkets and shopping malls rarely produce results.

Employment or home health aide agencies

Many communities have commercial employment agencies listed in the telephone Yellow Pages. These agencies, both public and private, function as brokers between people looking for jobs and employers offering jobs. General employment and temporary help agencies recruit many categories of workers, everyone from office secretaries to household handymen.

You should feel free to call a private employment agency to determine if it can help in finding either experienced aides or inexperienced-but-willing-to-learn folks to supply PA help. The agency would supply you with the names of people to interview, or arrange for interviews at their office. If you hire someone, you will receive billings from the agency and not from the person you hired.

Employment agencies should not be a high priority for you in recruiting PA help. Trained aides are more likely to register with a home health agency than with an employment agency. In fact, some employment agencies also operate a separate office that specializes as a home health aide agency. Both kinds of agencies will charge you an administrative fee in addition to the hourly salary paid to the aide. The home health aide agency might charge a higher fee; however, it will be responsible for screening, generically training, and scheduling the aides assigned to you; a general employment agency will not provide these services.

When you call, have a clear job description ready in case the agency requests it. In addition, you will be asked for the hourly salary you are willing to pay; be sure to ask about the schedule of fees that the agency additionally charges for its brokerage services. These employment agency or home health aide agency routes are usually the most costly ways of recruiting PAs.

Local medical facilities

Hospitals, rehabilitation centers, and nursing homes may have listings of home health aide agencies or individuals for hire, or they may provide a location where you can post your own recruiting notices.

These lists are used mainly by patients being discharged who will require assistance at home. However, hospitals are often willing to share these lists with anyone who needs assistance. If a facility does maintain lists of agencies or private aides, the lists are typically available from the facility's Office of Discharge Planning, Social Work, or a similar patient-service department.

Churches or civic organizations

Members of churches and community service groups will sometimes be interested in providing either volunteer respite help or paid PA work. Also inquire with one of "the flock" about the best way to post a bulletin board notice or newsletter ad, or have an announcement made at a meeting or gathering.

How to Advertise for Your Own PAs

Once you have identified your potential pool of PA applicants (your "fishing spot"), you need to find a way to attract them to your job offer and then motivate them to contact you for more details.

Using a few reliable tricks of the advertising trade, you too can find PA candidates through newspapers ads, college campus posting, and even the Internet. By making your ad appealing, you can increase the overall interest in your position, the number of applicants who contact you, and the eventual quality of your applicant pool. With more quality people making inquiries, you can be more selective during your screening process, and that means you can hire better PAs.

Secrets for attracting PAs to your ad or poster

First, let's review some basics used by expensive, professional ad agencies when they create spots for TV, magazines, and newspapers.

Picture yourself as someone looking for a job. You are flipping through the "Help Wanted" ads of today's paper or Web site, or checking out posters on a bulletin board. As you scan all the ads, you see two that offer PA jobs. You have never done PA work before, so you are reading the two ads to decide whether this kind of work might be interesting. Which of these sounds more attractive and friendly? To which would you apply first, and why?

```
Handicapped Needs Help Now
Part-time, must be flexible; state hours
available, reasons for wanting job, wage
desired, & references. Send resume to:
P.O. Box 297, Fonda, NY 12068.
```

Or

```
EARN $145 PER MONTH
for just 4 1/2 hours per week. Cool,
active guy in wheelchair needs help to
dress, shower, etc. M-W-F, 7-8:30 A.M.
Need help now, routine is easy, no
experience necessary. Please call Jim
today 583-1972.
```

The first ad is less appealing, in part, because it does not offer you any reason to want the job or to respond to the ad—sort of like fishing with a bare hook and no bait! It simply demands information from the reader, and gives the impression that the person who wrote the ad is very inflexible, demanding, uninteresting, and maybe even angry. The ad does not list any benefits; there is really no reason for you to respond. There seems to be no rush—maybe this is an old, ongoing ad. And is it easy to respond? Hardly. He wants you to go through the formality of mailing your resume. What's with this guy, anyway?

The much more attractive ad is the second one. That ad will probably get several responses. The individual who wrote it tried to make the ad, the job, and himself sound appealing and attractive to prospective PAs. He even sounds like a neat guy to work for, and you would be wise to call right away—it sounds like he will be filling the job right away.

The second ad illustrates several strategies on how to successfully convey basic job details, describe them in an interesting way, help the average reader feel qualified to do the work (and identify with doing the job), give the interested reader an impulse to act now, and provide an easy way for the reader to contact the sponsor. These basic strategies apply to most forms of advertising, including newspaper and Internet ads, posters, and index-card notices for bulletin boards.

It's a fact: Every day many companies and corporations waste advertising money on expensive ads that:

- fail to attract the desired type of customer, because the ad is in the wrong TV or radio slot, Internet Web site, magazine, newspaper, or newsletter

- are ignored by the target customers, because the ad's headline and text do not emphasize benefits that are attractive to those specific people

- make customers wonder what the job is about and lose their interest, because the job description is poorly written and important details are left out of the ad

- allow customers to put off responding and lose interest, because the ad does not urge the reader to act right away

- make it difficult for customers to contact the advertiser, because the contact information is confusing or requires too much effort and time.

To prevent losing good customers in those ways, here are six basic planning steps to think about before lifting a pen (or keyboard) to write your PA ad:

① Identify the types of people in your community who would be good help providers, and might be interested in doing your PA work.

These typically include college students, moonlighting aides who work for themselves or an agency, and working-age and retired people who might lack PA experience but be trainable.

② Identify the job benefits desired by these people that you can offer with your PA job. The most common benefits desired by college students, self-employed health aides, and mature adults are:

- an attractive, competitive salary, or the free room of a live-in position

- part-time hours
- interesting work that is not boring, or—for students— work that is related to their academic studies
- an interesting person to work for;
- work that gives the aide a sense of being important, needed, and appreciated
- job flexibility that enables time off for leisure activities, exam crunches, child care, and holidays
- a job location close to their residence.

③ Identify ways to advertise to the target people. Which newspapers, newsletters, job posting areas on bulletin boards, or Internet areas do these specific people read?

College students most often read the campus paper; others usually read a community-wide paper. If your city publishes several community papers, find out which one has the largest circulation, the best reputation for the best classifieds, and is read by the educated, capable people whom you want as aides. Given the choice, would you reach your desired reader from the community's well-respected, traditional paper (with ads that are a bit more expensive), or a "thrifty-nickel" or "penny-saver" rag that has less expensive ads and is circulated for free to readers?

In addition to traditional newspapers, college campuses and municipal communities are using the Internet to promote special-interest groups. These groups have traditionally printed periodic newsletters, and those newsletters are now increasingly being posted on group Web sites. Ask around, do some Web surfing, and find out which campus or community groups sponsor sites that could list your PA jobs or live-in positions. As yet another alternative, the buildings of colleges and health care facilities usually feature many kinds of hallway cork boards for tacking up posters and index-card notices. This chapter also provides strategies for creating eye-catching cork-board ads.

> *The golden rule for attracting PAs to your ads: Identify what benefits the potential PAs want, and then stress those job benefits in your ad's headline and lead line.*

④ Write your ad copy, following the five-part form listed later in this section.

⑤ When your ad or poster copy is complete, make sure its layout follows an easy-to-read format.

⑥ Get your ad posted, and be ready to receive inquiries from people who want to be your next PA!

How-to strategies for each of these steps are coming up in this chapter. However, before getting into details, let's check out a few concepts of marketing and advertising with a story told at a professional seminar for advertising agencies. The lecturer told us a story about her personal love for chocolate-covered ice cream bars.

> *I want to tell you how very much I love the taste of ice cream bars with that crunchy chocolate coating. You could even get me to go to my in-laws' for dinner if you promised me an ice cream bar for dessert. There are a lot of people like me who have a deep-seated passion for those things.*
>
> *In my spare time, I like to fish for trout and bass. When I was a kid, I figured that since I loved ice cream bars, the fish would also. I actually tried fishing with one on my hook one time and, of course, didn't attract any fish. Because to attract fish, you have to picture yourself as a fish for a moment and ask yourself, 'What food would attract me to risk getting caught on a fisherman's hook?' The answer is 'worms,' and you must use worms to attract a fish regardless of whether worms would appeal to you. The same lesson applies to how we word advertisements in order to attract customers to buy a product.*

The story emphasizes how important carefully chosen benefits are to attracting your aide applicants.

How do you put these benefits into an ad? What other details are important? Here is the classic, five-part, time-proven formula of essential elements for structuring an ad, poster, or index-card notice:

- **The attractive headline.** Use the most attractive benefit, or a title that describes the job, or a desirable type of applicant.
- **The lead line.** Provide more detail about the attractive benefits and introduce the type of job.
- **The brief job description.** Let the reader know a few details of what will have to be done.
- **The sense of urgency.** Tell them to apply now!
- **The contact details.** How do they reach you? Make it easy and fast, while protecting your privacy.

As your author, I have enjoyed putting these five parts together to create many different ads over the years. Of those, the following actual ad is one of my favorites, and has ben very successful. I have used it in both campus and community newspapers.

> **$9 for Help to Man with Disability**
> Get experience working with a
> disability. Cool, active guy who uses
> wheelchair needs help with living
> activities, 6-8 hrs weekly. Just 10 min
> from campus (car required), routine
> easy to learn. Needed now. Call Skip
> today & lv message, 555-3721.

The attractive headline. Professional advertising firms usually agree that the most important part of the entire commercial ad is the headline. If the headline does not hook readers, they won't read the rest of the ad. You will have lost them.

In your ad, poster, or index-card notice, this means catching the eye of prospects who are casually scanning an entire bulletin board full of notices (or the crowded classified ad page of a newspaper or Net bulletin board). It's a fact: Your headline has about one second to "hook and hold" the quickly scanning reader.

A general, dull heading of "Help Wanted," "Job," or "Handicapped Needs Help" will hardly be attractive enough to hook the reader or to differentiate your job from all the others in the "help wanted" area. Some readers will, indeed, be looking for a PA-like job, and will stop to read your ad only if its headline describes either a PA-type job or benefits that typical PAs want.

What makes the most powerful, magnetic headline? In simple terms, it states something the reader wants or needs—a benefit. The most common benefits sought by the type of person interested in PA work are a salary, a free room, or the experience in working with someone with a disability. If you will be advertising on a college campus, I strongly recommend a headline-and-lead-line combination that shouts salary plus disability experience. Career-related experience is often very attractive to a pre-med or therapy student. In addition, your offering the opportunity to work with someone with a disability attracts high-quality people who simply enjoy helping others.

Three categories of successful headlines that have actually worked in PA ads include the following:

General headlines. These bring the greatest number of inquiries, but require more screening from you to get to desirable applicants:

- Weekly Salary
- Earn $80 Per Month
- Earn $ Now
- Free Furn Apt
- Free Balcony Apt
- Free Apt & Utils

Job-specific headlines. These attract people specifically interested in aide-type work, especially med-oriented college students as well as aides who are either self employed or agency-employed and looking to moonlight in addition to their agency work:

- $$$ Help Man with Disability
- Help Woman with Disability
- Live-in Help to Disabled Man
- Salary for Help to Disabled Woman

Applicant-specific headlines. These are even more specific in attracting the people who are described (identify with) by the job-related titles; however, be careful not to be too specific:

- Home Health Aide
- Caregiver
- Personal Assistant
- Household Help
- Companion to Senior Citizen
- Nursing Student
- Pre-med Student

For any of these three types of headlines, the readers are briefly hooked and prompted to read further. Consequently, they step up to the ad or poster to get a closer look at the details. They read the rest of the ad to learn how to take advantage of the attractive benefits stated in the heading.

The lead line. After the large-print headline is the lead line. This is the first line or two of the ad's text, and includes details about additional benefits. Here the readers find more detail about the sweet deal promised in the heading, and they further develop an interest in the offer. There is purposely no mention yet of any obligation, only more details about benefits.

Later in this chapter, you will find many examples of ads and notices. In each example you will first find a successful headline. Right after the headline is the lead line, with more details about the benefit stated in the headline. Depending on the amount of space available for ad copy, the lead-line section might consist of a single phrase or several sentences.

The rate for a newspaper ad is based on the length of the ad. To save money, you might be tempted to omit the lead line and shorten the ad as much as possible. Remember: Do not make your ad so short that it is not effective. Run a longer, attractive ad a few times and be successful, instead of running a short, dull ad many times with no success.

The brief job description. This section is very brief, merely sketching out the "what, where, when, and how often" of what you want done. It should be fair and not sugarcoated, but its tone should continue to be pleasing and not harsh.

In a way, the ad's brief job description is the first step for screening readers. It should screen out people who are not interested in this type of work, as well as those who are put off by the schedule and residence location you specify. If this section is too vague, you will be answering unnecessary phone inquiries. For more examples of how this works, check out the sample ads later in this chapter.

The sense of urgency. Most TV, radio, and print ads try to create a sense of urgency so that the viewer, listener, or reader will "act fast" on the offer. In ads for merchandise, some examples include "Act Today," "This is a limited time offer," "Sale Ends Wednesday," or "Come in today, when this supply is gone… it's gone forever… do not be left out."

For PA recruiting, this "hard sell" might be too strong. More realistic examples would include "Help needed now," "Immediate need," "Call today for details," or, if part of your offer includes housing, "This apt will go fast." The objective is to get readers to move quickly to take advantage of the ad while they have the interest and consequent impulse. The "sense of urgency" phrase usually goes between the job description and the contact information.

The contact details. The most alluring, attractive ad is useless if information is not provided for contacting the ad's sponsor. The contact info should enable readers to quickly and easily take advantage of the offer while their interest is at a peak.

You have several choices in ways for a potential PA to contact you. The key is to make it quick and easy for readers to act on their impulse. At the same time, you also want to protect your privacy and the security of your possessions.

Do not *ever, ever* publish your last name, street address, or any other data that would enable an undesirable person to find out where you live. This very serious caution is addressed not only to women, but to anyone with (or without) a disability. There are drug addicts who want your prescription meds, thieves who want your expensive medical equipment, and other unpleasant people whom you have no desire to meet in the middle of the night. Protect your privacy when writing ads.

The best way is the easiest for the PA: by phone. If several folks use the phone number listed in the ad, you may wish to also list the first name of the individual who can answer questions. Brief the other people at your phone number about the importance of writing down names and phone numbers of ad respondents who might call in your absence.

You might be tempted to offer your e-mail address for inquiries. I would instead suggest, whenever possible, that you offer a phone number that will record calls on an answering machine or phone company voice mail.[3] There are considerable advantages in listening to and comparing the voices of callers, including your ability to evaluate both what is said and the caller's attitude behind how it is said.

However, if you are in a shared-phone residence, and you have concerns that roommates might lose messages, take inaccurate messages, or even somehow offend callers, then you might consider listing either a friend's phone or your e-mail address.

---

3. As discussed in chapter 📖 7, "Ten Steps to Getting All or Some of Your Help from Personally Employed Aides," your recording all ad inquiries will make screening the applicants much easier.

Newspaper, newsletter, and internet ads

A classified or display advertisement in a newspaper or at an organization's Web site can be very cost-effective. In addition to appearing on the printed page, many college campuses and other communities are sponsoring bulletin boards in cyberspace for posting notices.

By "cost-effective" we mean that you should consider two factors: the price of the ad and the number of potential PAs who can be reached by the ad. The paid ad might at first seem expensive, but it might provide you with the greatest number of responses for your costs in terms of money, time, and effort. If we divide the price of the ad by the number of people who read it, the "cost per PA inquiry" is usually very inexpensive.

For example, a newspaper or Internet ad that is run for five days in a large city might cost $50. If that ad is effectively worded and gets you 25 inquiries, then the "cost per inquiry" is just $2. Please also note that the $50 is probably deductible on your personal income taxes as a medically related expense. In addition, placing an ad is easier for you than creating, reproducing, and posting notices and posters.

Newsletters can also be effective ways of reaching the right kind of applicant. Check the local college campus or general community for clubs or organizations geared toward medical people. The drawback of newsletters is that they are less frequently published and often published on a sporadic schedule. You may submit an ad or notice to a newsletter and find that it is not published quickly enough to be of benefit to your time-sensitive need for help. The good news for you is that printed and mailed special-interest newsletters are rapidly being replaced by notices posted at group Web sites.

You can use newspaper or Internet ads to recruit PAs in the locale where you now live, as well as in a distant area to which you will soon be moving. You might find it necessary to move to a new part of the same city or even across the country because of changes in school, work, health, or vacation sites. When you are dependent upon PA help, sometimes it is essential to recruit help in advance of moving so that a new PA is hired and available when you arrive.

With a newspaper or Internet ad, a PA can be successfully recruited, interviewed, and hired—sight unseen—even from 3,000 miles away! The first step in long-distance hiring is to call ahead to the school you will attend, to a contact you have at your new place of work, or to any other contact in the new locale. Ask for the name and phone number of the one or two most widely read campus or community newspapers. Call that paper's classified ad office and explain that you would like details for placing an ad by phone.

This information is also usually available on the Web. On the Web, you can secure the details and specifications about placing printed ads in a college campus or community newspaper, or indeed, about placing an on-screen ad at an appropriate Web listing.

For approaching papers in a traditional way, sometimes it is helpful to get a recent issue to research the details, deadlines, rates, and forms of payment they will accept. Ask the particular newspaper about any discount they might offer with certain types or frequency of ads purchased. Also ask about which days of the week have the most and least number of readers. Thursday, Friday, Saturday, and Sunday are usually the days of heaviest readership for daily papers.

Some people are satisfied with simply dictating the contents of their ad over the phone, telling the clerk which dates the ad should run, and then finding out the price. Other folks prefer to write out their ad and experiment with attractive layouts that can be phoned, faxed, or e-mailed to the newspaper. Orders can usually be paid by credit card.

Of course, if you find an appropriate Web site through a search engine or word of mouth, getting your ad up and running is even easier and faster. The sites will post their own schedules and rates, and they usually employ essentially the same basics that have long been used by newspapers.

There are three basic layouts for ads: classified ads, display ads, and boxed classifieds.

Classified ads are the familiar ones that run, one after another, on newspaper pages. They are called "classified," because the newspaper organizes them into alphabetical classes or categories for easy reference. Examples include Apartments, Automotive, Employment, Help Wanted, and so on. The format for the text is usually a running series of phrases and sentences. Classified ads are usually billed by the number of words in your message, and they look like this:

Help Woman with Disability
$9/hr on campus, hours flexible to fit your schedule; female wheelchair student in SIU dorm seeks help in Tappan Hall with personal needs; immediate need; write Bx 110 c/o The Campus Times.

Live-in Help to Man with Disability
$8.50/hr at West Campus dorms this fall; male whlchr student will need help at Shelton Hall with living activities; mature M or F apply by 8/15; write Jim, Bx 403, Johnstown, NY 12069.

HOME HEALTH AIDE
Earn $8 w/flexible hours in Fonda; help senior in her home w/bathing, laundry, cleaning; please apply soon. Betty, 835-8562

FREE FURN APT
Boston in classic Back Bay, near campus, v-modern w/full kit & 2 bdrms; share in return for live-in help to male professor in whlchr (2-3 hrs/day); mature M only, need now; call Steve aft 6pm, 553-5354.

HEALTH AIDE
Earn $8 plus private room in farmhouse,
home-cooked meals, just 20 min from
downtown Omaha. Farm family needs
pm help to senior male parent. Flexible
schedule, 4 days weekly, will train.
Needed now, please; call Martha and lv
message. 555-3219.

Display ads are usually surrounded by a boxed border. The format inside the box can be anything you want it to be. It can look like a line-after-line classified ad, or you can include artistic headlines, logos, drawings, and photos like a poster. Display ads can take up an entire page, to sell cars or supermarket food, or they can be the smaller ads used by movie theaters and pizza joints.

You can sometimes get your display ad put in the classified section. However, displays are usually more expensive than a boxed classified of the same size. Display ads are usually sold by size, by the "column inch."

HELP WOMAN WITH DISABILITY

✔ **$8 hourly**
✔ **On campus**
✔ **Flexible hours to fit your schedule**

Female wheelchair student at SIU seeks help in Pierce Hall with personal needs; routine is easy to learn; immediate need; write Bx 110 c/o The Campus Times.

The third alternative, the **boxed classified**, is a sort of hybrid that combines a classified with a boxed border. This ad is run in the classified section, but its boxed structure makes it stick out in the crowd. You could say they are like a boxed display ad with only text (and not graphics) inside. This box, like a bold-printed headline, draws more attention to your ad. You will probably be billed for a classified ad (by word count) plus a bit extra for the border and bold headline.

Help Woman with Disability
$8/hr on campus, hours flexible to fit
your schedule; female wheelchair
student in SIU dorm seeks help in
Tappan Hall with personal needs;
immediate need; write Bx 110 c/o The
Campus Times.

Live-in Help to Man with Disability
$7.50/hr at West Campus dorms this
fall; male whlchr student will need
help at Shelton Hall with living
activities; mature M or F apply by
8/15; write Jim, Bx 403, Johnstown,
NY 12069.

HOME HEALTH AIDE
Earn $8 w/flexible hours in Fonda;
help senior in her home w/bathing,
laundry, cleaning; please apply soon.
Betty, 835-8562

My suggestion is to write out your ad and get it to the newspaper by fax, e-mail, or dictating it over the phone. Of course, bringing in a handwritten copy is also an option! Printing the ad on your computer ahead of time lets you experiment with the headline and wording. A bold-headline, boxed classified can be very effective in getting your ad noticed within a page of others. If the paper will not allow that, at least be sure your ad has a bold headline.

Bulletin board posters and index cards

A truly inexpensive way to advertise your own PA job is by putting up posters or index-card notices in areas frequented by people who might be interested in a PA job. These areas include college campuses, medical facilities, and, much less successfully, community bulletin boards found in supermarkets and other general public places. Not only can posted notices be less expensive than newspaper ads, but in some places they can be much faster in getting results. If you are in a crisis and must "speed-recruit" a new PA in a matter of hours—even before the next newspaper comes out—then a mess of posters might do the job.

Here is a true story of mine to show you how quickly you can recruit a replacement PA when necessary.

> *When I was an undergrad college student, I lived in a dorm room.
> I had arranged through the housing office to have my student aide
> as my roommate. One morning during the turbulent '60s, my
> roommate-aide suddenly informed me that he had decided to pack
> his belongings, load his car, and move to Canada that same day. He
> wished me luck in finding a new aide.*

It was 6 A.M., he was wired, and I was still in bed. He went to the wall phone in our room, lifted the receiver, and told me that he didn't have time to get me up. He further informed me that he would make one phone call for me. I quickly went into a calming "psychologist mode" and talked him into getting me dressed and out of bed.

At 7:30, as he headed for his '64 Mustang and the Canadian border, I rushed to create a poster master on my typewriter (remember typewriters?). I then wheeled to the nearest campus copy machine, made photocopies, and hand-lettered colored headlines with a marker pen on each poster copy.

I offered a six-pack of beer to a dorm buddy if he would help me put up my posters. We walked through the 11 nearby residence halls, and he stapled a poster to each floor's cork board.

I was a 19-year-old quad and sophomore, and in a survival frame of mind. This was all accomplished by noon. I then baby-sat my room phone to receive replies, and had a replacement hired and moved in by that evening. Ah, the power of positive thinking!

The objective of posting any notice is to maximize the number of applications you receive, by increasing the chances that many people will read the notice. Here are some advertising strategies that I used in my true story, and that have been proven by others to get your poster noticed.

Make your poster colorful, attractive, and easy to read

Choose paper colors, print colors, headings, and an overall design that will attract readers and make your message easy to read quickly. The next time you pass by a crowded bulletin board, take a moment to see which posters stand out from the others and, in contrast, which ones blend together and are difficult to find. The following features make posters and index-card notices more vivid.

Bright-colored paper. Poster cardboard, computer and photocopy paper, and index cards all come in a wide variety of bright colors, usually at little or no additional cost over plain white. Choose a color that is bright and yet sufficiently light to show black or dark-colored printing.

Wide, dark headings of sufficient size. If, for example, you have chosen a bright yellow paper, consider a large heading clearly printed with a red marker pen. The headline should be clearly printed (avoid script or fancy calligraphy), and in sufficiently wide and tall letters to be seen from at least six feet away. Avoid letters that are the skinny width of pencil or pen. For lettering, use a color of ink that contrasts—loudly clashes—with the light color of your poster paper. For example, avoid using a dark-blue marker heading on a blue paper. Never use yellow or a similar light, faint color for any lettering.

Of course, the quicker alternative to hand-lettering a colored headline is to use a computer. Choose a sans-serif font (like Helvetica or Universe) for headlines; use serif fonts (like Times) for the poster body. Sans-serif letters are plainer and easier to read at a distance for short headlines. However, serif letters—like the text of this book—make the longer text of the body of your poster easier to read.

Neatly lettered body. After the large heading, the body of the poster should be neatly lettered. The main body should not be handwritten unless the handwriting is exceptionally neat and clear. On a computer, consider 14- or 16-point type size and a typeface such as Times. Details are easily read when they are broken up into several separate phrases, sentences, or paragraphs. Prefacing each item with a graphic number ❹ , bullet (•), or symbol (✔) helps to emphasize it (see the poster example).

Think "utility," not "art contest." The purpose of a poster is to sell someone on being your PA, not to win an art contest. A poster can be artistic and attractive as long as it is easily and quickly readable and does its job. If readers step up to the poster or card and find the message difficult to read, they will quit and walk on.

Follow these steps for quickly making a quantity of posters

- When you need a quantity of posters in a hurry, start by making a clear master by hand or on a typewriter or computer. The large, preprinted headline can be included on the master, or a space can be left for hand-lettering a headline on each poster copy with a bright-colored marker.

- Along the poster bottom, write several tear tabs with your phone number and first name. These should be lettered sideways (see the poster example). These tabs will make it easy for someone who is interested in your PA job to rip off a tab and call you later. The unfortunate alternative is the reader taking your entire poster just for its phone number or inaccurately copying your phone number. Be sure to include your name and even a phrase like "PA JOB" with your phone number on each tear tab; otherwise, a reader could later find a tear tab with only a phone number in his pocket and forget its purpose.

- Make copies on a photocopier or computer printer using bright-colored paper such as yellow, orange, pink, or lime green.

- For each poster copy, use scissors to cut slits between each of the contact-information tear tabs along the bottom edge.

- Put up the posters in effective locations with a stapler, as discussed in the subsections.

Choose posting areas or bulletin boards that have a reputation for being read routinely by many people

If the building where you wish to post a notice offers only one or two bulletin boards, you will not have much problem choosing which boards to use. However, you might be advertising your PA position on a college campus or in an entire community where a hundred or more boards might be available. In that case, it is wise to decide which locations have the most marketing potential.

Instead of advertising throughout an entire campus or community, identify the boards that are read primarily by a specific type of person. For example, if your college offers a nursing program and you believe nursing students would make good PAs, then find a bulletin board they are likely to read. This might be in the hallway of the building where nursing classes are held, or in the residence hall where nursing students live.

In addition, choose boards in areas where people stand or sit to wait for something. A hallway or lobby area where people wait for elevator cars to arrive, inside the elevator car where people ride, along a cafeteria line, or in a lounge or reception area are good places. When folks have to pass time in an area, they tend to be bored and will read anything they can find—especially attractive notices about benefits that they need. As another strategy, choose boards that directly face people who walk by, sit, or wait in line.

Honor restrictions regarding posting notices and posters

When information is to be posted on a bulletin board on a college campus, personnel office, shopping mall, supermarket, or similar area, sometimes there are clearly printed restrictions regarding the type of notice and its size. If the posting area is small, posters are often not allowed and notices must be printed on index cards. There might also be restrictions regarding the type of messages permitted to be posted, such as "Ride Notices Only," "Housing Notices Only," or "Psychology Department News Only." The sponsor of a board may even require that all notices be taken to a specific office to receive an approval stamp. If any of these restrictions are in effect where you wish to post notices, it is wise to honor the restrictions or your notice might soon be torn down.

Locate your poster or notice card so it can be seen easily

Your message will be read by more people if it is not lost within a sea of other notices on a crowded cork board. "Bulletin board ethics" hold that removing other notices is okay if they have expired. To make space for your notice, you may remove other notices announcing events that have already occurred. Additionally, your poster should be mounted without covering that of someone else. Try to clear sufficient space so that at least a half-inch border of clean bulletin board appears on all sides of your poster; it will stand out better in the crowd.

When mounting posters or index cards, bring a stapler

Mount your notices securely on the cork boards. Bring a loaded stapler and staple your poster in each of the four corners. Do not use tape or thumbtacks to mount your posters. If the next guy wants to mount his notice and hasn't brought a tack or stapler, he might be tempted to tear down your notice in order to use your thumbtack. He might also remove your thumbtack, cover your notice with his, and replace the tack through both notices without yours showing. It happens often.

Figures 8-1 and *8-2* show examples of effective posters and bulletin board notices.

Figure 8-1: **Sample poster**

FREE FURNISHED APARTMENT

• Boston, in classic Coolidge Corner, within qtr block of Beacon trolley stop

• Very modern, full kitchen, 8th floor, north & west balcony views

• Share in return for live-in help to working, college-age male of wheelchair mobility (2-3 hrs/day)

• Mature males only, non-smoking, no drugs

• No experience necessary – Needed right away!!!

Please call Earl after 6pm for details, 277-7033

| Earl after 6pm 277-7033 | Earl after 6pm 277-7033 | Earl after 6pm 277-7033 | Earl after 6pm 277-7033 | Earl after 6pm 277-7033 | Earl after 6pm 277-7033 | Earl after 6pm 277-7033 | Earl after 6pm 277-7033 |

(Make vertical cuts between tear tabs)

Figure 8-2: **Sample index-card notice**

$160 per Month - Help Woman in Wheelchair

- $9 per hour for interesting & appreciated work

- Just 5 hours each week—M-W-F, 7-8:30 a.m.

- We live just 5 mins from downtown Seattle

- Mature, dependable female, please

- No experience necessary

- Help needed now, please

- Call Candice, leave message if not in—555-6038

(Message is typed onto a bright-colored index card)

Chapter 9
Initial Training and Ongoing Management of Aides and PAs

Why is it important for you, or someone you trust, to train and manage the PAs you use?

To *manage* is to "supervise, take charge of, or control." It is very important that you be in control of the activities, schedule, and quality of your daily lifestyle—doing what you want to do, when you want to, and in the way you want to.

Because you are dependent on help from others, it is important that you maintain a feeling of control within yourself, an image of control in the eyes of your PAs, and the function of control in accomplishing your lifestyle. The first speaks to the importance to yourself of your sense of empowerment; the second addresses the importance to your PAs of your image or appearance of knowing what you need and how to accomplish it; and the third underscores the importance of your actually being in control as a way of achieving your chosen lifestyle.

Someone must make these decisions, direct and instruct PAs in providing help, and consequently be in control of your lifestyle. If you do not make these decisions, your PAs will, and consequently they could control your lifestyle!

Sometimes having someone else make these decisions and manage the assistants who give help is both necessary and desirable. These are the times when the help recipient is either unable or unwilling to make decisions and be in control. In these cases, that "someone else" must be very carefully chosen, so that he or she will accurately represent and conscientiously maintain your lifestyle. It can be a family member, a managing coordinator from among your PAs, a home health aide agency supervisor, or the staff at a residence care facility.

Sometimes the people in charge are the aides or PAs themselves. Many ethical and caring aides succeed in looking out for the best interests of the help recipient. In contrast, other aides take unfair advantage of the situation. Here the people providing help are also deciding how and when it should be provided. When used to unfair advantage, this conflict of interest is the same as the old adage: of "putting the fox in charge of the henhouse." As illogical as that sounds, your PAs will be in control of, and managing, your lifestyle—sometimes more for their interests than for yours—unless you, or someone else you select, effectively manages them.

These training and management principles universally apply to all categories of providers. For regardless of the type of provider, and their degree of training and experience, each will greet you on your first work day by saying, "Hello, I am Sam. I will be glad to help you as soon as you tell me what help you need, as well as how and when you need it."

At that moment, aide after aide, year after year, you or your trusted representative becomes a trainer and manager.

There are four primary factors to training and managing PAs. First, you should use the qualities and strategies of a good manager. Second, you should make decisions about who helps you, what help they provide, how the help is provided, and when the help is provided. Third, follow the three-step training method explained below, and provide clear initial training instructions. Finally, provide each PA with good ongoing management and appreciation.

> *Just as a building contractor requires blueprints before hiring carpenters and ordering lumber, you should organize your needs for assistance before trying to hire, train, and manage PAs.*

Use the qualities and strategies of a good manager

Being a good trainer and manager is perhaps 50 percent preparation before the first PA begins to assist you, and 50 percent good day-to-day training and management practices.

To help you prepare to be a good manager, you might want to review the main points of these chapters. You might either take a block of time to formally study them, or take three minutes now just to read through this list of topics. A quick read-through will assure you that these topics are discussed in this reference book, and are readily available for your on-the-spot referencing when specific problems occur in the future.

- Respecting the human rights that apply to both you and the help providers, chapter 📖 **22 "A Bill of Rights for You as a Help Recipient, Caregiver, or Paid Provider."**

- Understanding and respecting the personal concerns of three types of help recipients and providers, chapters 📖 **23 "Your Personal Concerns as a Help Recipient,"** 📖 **24 "Your Personal Concerns as a Family Caregiver,"** and 📖 **25 "Your Personal Concerns as a Paid Help Provider, plus Ten Reasons Why PAs Quit and Are Fired."**

- Knowing how to find and appropriately use PA help in various settings, chapter 📖 4 **"Settings Where You Use Help."**

- Knowing about the different types of PA help that are available, and your role in using each type, chapter 📖 1 **"Beyond Family Caregivers: Options and Settings for Finding Outside Assistance."**

- Using the qualities and strategies of a good manager, chapter 📖 15 **"Your Qualities and Strategies as a Good PA Manager."**

- Using an assertive communication style and avoiding styles that are weakly passive or abusively aggressive, chapter 📖 14 **"Say It, Ask for It, and Act—Assertively!"**

- Providing a pleasant, work-efficient environment with adequate supplies, chapter 📖 17 **"Setting Up Efficient Work Areas and Maintaining Adequate Supplies."**

Make decisions

It is important for you to decide what help you need and how PAs will provide it before you attempt to recruit, interview, and train them. As discussed earlier in this chapter, you—or someone close to you, whom you trust—should make these decisions so that you stay in control of your lifestyle.

Make decisions about the following:

- Who helps you—choose quality PAs who are honest, reliable, responsible, and able to provide you with quality help.

- What help you need—provide a list of specific tasks necessary for your chosen lifestyle.

- How that help is provided—tell PAs how you prefer that help be provided so your specific needs are accommodated.

- When the help is provided—give PAs clear time guidelines for your daily schedule of when you need help.

To help you identify your needs for assistance and how that assistance should be provided, you might want to review these topics and chapters:

- How to avoid abusing PAs with inappropriate requests for help, 📖 11 **"When It Is, and Is Not, Okay to Ask for Help."**

- Making a master list and schedule of your needs for assistance, 📖 13 **"Defining and Describing Your Help Needs."**

- The advantages of employing several part-time PAs, 📖 16 **"Dividing Your Needs, and Assigning Work Shifts, Among Several PAs."**

- The power and importance of paying a kind of salary that costs you nothing—routinely expressing appreciation to PAs, chapter 📖 15 **"Your Qualities and Strategies as a Good PA Manager."**

Follow the three-step training method and provide clear initial training instructions

There are a number of factors that make teaching easier for you, and learning easier for the new PAs. If the training system cited here needs modification—especially to accommodate your limitations—you should feel free to do so.

> *Hannah's primary and secondary disabilities include her inability to speak detailed training descriptions. Diane, her mother and family caregiver—or a currently hired PA—would traditionally provide a training narration to each and every new PA.*
>
> *To save everyone's vocal cords, Hannah and her Mom enlisted technical help from friends in video taping Hannah's ADL routine on three 10-minute tapes. Newly hired PAs are asked to review the tapes at home and to arrive on the first day of live training with a headstart!*
>
> *When asked about the steps in inexpensively making one or more training tapes, I was advised to start by writing out a list of scenes to be taped. Next, the "speaking script" could be either very detailed or just a handwritten list of objectives. Finally, put a video camera on a tripod and have a family caregiver or quality PA demonstrate <u>what</u> needs to be done while narrating <u>how</u> to do it. Make, or have made, three or four copies for returnable handouts to the trainees.*

What follows is a simple, three-step process that will smooth the training transition and ensure that your new PAs become competent and confident providers of help. The main steps to training new PAs are:

- Schedule the new PAs to watch a current PA perform each part of your routine.

- Have the new PAs do the routine once (for the simpler tasks) or twice (for the more complex tasks) while a current PA stands by.

- Finish their training by having the new PAs work with you, while receiving your occasional reminders and lots of patience.

The first training step: The new PA observes you and a current PA

Begin by scheduling the new PAs to watch a current PA perform each part of your routine. This demonstration strategy saves you enormous time and energy. Each task that a current PA demonstrates truly is worth a thousand words for you. The alternative to having a current aide help with training is for you, alone, to attempt to describe each task and the way it should be performed. It is possible to train this way, but it is a tiring, inefficient method.

As years go by, and your routine becomes increasingly detailed, this strategy becomes increasingly important to both you and each new aide. For you, as your routine becomes more complex, an attempt to describe and train on each detail by yourself would become truly exhausting. As you become tired—and consequently uptight—the training process for both you and the new PA turns into a less-than-enjoyable process. It is not uncommon for a new aide to resign during training if the process becomes sufficiently stressful. So although you will briefly be paying two salaries—for the current and the new aides—during training, the multiple advantages make the extra cost worthwhile.

If you already employ more than one part-time PA, be careful in selecting which one to use, during early interviews and demonstrations as well as during these post-hiring demonstrations and training. Choose a current aide who has the personal qualities and work habits closest to those that you want the new people to adopt. The new folks will tend to model what they see in the current PA.

The new PAs will learn more quickly when parts of the three-step training are held close together, perhaps within a seven- to ten-day period. If the sessions are spread further apart, the new aides will tend to forget, and thus need to relearn, some details.

Please note that this demo step can be skipped for any part of your routine that was demonstrated a few days ago when this new PA interviewed with you. If you are following chapter 📖 **7, "Ten Steps to Getting All or Some of Your Help from Personally Employed Aides,"** you will have already conducted an interview and demo of your routine with each applicant. It is not necessary now to repeat the demo for any part of your routine that this new PA saw then.

The second training step: The new PA performs with you and a current PA
Next, have the new PAs do the routine once (for the simpler tasks) or twice (for the more complex tasks) while a current PA stands by. As the current aide initially demonstrates the routine, and later watches the new people, her primary role is to narrate what she is doing and how she is doing it. These are the parts that she knows best, and she can demonstrate and explain as she provides you help.

Your role during training is to fill in the part that you uniquely understand—the reasons why each "what and how" are important. Of course, you will also be supplying any details that are left out by your aide. Your preferences are very important to your independence and safety, and to saving everyone time and effort.

> *An already nervous, new aide*
> + *Unnecessary training stress*
> = *Bye, bye!*

Allow extra time for the completion of each part of your routine while new aides are learning. New PAs cannot be expected to be as efficient and fast as your veterans. The learning process requires extra schedule time, sometimes twice the usual allotment. A two-hour "veteran" routine can sometimes take a "newbie" up to three or four hours for the first one or two runs (although other new folks will be naturally quicker to catch on). Avoid training on tight-schedule mornings, and either start your routine earlier or count on staying longer. Please remember that new PAs who are struggling to learn the details of your routine are taking that extra learning time because they are afraid of doing something wrong and hurting you; they want to learn to do each task the right way, and want to please you. In return, be patient with them.

In allowing that extra learning time for new PAs, you are wise to delay bringing them up to speed on your usual schedule until they have pretty much mastered your routine. This is a new job, and new PAs are understandably nervous about memorizing all those hundreds of details, and then doing them correctly. Pushing new aides to perform faster before they are capable can be summarized in two words: stress and tension. It is not uncommon, when an already nervous new aide is pushed too fast and too soon, for that new PA to resign. You have invested a lot of money, time, and effort recruiting, interviewing, and hiring a new aide. It would be a shame to unnecessarily lose him or her halfway through training!

In addition to teaching aides tasks where you need physical help, instruct them about your other expectations. Be clear about when you want your PA to arrive each day and by what time you need to finish so that you, in turn, can meet your daily schedule of appointments, meetings, and activities. Again, aides will better remember your preferences if they understand the reasons why they are important to you.[1]

The third training step: The new PA begins working with you, alone

Finish the training by having the new PAs work directly with you, while receiving your occasional reminders and lots of patience.

Be yourself and be pleasant. Forget about thinking of yourself as a supervisor, boss, or employer who must command respect. Instead, think of the new PAs as friends who are probably quite nervous about the first few times of helping you. Think of them as teammates. They work not as much *for* you as *with* you.

Speak clearly and at a comfortable rate. New PAs cannot learn what they cannot hear. Give clear, logical instructions. Before you begin teaching, be sure your routine follows an order that is both logical and efficient for your aides to follow. Efficient means that the steps of the routine do not waste time or energy. In short, design the routine to get all your needs met while making the work as easy as possible for the provider.

Invite questions about anything that is not understood. Be consistent each time in the order of steps and the way each is performed. Do not allow PAs to perform a duty in a wrong way and begin bad habits. Do yourself and the PAs a favor: Insist that they do tasks correctly the first time, and politely tell them why your way is important.

As you provide initial training to new PAs, there is a fine boundary line between the stage where they are still learning and need instruction, and the sudden transition to where they have sufficiently learned the routine, prefer to independently generate their own "what's next" from memory, and actually resent your additional instruction. Let them do it as soon as they can—unless, of course, they forget a step of your routine. Then it's okay for you to remind them only of the forgotten step!

What advice is there to guide good PA managers among these gray boundaries?

After a new PA has performed your tasks once or twice, she will begin to remember the steps. As soon as you sense that she can do parts of the routine from her own memory, stop supplying her with the step-by-step training instructions.

---

1. For more detail about why your preferences are important, and how to convey that importance to help providers, please see chapter 📖 **12, "Getting It Done—Your Way!"**

She will learn more quickly and establish a firmer memory of the details when she is forced to use that memory. In contrast, you will foster her dependence on your instructions when you deny her the chance to work from her own memory.

In addition, most people enjoy being independent, working at their own speed, and working with a minimum of control and evaluative supervision from others. When a PA has learned your routine, she will usually resent unnecessary reminders from you.

However, you should not expect that any PA will remember every step of a routine without mistakes and memory lapses. The objective of training should not be perfect memorization. During the daily repetition of your routine, even the best PAs will occasionally and randomly space out what comes next. These tiny lapses in memory are to be expected several times in each work shift. None of your aides should be expected to flawlessly memorize the whole routine, although a rare few might delight you by doing so.

As the weeks pass and you go through each routine with a provider, be ready to fill in her memory lapses whenever necessary. She will unknowingly prompt you with any of three indicators:

- she pauses, and has obviously forgotten what comes next
- she starts to do the wrong task
- she asks you for a reminder of what comes next.

When you fill in a PA's memory lapse, provide her with only as much instruction as she needs to get back on track. If she is halfway through helping you get dressed, and spaces out "step 23," then remind her of just step 23. She probably will not need 21, 22, 24, 25, and 26—just 23.

However, if she is tired, not feeling well, nursing a hangover, or otherwise having a forgetful day, she might need more detailed reminders. There will be days when a PA simply forgets most of your routine. She is willing to help you, but her memory has turned into mush. Instead of single-step reminders, she will need a complete, step-by-step narration of the whole thing. Be patient; this tedious sort of day is rare and will pass.

During the initial training or "detailed reminder days," you might try providing groups of two or three steps at a time. Studies show that people can often remember data and follow steps that are packaged in groups of two, three, and four items. That is why phone numbers, (xxx) xxx-xxxx, social security numbers, xxx-xx-xxxx, and nine-digit postal Zip Codes (xxxxx-xxxx) are packaged in bite-sized groups.

As necessary, supply the next forgotten step of a task, or a reminder of the reasoning behind a forgotten preference. After running through your routine a few times with each new PA, the two of you will develop a rhythm—a dance. When you sense that your dancing partner has forgotten a step, provide as small a reminder as possible—one, sometimes two softly spoken words—that will get your partner back into step without interrupting the dance's rhythm. Your objective is not to reprimand, punish, or demonstrate your authority. It is simply to remind your partner of a forgotten step so you can continue dancing (here, "dancing" equates to your conversation, your both watching a TV program or listening to a CD, or your shared quiet time).

How subtle should the reminder be? When I am working with a current PA in providing a two-hour demo of my routine to three or four PA applicants, I might give my PA a dozen, one- or two-word reminders that are so subtle that none of the applicants ever notices. I can often carry on a conversation with an applicant, break off for a split second with a quiet reminder to my PA, and continue my applicant conversation without the applicant realizing what is happening. If the applicant hears anything, she might suspect that I took a second to clear my throat. That is how subtle reminders can be.

Why be subtle in bridging memory lapses? Your current PAs, as well as PA applicants, are typically nervous about making a mistake, doing something wrong, or forgetting details. The prime reason why these innocent mistakes make them nervous is their concern as to how you will react. You could get angry, show disappointment, and become frustrated—or show them that reasonable mistakes are a routine expectation and therefore not a big deal. The result is that your PAs will be more comfortable while working with you, and will want to keep the job longer. And that is one of your primary objectives as a first-class PA manager!

Be patient, tolerant, and understanding of mistakes. Mistakes and lapses of memory can be expected both during the learning period and afterward.

A bonus of this third training step is that it acts as an eighth screening step in your hiring process. With a rare, 1 or 2 percent of freshly hired PAs (with 1 in 50 or 100 new PAs), an eighth screening takes place during the first or second training session.

Here, your current PA appears on schedule, but the new aide does not. There are equal chances that the newbie has not yet adjusted to the new schedule, or has suddenly decided to quit when faced with the cold reality of the first actual work shift. If you follow the three-step training process, you are protected by having also scheduled a current aide for these initial shifts.

Provide good ongoing management and appreciation

Once you have hired and initially trained new PAs, you next begin their ongoing care and feeding. There are thousands of theories and books on managing employees. However, as a PA user and manager, most of what you need to know is summarized here.

Routinely show enthusiasm both when a PA arrives for work and leaves at the end of a shift. Greet her arrival with a smile, eye contact, and a happy "Hello." As she is about to leave at the end of a shift, tell her that you are looking forward to seeing her the next time. Each PA will quickly begin to associate arriving at work with feeling good. As several aides have told your author over the years, "I like coming here. You are usually glad to see me. I can be having a crummy day, but I look forward to coming here."

The greeting can be as simple as a ten-second smile and, "Hey, there's Megan. How is everything with you today?" As she is about to leave at the end of her shift, "Gee, Megs, thanks so much for your help tonight. I will look forward to seeing you on Thursday."

Routinely show appreciation when the help you receive merits it. Your expressing appreciation to PAs is a very effective way to keep them happy. Some volunteers are especially faithful and loyal to their duties for years, because of the appreciation they receive. Pay your PAs with both routine appreciation and a weekly salary.

Appreciation provides at least six advantages for you:

- it speeds the initial learning process
- it reinforces on-going, high quality work
- it keeps PAs happy and fuels their desire to keep your job longer
- it results in a closer relationship, increased trust, and more open communication between you and PAs so that you will better know about their concerns and problems, and be better able to resolve those that are work-related
- it prompts PAs to like you and show you appreciation in return
- it earns your PAs' respect and loyalty, for a better routine attendance record and a smoother transition when they eventually resign.

For detail about the importance and power of appreciation, as well as ways to effectively express it, see chapter 📖 **15, "Your Qualities and Strategies as a Good PA Manager."**

Routinely show sincere interest and caring for the personal issues and events that each PA considers important. The logic is simple and very powerful: If you care about what is important to your PAs, they will care about what is important to you. You need not become a therapist, but in normal conversation, find out about each PA's likes, dislikes, interests, hobbies, concerns, and birth date. During today's shift, discover at least one current concern or event for each PA. When greeting the PA's next arrival, simply ask about yesterday's concern. Then, during today's conversation, discover a new concern to ask about tomorrow. On their birthdays, be ready to hand them a birthday card—or better yet, a pint of Ben and Jerry's to bring home!

Routinely correct poor job performance and personal habits quickly. Do not let them become firmly established. Speak with the PA about problems in a clear, direct, assertive manner.[2]

Provide a minimum amount of supervision and reminders of task details. No employee likes unnecessarily tight and constant supervision while he is doing a good job. The best PAs remember tasks and complete them without being reminded. You can encourage this by supervising and reminding only when necessary, and by expressing appreciation to reinforce each good habit.

"Jeff, I would like to tell you how much I appreciate your remembering to water the plants on Monday and Thursdays. Thanks." You can probably bet money that Jeff will now take pride in remembering to water the plants, especially if you continue to thank him for it!

---

2. For detail about what is assertive communication, and how to use it to your advantage, please see chapter 📖 **14, "Say It, Ask for It, and Act—Assertively!"**

Respect an employee who states or shows that she no longer wants the job, and part ways with her in a manner appropriate to the situation.

It was once said that trying to keep a dying romance alive is like trying to re-heat and eat cold mashed potatoes. No matter how much you try, the results will not be what you had hoped for. The same holds true for trying to keep alive a failing PA relationship. If a PA wants out, respect her decision and begin planning with her to recruit a replacement and schedule her departure in a smooth transition.[3]

Of course, there is much more to the comprehensive skills of initial training and ongoing management than the brief outline presented here. Combine this information with the other chapter topics of this book, and you will have a solid foundation for efficiently training and effectively managing your PAs so you get a high quality of help, and keep it longer.

---

3. For discussions about how to recognize PA problems early on—and either remedy them and keep the PA, or prepare for the PA's departure—please see chapter 📖 10, "Recognizing and Resolving Your PA Problems, or Parting Ways."

Chapter 10

Recognizing and Resolving Your PA Problems, or Parting Ways

No paid provider is permanent. Each one will leave you eventually, either by resigning or being fired. Sooner or later, you will face the situation of replacing a current PA with a new one, and then parting ways with the current one (one hopes that it occurs in that order). This chapter will give you the skills to implement that smooth transition.

An aide's resignation causes two reactions: You feel and cope with several emotions, and then you recruit the PA's replacement and go on with life. There are several reasons why a trusted PA's departure often stirs more feelings of personal loss than would the resignation of an ordinary employee. However, this is not a time to react emotionally; instead, it is a time to rationally plan and survive. By concentrating on the positive action of recruiting a new PA, it is easier to cope with any negative emotions about losing the current one, and you promptly progress—as you must—toward getting your daily life and schedule back to normal.

At the time she was hired, she agreed to be with you for at least ten months. Great! The stress associated with your recurring RISHTMP cycle (the cycle of recruiting, interviewing, screening, hiring, training, managing, and parting ways) could again be put aside for almost a year, and you could get back to other, more fun things. Your built-in defenses relaxed as they do when the dentist tells you he is finished with the drilling stage of filling your tooth.

Then this morning, just two months after that hiring, she informed you of her need to leave you in just two weeks. Several emotions kicked into gear inside you; the dentist had suddenly picked up his drill again!

The emotions that you feel when a PA announces an early resignation can include anger, disappointment, depression, and uncertainty about having to gear up to go through another cycle. The feeling can be mild or severe, and equally affects new PA managers and seasoned veterans of many years.

If we recognize this feeling as chiefly a loss of a reliable source of help, then we can also recognize that the best strategy for minimizing the feeling is to have reliable replacement help trained and ready to arrive as the former help departs. The feeling of emptiness is considerably more severe if she was your one-and-only aide, and you have no immediate replacement lined up. We discuss the emotions associated with resignations in the second section of this chapter.

But for now, there is another side to the issue. Is there anything you could have done to prevent the resignation? In some cases, the answer clearly is "no." In many situations, through, problems can be identified and resolved at an early stage, long before they result in a sudden resignation or require a quick termination.

Keeping it together: Recognizing and resolving PA problems

Your PAs are an investment. You have spent a lot of time and effort to find them, screen them, hire them, and train them. Like any investment, you want to maximize your return, and that means keeping them as PAs for as long as possible.

But these are not stocks or bonds, they are people. They have needs and desires of their own, aside from the responsibilities they were hired to fulfill. They will have good days and bad days, both at home and at work, just like you. Like any good manager, you will have to be on the lookout for indications of upcoming trouble and take direct steps to address any problems. That way you can avoid unnecessary resignations or terminations, and the stress that accompanies them.

Signs of a healthy job relationship

It is easy to spot workers who are happy with their jobs. They seem to like the work, enjoy working for you, and have no personal problems that negatively affect work. They show this healthy relationship with work in the following ways:

- By arriving at, or a few minutes in advance of, the scheduled arrival time.
- By arriving with a reasonably pleasant attitude, being friendly, and often smiling at you.
- By showing interest in you and your concerns or well-being.
- By showing interest and pride in pleasing you by performing quality work for you. They ask how you prefer tasks to be done and then enjoy receiving your appreciation; they want to please you and are bothered when they are unable to do so.
- By being reasonably neat and clean in appearance.
- By working steadily and seeing duties through to completion.
- By remembering most details of the duties as well as your preferences as to the ways the details are performed.
- By speaking clearly and making good eye contact with you while performing many duties.
- By being willing to work until, and occasionally a bit beyond, the scheduled departure time.
- By often asking, when leaving, whether there is anything else they can do for you.
- By showing some degree of enthusiasm about seeing you next time.
- By faithfully calling you as much in advance as possible when they find that they will be late in arriving or will be unable to arrive at all.
- By never arriving under the influence of alcohol or drugs.

Signs of an unhealthy job relationship

It is often more difficult to spot workers who are unhappy with their jobs than those who are happy. The unhappy worker is often passive about expressing dissatisfaction. The dissatisfaction might arise from not liking the job or the employer, or from a personal problem that is completely unrelated to the job but does affect job performance. Unhappy campers show this unhealthy outlook in the following ways:

- By often arriving late, calling in sick, or just not showing up for scheduled work. They seem not to care about any negative consequences of their habits.

- By frequently arriving with an unpleasant or negative attitude, which can range from being unfriendly to arrogant or abusive toward you.

- By having little interest in you and your concerns or well-being, and seldom initiating (and often refusing) to participate in friendly discussion or conversation.

- By having very little interest or pride in performing high-quality work for you, and not caring whether you are pleased with the quality of their work.

- By often arriving with a sloppy appearance in clothing and personal grooming.

- By working slowly or sporadically with many rest periods and being easily distracted from work by your TV, magazines, use of your bathroom for prolonged times, or personal phone calls.

- By rushing to accomplish job duties, with details left unfinished, so they can leave early.

- By mumbling partial communications with you while avoiding eye contact and seemingly not wanting to be near you.

- By cutting duties short and attempting to leave before the scheduled departure time.

- By not caring enough to say "good-bye," and seeming to be bothered by the painful thought of the next scheduled work shift.

- By seeming to not care whether they arrive on time, and giving you no advance notice of expected lateness or inability to work.

- By arriving under the influence of drugs or alcohol.

Common reasons behind negative symptoms

These unhealthy job symptoms are outward signs of an inner problem. The problem may or may not be work-related, and may or may not be resolvable. Some common reasons for outward symptoms of an unhealthy relationship with the PA job can include the following:

- You failed—or at least are accused of failing—to provide a complete list of all the expected duties at the time the PA was hired, and you often add new, unexpected duties.

- You frequently change the listing of the duties or the order in which they are to be performed.

- You often change the expected arrival or departure times, and the duties frequently last beyond the scheduled departure time.

- You have poorly organized the work area and the duties often waste the PA's time and energy.

- You are overly critical of the PA's work, and fail to routinely pay the essential dual salary of appreciation and money.

- You communicate with a negative, aggressive attitude or engage in other poor employer practices detailed in other parts of this book.

- When you employ several PAs, you obviously play favorites by unfairly distributing the work load (or undesirable tasks) to one or two aides, or gossiping to one aide about another's personal problems.

- The PAs do not like the personal nature of the work.

- They dislike the continuous responsibility of the job.

- They dislike the hours or days of the job.

- The salary is inadequate for their needs.

- They dislike the commuting distance to the job.

- They lack the strength or stamina required for the job.

- They have developed new health or stamina problems.

- The job interferes with their other responsibilities or interests: personal, family problems, academic studies, career responsibilities, and so on.

- They have found another job that is more desirable: preferred days or hours, closer to home, higher salary, preferred type of work, or the like.

- They have performed the job for a short or long period, and have become tired of you or this type of work.

Steps for resolving problems and decreasing resignations

There are two primary avenues to take when significant problems are causing negative symptoms to appear:

- To avoid premature, early PA resignations by discussing their concerns and resolving the issues

- To prepare to replace them (by firing them or accepting their resignation) if the problem cannot be corrected and the symptoms are of a type or severity that cannot be tolerated by you or the PA.

If the PAs are good employees and you want to keep them longer, then watch for the first signs of unhealthy symptoms and take prompt action. Some steps include:

- Identify to yourself the unhealthy, negative symptoms the aide is showing.

- Ask yourself whether this seems to be a short-term personal problem that is not related to you or the job, or whether it is job-related and is therefore a valid concern to you.

- If the concern is personal and not related to you, empathize with the PA's feelings by telling her that you care. Be a good listener and prove that your support for the PA is not merely job-related. You will earn considerable respect and loyalty from many aides this way.

- In contrast, if the symptom seems to be related to a problem with you or the job, pick a good time to speak with your aide. Identify the symptom that you have recently noticed, remind the aide how important he or she is, and ask in a pleasant, helpful tone whether anything is wrong with which you can help.

- In either case, listen carefully to the response to determine what, if anything, you can do to assist in relieving the problem.

- If the problem is job-related, be sincere in wanting to make reasonable changes to improve the situation.

- Remember that some problems simply do not have solutions, and that you will not be able to save each PA situation. However, the action that you can always take is to be a good listener.

- When negative symptoms persist and seem not to be resolvable, start looking at your other current providers for their additional potential as temporary replacements in case the ailing aide must suddenly resign. If the ailing aide suddenly leaves, can your other aides fill in a few extra hours while you recruit a formal replacement, or will you be alone? The bottom-line question here is, "Do I have my needs covered, or am I headed for a crisis?" In either case, you are always wise to take early, positive, and constructive action to minimize any losses.

> *When you sense that PAs are feeling the weight of a problem, and you want to get them to open up, a classic phrase to consider is, "Candice, you don't seem to be yourself—is everything okay?"*

Do not rely on PAs to take the initiative to bring a problem to your attention and to propose possible remedies. As the PA manager, that is your job. Often, you will be able to spot the symptoms of a problem before the PAs realize that a problem exists, or before they have the courage to speak with you.

Remember that you are attempting to resolve the problem that is causing the negative symptom, and not to scold or punish the aides for showing negative symptoms. If you reprimand them for negative behavior, you are ignoring the reason behind the behavior. The source of dissatisfaction will still exist and will eventually require attention, perhaps after an unnecessary, early resignation.

Reducing resignations by taking preventative steps

There are at least four steps you can take to minimize being surprised by problems, or to minimize the effect of unavoidable resignations.

Stay close to your aides and their concerns

To minimize the opportunity for sudden departures, do your best to maintain open daily communication with PAs. Ways of communicating include the routine "small talk" of asking about the day-to-day personal events that are important to each aide. In addition, periodically ask about any problems or concerns that might, or might not, be job-related.

The strategy for getting inside the loop of some of each aide's concerns can be very simple. When Suzy arrives today for her PA shift, greet her with a reasonable smile and ask, "What's new?" In her answer will naturally be three or four topics, events, or personal concerns that are important to her. Whether or not you engage in a long conversation today, you should remember one or two of today's topics that were apparently important to her. Tomorrow when she again arrives, ask for an update on one or two of yesterday's topics—while remembering, in turn, today's topics for tomorrow's conversation. After a few days of your carrying on this conversational chain with aides, they will feel that you really care about what is important to them. They will care more about you and will begin to trust you. If their concerns start to include PA job concerns, you will soon hear the news because you have stayed in touch.

Your objectives in "staying in touch" with aides include increasing your ability to recognize job dissatisfaction early; to remedy problems before they prompt resignations; and consequently to avoid completely unforeseen, surprise resignations. Surprise resignations often occur during a PA's personal crisis, and sometimes mean that he must quit and leave right away, without time for you to first hire a replacement.

> *You will usually know—long before the PA does—that she is becoming dissatisfied with, or simply unable to continue, her job. Be observant and be a good listener.*

When an aide shows symptoms of discontent, but denies that anything is wrong, trust your intuition and be patient. It is not uncommon for you to recognize outward symptoms of either personal problems or job dissatisfaction before the PA does. Often your inquiry will prompt the aide to do some soul-searching and subsequently identify the source of the symptoms you have observed. Keep showing that you care. Often the PA will approach you a few days later to discuss newfound concerns.

If the discontent cannot be remedied, be prepared for a resignation. In fact, you should always be prepared for resignations. Whether or not you see it coming, be prepared for its inevitability. When an aide does deliver the news, do not outwardly react, but instead quietly think carefully and plan your next move. Keep your cool. You will show power in resisting an automatic reaction to a resignation announcement, and having the wisdom to make decisions and plan before speaking. This stay-cool strategy is discussed in more detail later in this chapter.

Divide your needs among several part-time PAs

You should seriously consider dividing your needs among several part-time aides. When you employ two or more PAs, you decrease the frequency of early resignations. In addition, the sudden departure of one has less of a negative effect.

Remember that it costs no more to employ three aides than one, for the same total of hours. If one suddenly becomes undesirable or breaks a leg, she is replaceable because you have two or more instant backups. Here is a brief listing of the advantages:

- When you have a variety of needs, your PAs should have a variety of skills. For example, your needs might include personal hygiene, occasional wheelchair repair, and occasional clothes mending. It is rare to find one PA who has skills for hygiene, mechanical repairs, and sewing. However, if you get help from two or more, you will have a better variety of skills to choose from when making assignments.

- When your schedule of needs is varied, two or more PAs can better accommodate several days and times of needs.

- With two or more PAs, you have instant, trained backups when one aide is suddenly sick or unable to work.

- When one provider needs vacation time, the second or third can fill in.

- You have more time and less stress for recruiting, hiring, and training new PAs. Few, if any, PAs will work for you permanently. Each will resign at some time. That transition period between resignation and recruiting, hiring, and training a replacement can be stressful. With two or more PAs, you never feel the anxiety of, "Will I find a quality replacement before my one-and-only PA leaves?"

- You avoid the situation of being totally dependent on a single PA. Such a person consequently has a lot of power that is too often unfairly used to advantage over the help recipient.

- You will be reducing the incidence of PA burnout, and keeping PAs longer. A single PA will burn out more easily than one who works as part of a team—ask any family caregiver who works alone.

- Your PA job is more attractive to applicants.

- You have several people, and not just you, scrutinizing your schedule and supply of continuous help, and there is less chance of a no-show gap for a shift.

- You enjoy and benefit from a variety of people, cultures, conversations, and problem-solving ideas.[1]

Request realistic work commitments from new PAs

Although many PAs are hired from the general community, if you live near a college or university you should also consider recruiting from the campus community. People in the general community plans their schedule around a 12-month calendar, but college students plan in terms of semesters. Most colleges divide the year into three semesters:

- fall semester (September through mid-December)

- spring (mid-January through mid-May)

- summer (mid-May through August).

Most students attend classes during fall and spring semesters, taking off for the summer. However, about 25 percent of students do take summer courses, so there are still plenty of potential PAs to answer your recruiting ads.

When you are interviewing PA applicants from either the general or campus community, be sure to tell them of the minimum period of time that you want them to work for you. (I regret to confirm that few aides will be willing to commit to "forever.")

Ideally, you would like to sign up each new aide for at least a 12-month (1 year) period. In reality, most people cannot plan that far in advance, and their commitment that far into the future would be meaningless. Instead, ask for one bite-sized commitment at a time: four-, six-, or eight-month stretches.

- When hiring PAs from the general community, request a minimum six-month commitment from the hiring date.

- When hiring college-student aides who begin work:
  - ▸ With the fall semester (September), tell them that you would like a commitment through at least May, the end of spring semester.
  - ▸ With the spring semester (January), cite the same minimum May commitment.
  - ▸ With the summer semester (May), request a minimum commitment through at least mid-August, the semester's end. Because summer students often continue studies into the fall and spring semesters, periodically ask about a summer PA's interest in continuing through the fall semester (until mid-December) or the spring semester (through mid May).

---

1. For more detail about why and how to use two or more part-timers, please see chapter 📖 **16,** **"Dividing Your Needs, and Assigning Work Shifts, Among Several PAs."**

Request advance notice for resignations

In addition to this work commitment, tell applicants that in the rare event it becomes necessary to resign before that time, you need at least a four- to six-week advance notice in order to replace them.

Use the term *rare* to imply that an early departure is not a common event (although, sadly, it is). If each PA believes that almost all of your aides work for the entire duration of their original commitment, then most aides:

- will make an extra effort to complete their commitment

- if resigning early, will feel guilty in doing so. This usually buys you their extra time and assistance while you recruit, interview, hire, and train a replacement.

For job applicants to take this minimum employment commitment and advance resignation notice seriously, tell them why each is important to you. My personal approach is to deliver a mini-lecture during the initial staff meeting whenever I have hired new PAs. I tell them how carefully I selected them for their dependability and responsibility (true). I cite my hope that we will still all be together at the end of their commitment, six or eight months from now. Then I briefly outline the recruiting and training costs to me of money, time, effort, and trust. I ask that the PAs let me know if the hours, shifts, or my personality start to disappoint anyone. That way we can resolve the problems instead having a PA quit. This technique will have an advantageous effect on probably 75 percent of your PAs—the ones with a conscience.

Remember that your goal in resolving problems cannot realistically be to avoid all resignations, but merely to delay them. Almost every help provider will to resign and move on at some point. In accepting that resignations are inevitable, you should become comfortable with them. You can practice coping with the disappointments that resignations cause, and then take constructive steps to replace the resigning PA and get on with your life. And that is the topic of the next, specialized part of this chapter.

Parting ways: PA resignations and terminations

If the problems cannot be corrected, and the negative symptoms shown by PAs are of a type or severity that cannot be tolerated, then the PAs' replacement—by resignation or firing—probably cannot be avoided. You should begin early with the process of negotiating their resignations and recruiting their replacements.

The simple facts behind a PA departure

There are several common reasons for parting ways with a PA.[2] Regardless of the actual reason, most PAs will eventually leave you either by their resignation or, rarely, by your firing them. Resignations occur in two ways:

---

2. These are detailed in chapter 📖 25, "Your Personal Concerns as a Paid Help Provider, plus Ten Reasons Why PAs Quit and Are Fired."

- PAs work through the full term of their original commitment, and their departures and replacements are foreseeable and well scheduled

- PAs announce an early resignation before the natural end of their original commitment, and recruiting and hiring a replacement are accomplished as soon as possible.

Because your requirement for PA assistance is usually continuous and does not permit interruption, it is wise, whenever possible, to make each PA departure a well-planned event and to avoid abrupt resignations and firings.

How do resignations happen?

At hiring, most PAs will promise you a long term of employment. Hearing this initial commitment, you feel optimistic and trust that your PA recruiting and hiring are finished for a while. Over the ensuing days or weeks of working with the aide, you become friends, develop trust, and feel comfort in believing that you can count on this PA's help for the next six months. So much of your lifestyle with a disability involves one unpredictable crisis after another, sometimes with hourly frequency. The loyal help from this high-quality PA provides an appreciated, and often essential, counterbalance of dependability, security, and stability.

Then, at the end of a Friday evening shift of working with you, this PA takes a little longer than usual at your bedroom door to reach for her car keys. You take advantage of her delay to tell her one more time how much you appreciate her help: "Hey, Lauren, thanks so much for another great week of help. You're fun to work with. I hope you have a great weekend, and I will look forward to seeing you on Monday morning."

She tries to smile, looks down at her feet, and speaks in a low, depressed voice: "Walter, I need to tell you something. I know I have worked only a month toward our six-month agreement, but I have been offered a half-time internship at the campus. I could not accept it in addition to continuing my work with you. This is a rare, student internship in my major, and I cannot pass it up. I am very sorry."

She looks nervously at the floor, the wall, and then at you. It is common that someone who feels very sorry and guilty about resigning lacks the courage to deliver the concluding message, "and therefore, I have to resign from working with you."

You are unable to speak or react as you feel a rush of several emotions (see the discussion, later in this section) that usually begins with disbelief.

How often do resignations occur?

In reality, about 50-plus percent of PAs will work for the entire duration of their original commitment, and then they will resign. If you do a good job of recruiting and screening applicants, and weeding out undesirable people before they are hired, firing a PA will be a rare event. Typically, there will be one firing for each 75-or-so quality PAs who will eventually resign.

Of a typical 75 PAs hired:

- 1 will become sufficiently undesirable to require firing
- 35 will resign before working for the duration of their original time commitment
- 39 will work through, and possibly beyond, their commitment. In more than 30 years of managing my own PAs, your author has interviewed and screened more than 1,500 applicants, hired about 350 PAs, and found it necessary to fire fewer than 6! Of those 344 quality aides, perhaps 200 have worked the duration of their initial commitment. Consequently, I guess I have heard about 150 reasons for aides resigning ahead of time. Each resigning aide undoubtedly believed his or her reason to be unique.

In all of those years, I have tried to find a pattern or formula so I could spot early resignations coming. I have examined anything that might contribute to my predicting and reducing the frequency of PAs leaving early. I have concluded simply that personal attitudes, opinions, and plans often change.

In today's quickly changing lifestyle, many people can make commitments for only a few months into the future. Consequently, as PA managers, we can reduce early resignations by reducing the size of the employment commitments we request. If we ask for a year-long commitment from newly hired PAs, but find that most PAs resign after six months, then we should revise our expectations and request "renewable commitments" that do not exceed six months. That way, there are fewer surprise, early departures and more that are foreseeable and planned.

How do PAs deliver the news?

Although the circumstances around resignations vary, there are some interesting consistencies.

Most PAs will inform you of their need to resign during the final five minutes of a work shift. This usually occurs with the PAs who feel sorry and guilty about leaving you. They might tell you that they waited until your routine was finished because they wanted to spare your feelings. In truth, they were sparing their own. They wanted to drop the news and leave their shift.

When stating why they must resign, almost all will want to convince you that they have no choice in the matter. "I really want to continue my work with you, but this new job is forcing me to leave." What the guilt-ridden PA really means is, "I have enjoyed working with you, but I have decided to leave you in favor of another job that is more attractive, pays more than yours, or provides me with more opportunities for improving my social life."

At the end of the resignation speech, most will try to alleviate their guilt by offering to work until you recruit a replacement. "I really feel badly about your need to recruit my replacement. I will work as long as I can while you find someone. After that, I will be glad to be available whenever you need an emergency fill-in."

These promises are made primarily to alleviate guilt. The PA will usually work a reasonable extension while you recruit, but once he has left your job, he will rarely be further available for fill-ins. In contrast, other PAs, who are quitting because they are angry with you or tired of the job, will not care enough even to make these offers.

Reasons for depression regarding a good PA's departure

A PA's departure often brings up a mixture of emotions in you. For you, a PA's departure has many more consequences than, say, the departure of a cashier from a grocery store. You are far more dependent on a PA than is the grocery store on the cashier.

You have usually become comfortable with and trusting in the relationship. There is the feeling of loss of a known and somewhat predictable personality, along with the additional uncertainty about the kind of individual the new PA will be.

It is a fact that life with a disability is quite unpredictable: there are always possibilities for illnesses, bone breaks, bowel and urine accidents, and the mechanical breakdowns of mobility and medical equipment. You are dependent on so many factors each day: mobility aids, architectural accessibility, prescription medications, and assistance from caregivers or PAs. Each time any one of these malfunctions or fails, you are suddenly unable to do something—something that only a few seconds ago seemed to be a certain, easy activity.

With such an abundance of variables that cause sudden change, we are often attracted to elements that provide supplemental stability and security. Have you ever wondered why you might prefer or enjoy:

- keeping some standard parts of your daily schedule unchanged and consistent from day to day?

- keeping items in your activity areas (grooming items around the bathroom sink, computer accessories and work files in your desk area, and books or hobby items in a leisure area) in consistent, standard locations?

- dedicating certain parts of your weekend to routine, predictable activities?

- keeping annual family traditions around holidays?

- after getting into bed at night, enjoying at least a brief, routine period of silence and tranquility when you do not have to manage any PAs, there is little chance for anything to malfunction or break down, and you can enjoy some privacy?

- maintaining most types of relationships for as long as possible?

In a similar way, good caregivers or PAs do much more for you than just provide physical assistance. They provide a dependable, reliable element of consistent support and help. When you are with trustworthy PAs who know your routine, you feel a bit more safe, secure, and protected and a little less limited, unable, and vulnerable. You feel less disabled because the aide with you readily bridges the gap of things you cannot do easily, quickly, and safely when alone.

In addition, good PAs are often good friends, regardless of differences in age, culture, and other demographics. Some of the friendship is based on the usual factors of shared interests and values; however, your feeling of attraction and bond to aides is often stronger than theirs toward you. In reality, you usually have an additional attraction to the functional role of an assistance-providing aide, and secondarily toward him or her as a special person. This weighted relationship becomes increasingly evident as someone lives longer with a disability and experiences a number of aide relationships over time.

Your dependence on aides has resulted in a unique trust: your trust that they will continue to provide help whenever, wherever, and however you need it. This happens each time without fail—the pinnacle of loyalty.

Indeed, aides can provide a sense of security, stability, and comfort in your life from both their physical assistance and their image. They represent an icon of something you can depend on.

So, regardless of whether you value primarily the person or the function of meeting dependent needs, a PA's departure often causes a variety of losses and a mixture of emotions.

Emotions regarding PA departures will vary

The emotions you feel toward PAs who surprise you by quitting early will differ from feelings toward those who resign on schedule, according to their original commitment. Consequently, whether you associate a particular early departure with "quitting" or "resigning" is primarily an emotional factor of whether you are angry about it!

When a trusted PA suddenly delivers his unexpected, early resignation, anger is only one of several emotions often involved at different stages. Other emotions that contribute to your initial feeling of shock can include:

- disbelief
- surprise
- disappointment
- frustration
- anger
- rejection
- abandonment
- depression
- despair
- guilt about possibly causing the PA's early departure
- worry that no future applicants will be interested in helping you
- worry that no future applicants will equal the high quality of the long-term caregiver or PA who is leaving you
- a lack of desire, energy, or trust to recruit future aides, and then to cope with their many, frequent disappointments.

Indeed, the last emotion in the list—the lack of desire to trust in future PAs after being hurt by a currently departing one—contributes an ongoing, bittersweet feeling to our lives. It is more frequent and more routinely integrated into our lifestyle than the occasional romantic sentiment of our able-bodied peers who suffer from having "loved and lost."

Those of us with disabilities have found that those certainties on which we must depend and trust one moment might suddenly disappear in the next moment. To cope with so much uncertainty, we have learned to expect that most of the relationships we have with our environment are temporally limited. Perhaps the epitome of this viewpoint comes from a friend of your author, who succinctly states, "We live with the expectation of dying."

Thus, at the moment a PA unexpectedly announces her need to resign, you might feel a mixture of emotions. These emotions are usually unavoidable, but they can be kept very private from the departing PA if you choose. At the instant paid PAs deliver the news to you that they intend to leave, why should you be concerned about whether you show your emotions? In one word it is power.

Reacting constructively to resignations

In the few seconds after a PA drops the bomb of resigning or quitting, your initial outward reaction is very important and should be carefully selected. At the time PAs make the initial announcement, they are either:

- unconcerned about quitting and its consequences for you
- feeling at least some degree of caring, sorrow, and guilt.

If your relationship has been a good one, then the PA will be concerned and willing to reasonably help you through the transition of finding and training a replacement. In contrast, if working with the PA has been the pits—and quitting is really a blessing—then you are best to part ways as soon as is practical for you.

At the moment they get the news of the resignation, the initial reaction from some help recipients is either to vent anger or to cry. This is not a time to react emotionally. Instead, it is a time to carefully and quietly plan—and survive.

Your primary concern right now is having the current PA continue to help you until you can recruit, interview, screen, hire, and train a replacement. You want help available tonight, so you can get into bed, and you want help in the morning, so you can get out of bed. There cannot be any gaps in assistance availability.

If the resigning PA already understands your concern and is willing to bridge the gap to a replacement, you should feel fortunate. This does not mean that you are not entitled to feel disappointed about the inconvenient departure. However, if you are selecting which emotions to reveal to the PA, show disappointment in the departure and appreciation that she has agreed to delay her departure, instead of anger that she is inconveniencing you.

In contrast, a resigning, selfish aide might be thinking only of her own needs. She intends to leave in a week or so, and that might not provide you enough replacement time. Your immediate goal is to educate her about your needs, and then to negotiate a later departure. The emotions to show her include disappointment and worry about not being able to find a replacement before she leaves. Again, try to contain the bubbling anger; it will be counterproductive to getting her to empathize with your concern. Appear to her to be very worried, and tell her why as well as what you need from her.

So, are you putting on an act with the intent to manipulate your PA into providing you with what you need to survive? You bet you are. Empathy and guilt have a good chance of getting you what you need. Anger, with the intent to "make her sorry that she is quitting," is juvenile, ineffective, and actually counterproductive to what you want.

Your course of action: Recruit and replace, now!

Regardless of whether the departing PA is supportive, your next goal is to recruit, interview, screen, hire, and train a replacement as soon as possible. Get your PA ad back into the newspaper or Internet and/or your posters onto bulletin boards.

I recall one time when a departing PA gave me only a few hours to find a replacement.[3] I was a 19-year-old college sophomore living in a residence hall. My live-in PA resigned in the morning, and I had a replacement hired and moved in by dinner time! "Express recruiting" can be accomplished in very little time.

So if a departing PA simply wants out, do not waste time getting angry or begging him to stay. Instead, direct that energy into constructive action. Get going with your PA ad and then follow one of this book's three, ten-step procedures. Please see chapters 📖 5, **"Ten Steps to Getting All or Some of Your Help from Family Caregivers,"** 📖 6, **"Ten Steps to Getting All or Some of Your Help from Agency-Employed Aides,"** or 📖 7, **"Ten Steps to Getting All or Some of Your Help from Personally Employed Aides."**

Although the average time for personal recruiting is 5 days, the process can be compressed to 24 hours or less. You are not alone in a hopeless situation. Select one of those three chapters and get going.

Firing a PA requires courage and careful planning

A manager will encounter few duties that are as emotionally difficult as firing an employee. Most of us, by nature, enjoy being liked. We do not look forward to delivering bad news, and often avoid firing because of the expectation of an angry reaction. To avoid facing the issue, a few managers will even resort to making life so miserable for an employee that they will quit as a substitute strategy for having the courage to fire an undesirable employee.

Though firing an employee cannot be made easy, knowing some basic procedural "dos and don'ts" can minimize the difficulty. And once more, because your requirement for PA assistance is usually continuous and does not permit interruption, it is wise to make each PA parting an advance-scheduled and well-planned event. Avoid abrupt, dramatic firing whenever possible.[4]

Your decision: Keep or fire the aide?

Before speaking, you should decide between two basic choices: Do you want to keep this aide, or fire her?

---

3. This is related in chapter 📖 8, **"Where and How to Advertise for Your Own PAs."**

4. For additional notes about criteria to consider when wanting to fire PAs, please see chapter 📖 18, **"Coping with and Reacting to PA Failures."**

As the saying goes, "Good help is hard to find." Each of the aides who helps you has cost you a considerable amount of time, physical and emotional energy, and advertising costs. Each time an aide leaves, through her resignation or your firing, a lot of your time and money goes out the door. More important is the loss of one of your most valued assets: dependable, trustworthy, and trained help to your dependent needs.

There is no question: PAs who have seriously bad habits that cannot be corrected must be fired, if they will not resign on their own. Ignoring untrustworthy employees can further cost you your possessions, the resignation of other PAs, or even your health or life.

However, if you are careful while hiring, there will rarely be a need for a firing. Indeed, a well-designed hiring process, such as the ten-step procedures found in this reference, includes steps that will screen out the majority of undesirable applicants before they can be hired.

This is not to say that carefully screened PAs are flawless. Everyone has bad habits, but those that truly merit firing should be both serious and not correctable. In more than 30 years of hiring and managing more than 350 of his own PAs, your author can count on one hand those he has been forced to fire.

"If in doubt—don't," is an adage that should be wisely applied to perhaps 99 percent of your impulses to fire someone. Most of these impulses occur during short, temporary, emotional crises. Given the benefit of taking an hour-long walk, a good night's sleep, or talking with a friend over a cup of coffee, most emotional impulses to fire a PA will cool down to expose merely differences in opinion or style between two people. Too often, firing a PA is a poorly selected way of merely expressing anger. The unnecessary, irreversible firing of a PA is analogous to suicide—each is the permanent solution to a temporary problem. When considering the firing of a PA, first be sure that you are dealing with a permanent, irresolvable problem.

For example, let's return to the question of whether to fire a PA who didn't appear on time this morning for work. Ask yourself the following questions. If the majority are answered with "yes," then firing this otherwise high-quality aide might be a regrettable mistake:

- Has the aide been consistently providing you with quality help?

- Has the aide had a good attitude toward you, respecting both you and your possessions?

- Was there an excusable reason, truly beyond the aide's fault or control, for the aide's failure to appear on time?

- Was today's failure a sharp departure from a usually dependable and punctual style; is this the first time this has happened?

- Does the aide seem to sincerely regret today's failure, and be taking steps to avoid a recurrence?

- If you have decided to keep the aide, does the aide need a punishing reprimand, or just your very serious request to avoid any chance of a recurrence?

In contrast, carefully consider firing if the aide:

- has not previously provided you with quality help
- has proven not to be responsible, dependable, or punctual
- has often had a "bad attitude" in not respecting you or your possessions
- does not have a good reason for this morning's failure, and does not seem to care
- does not seem to care about negative consequences for you
- does not seem eager to immediately take steps to prevent a recurrence
- has often shown you some of the other negative traits listed in a later chapter of this reference.[5]

In addition to carefully weighing the factual answers, use your intuition—your gut reaction—to identify any hidden messages. If the aide is favorably answering your questions, does your sixth sense tell you the aide is being honest and sincere? While the aide answers your questions, watch for the following body-language contradictions to what you hear:

- Does the aide make good eye contact with you, or look off to one side?
- Is the tone of voice warm, apologetic, and a bit nervous (consistent with the sincerity of genuine apologies), or is it somewhat arrogant (perhaps trying to hide anger toward you)?
- Is your overall impression that she is sincerely sorry about her failure, or is she instead struggling through anger and impatience to tell you whatever you want to hear?

With PA abuse, just one strike can make an out

There are some situations when a sudden, crisis firing is appropriate. These include any violent or potentially violent situations involving physical abuse, sexual abuse, abuse or carelessness because of heavy use of drugs or alcohol, or any other situations that create immediate danger to your health, safety, or possessions. It is rare that these will occur between you and a PA, but you should know that if any do occur, you are justified in a sudden firing.

It is amazing how some recipients of help will tolerate, support, and even defend abuse from PAs. A friend once spoke about a PA who routinely stole his money, medications, and even a girlfriend. My friend had learned to live with the situation, thinking that he could not fire the abuser, because he believed that good aides were too hard to find. When confronted with obvious evidence that his aide was acting in a criminal way, my friend would flatly deny to me—and to himself—that he was being deceived. He did not want to admit the problem, primarily because he was afraid of the consequences of firing the person upon whom he was dependent. He lacked the skills that you, the reader, are now mastering.

---

5. Please see chapter 📖 25, "Your Personal Concerns as a Paid Help Provider, plus Ten Reasons Why PAs Quit and Are Fired."

It is essential that each of us maintain control over our lifestyle. When PA abuse happens in any form, the primary damage is not in his actual abuse, but in his stealing our control—our spirit. The abuser has taken control when we live each hour in defending our possessions, safety, sexuality, or lifestyle. No PA is worth that kind of fearful living.

The reason this story hits home is that so many of us have been there. A PA has enormous power, control, and potential for abusing us, especially a one-and-only PA. We become totally dependent on and vulnerable to, that one person. The preventative remedy? In one word, *diversify*.

Instead of hiring just one PA, hire at least two part-timers. Divide your needs among as many PAs as possible. Your author averages 40 hours of weekly need, uses college students as aides, and maintains a continuous team of six or seven part-time PAs. The primary limitation on number is that each aide must have enough weekly hours to fulfill his or her salary expectations.[6]

Additionally, we are often reluctant to replace a high-quality aide because we cannot imagine finding a replacement of equal quality. Be assured, a carefully designed procedure for recruiting and screening will routinely (though not continually) find PAs who will be equal to or better than your current "jewel." No PA is permanent; each one will eventually leave, including your one-and-only jewel. By firing the deceitful aide now, you would not be changing the future course of destiny, but merely speeding the process while weighting it in your favor.

A final frequent question is, "How many serious failures should I allow? How many times will I forgive him for being late, for requiring me to phone with wake-up calls, for stealing my possessions, or for continuing other bad traits?

Indeed, in the PA ball game, just two strikes (of serious abuse) should make an out—and in some extreme cases, two strikes is being too generous. Most people should be allowed to screw up once. If they steal or fail to show up a second time, then they will do it repeatedly. They must be replaced—now. For even more serious problems, such as physical abuse or major theft, there should not be a second chance. At the first occurrence, you should immediately decide to fire the aide, and actually do so as soon as circumstances permit. A good PA is not *that* hard to find!

Measure twice, fire once: The careful art of firing

Carpenters have a saying, "Measure twice and cut once." Carpenters know that once a quality piece of wood is cut, the action cannot be undone. The cautionary wisdom can also be applied to our current topic of whether to fire a PA, and how to do it appropriately.

If you routinely do a thorough job of screening PA applicants before you hire them, having to fire an undesirable aide will truly be a rare event.[7]

---

6. For more detail about the advantages of using multiple aides, please see chapter 📖 **16, "Dividing Your Needs, and Assigning Work Shift, Among Several PAs."**

7. For a comprehensive outline and discussion that includes recruiting, interviewing, screening, and hiring, please see chapter 📖 **7, "Ten Steps to Getting All or Some of Your Help from Personally Employed Aides."**

You should rarely, if ever, fire a PA during a time when you are emotionally upset. The firing of a PA should usually be carefully planned. In the preceding section, we discussed whether a PA should get two chances or just one, depending on the severity of the undesirable behavior or abuse. Tailor the time frame for the following procedure according to whether you are in a one- or two-strike situation or crisis.

When you are tempted to fire a PA, go off by yourself for a while and do the following:

- Ask yourself for a list of rational, factual reasons for wanting to fire the PA ("I just hate his guts" is neither sufficient nor appropriate).

- Ask yourself whether these reasons or problems can be resolved, or whether they truly warrant a firing.

- Ask yourself whether the non-resolvable reasons are of a type and severity that actually jeopardize your health, safety, or security, or whether they are just based on differences in personality or styles.

> *In more than 30 years of managing the PAs I have used, your author has hired more than 350 PAs and found it necessary to fire fewer than a half dozen!*

After these decisions are made, if at all possible, wait at least 24 hours (sleep on your decision) and then review your answers to the questions in the first step. This will help cool any tendency to fire someone based on your emotional impulses. If, however, the problems are of a valid, well-established nature, the rationale for the upcoming PA firing will easily endure a 24-hour wait.

If your two or three reviews indicate that a firing is still warranted, it is wise to begin planning for the replacement PA before the actual firing. Decide which methods and resources you will use as well as how long the process will take. If possible without your current PA's knowledge, at least begin the process of recruiting, screening, and hiring the replacement PA before you fire your current PA.

If your decision is firmly and rationally based on valid reasons, then go forcefully ahead with your plans and do not allow yourself to back down. Here are some tips:

- Perform the firing at the end of the PA's shift, to minimize any negative "payback" during your routine and to ensure that your basic needs have been met in case the PA actually walks out after hearing your news.

- Perform the firing without the additional embarrassment to the PA of having others present, unless you believe that the PA might become physically abusive upon hearing the news.

- Before the PA arrives on the day of the firing, firmly review the list of reasons that have made the firing absolutely necessary. Write out the list if you fear that your mind might go blank during the upcoming confrontation. Many folks actually practice their verbal delivery of the firing several times while alone and facing a mirror.

- Convince yourself that you will not give the PA a second chance, regardless of any excuses, whining, or anger you may hear. If you have given the matter very careful thought, then you have probably considered and dismissed any reasons why the PA should not be fired.

- When addressing the PA:

  ▶ Introduce your need to speak with her and ask her to sit down, "Mary, I would like to speak with you for a minute; please have a seat."

  ▶ Position yourself squarely in front of her, face her, make good eye contact with her face and eyes, speak clearly, and use a firm and caring, but not loud or arrogant tone of voice.

  ▶ **Do not** begin your delivery with an apology—you will be doing nothing for which you should be sorry. On the contrary, you will probably be glad and relieved when the task is over, and perhaps the PA will also feel that way!

  ▶ With the stage set for you to deliver the news, you might decide to introduce the upcoming message with the classic, pre-firing phrase, "Mary, your employment is not working well."

  ▶ Next, give straightforward, honest, and clear reasons for the firing. Make this presentation directly to the point. "Mary, for some time now you have been coming to work late, either drunk or stoned, and you have almost dropped me twice in performing transfers. The situation is getting steadily worse."

  ▶ Before the PA can reply to these reasons, follow this statement of rationale with a firm, unemotional statement of actual firing. Without this statement, the PA will think you are just complaining or reprimanding, and won't understand that she is being fired. The statement of firing can be phrased several different ways.
  "Mary, based on these reasons,
    ▼ "I believe it is best if we part ways
    ▼ "I have decided to dismiss you
    ▼ "I have decided to replace you
    ▼ "I have decided that I will no longer need your help
    ▼ "I will no longer be asking you to help me
    ▼ "I have decided to let you go
    ▼ "I am firing you."

  ▶ Following this statement of firing, clearly indicate your intended time frame.
    ▼ If the firing is effective immediately, "Mary, please consider this to be your last day. I will send you your final paycheck tomorrow."
    ▼ If you are giving the PA a period of time to find new employment, "Mary, if you wish I will be glad to keep you for up to two weeks until you find new employment."

▾ If you are requesting the PA to stay a specific amount of time to help while you find and train a replacement, "Mary, I would appreciate your working for two more weeks while I find and train a replacement. This will also give you time to find another job."

▸ Do not allow yourself to be drawn into an argument or to react to any arrogant or nasty comments from the PA. Keep a straight, firm, and pleasant face. If a reply to a nasty response is required, many managers simply state (and perhaps have to repeat), "Mary, I'm sorry (or regret) that you feel that way."

▸ Be sure to collect any house keys or borrowed items at an appropriate time. If the PA refuses to return keys and you feel that your safety or possessions are threatened, promptly call a locksmith and have your key cores changed. The cost of a locksmith can be significant, but it is cheap when compared to the value of a few stolen goods if your PA becomes vengeful.

Though it is not uncommon for a fired PA to become defensive or angry on hearing the news, some PAs will be relieved and pleased. If a work relationship has become steadily worse, then the work has become a strongly negative situation for both of you. It is surprisingly common for a PA to thank you for firing him. He might even state that he is relieved because you had the courage to fire him, since he lacked the courage to simply quit. Both of you may experience relief after you have had the courage to finally terminate the unpleasant situation.

Part IV

Taking Control of Your Help Needs

Part IV

Taking Control of Your Help Needs

Parts II and III guided you in securing the help providers you use. Part IV will address your being in maximum control of what help you need, as well as when, where, and how you prefer to receive it.

Part IV advises you about identifying, listing, and evaluating your various needs for help. There is more to managing your help needs than simply scribbling out a list of tasks, and these four chapters provide you with a comprehensive game plan.

Before you list your help needs, you might have wondered whether there are guidelines about which tasks qualify for PA help. Do you simply have a free rein to ask your providers for whatever help you seem to require? Or, as for most matters that involve interpersonal relations, are there boundaries of some sort that should be respected? Indeed, there are guidelines, and these are outlined in chapter ⌨ **11, "When It Is, and Is Not, Okay to Ask for Help."**

When most of us first began to state our help needs, we probably started with an informal grocery list of items. As we used that memorized or written list for training PAs, we realized that a list of task names, by themselves, represented only part of our needs. In addition to identifying the names of tasks that require PA assistance, providers should know when, where, and how you prefer to receive their help. Your preferences will not always be popular with providers, who will often question why you want help provided in a certain way—especially when the PA's own preferences take less time and effort. Chapter ⌨ **12, "Getting It Done—Your Way!"** first assures you that most of your preferences are essential to your independence, health, and safety. Next, you will find a plan for convincing PAs of the importance of your preferences, and then for teaching your preferences so that PAs will remember them.

Help providers additionally need to know details about your scheduling and time expectations: when they should arrive to start work, how much time each group of tasks should require, and by what time each work shift should be wrapping up. In chapter ⌨ **13, "Defining and Describing Your Help Needs,"** you will find "how-to" tips on integrating your list of tasks with preferences, time frames, and the guidelines about which tasks qualify for help requests. Once your list is complete—whether you memorize it, hand-write it, or computer-print it—you should next get ready to verbally describe both your needs and your PA job. During PA phone inquiries, interviews, and training sessions, you will be reciting these details hundreds of times over the years. This chapter will coach you in delivering short and long versions, for different applications, so you will quickly impress PA applicants as being organized, structured, and in control.

Because of your dependence on physical assistance from providers, a good part of each day is spent in requesting help and then supervising the quality of help that you receive. Although you are ultimately dependent on receiving the assistance, you are first dependent on clearly communicating your needs. PAs cannot accommodate needs that they do not understand.

The final chapter of Part IV provides methods for effectively requesting help from PAs. Chapter 📖 14, "Say It, Ask for It, and Act—Assertively!," outlines the differences among passive, passive-aggressive, assertive, and aggressive styles, and then shows why the assertive style will maximize your ability to get the help you need.

After using Part IV for organizing your help needs, it will be time to move on to Part V, "Strategies for Being a Good Manager." You might imagine that you are currently building a machine that will mass-produce help to your needs. In Parts II and III, you brought help providers to the factory site and trained them, and in Part IV you identified and organized your needs for help. The upcoming Part V will provide blueprints for tooling the efficient machine that combines help providers with help needs to produce a steady output of assistance.

A common mechanic can initially assemble a simple, working mechanism. However, it requires a skilled engineer—a good PA manager—to design and fine-tune the machine's cogs so it operates smoothly and is not inclined to frequent breakdowns. The five chapters of Part V provide details for transforming mechanics into managers.

Part V Strategies for Being a Good Manager

Chapter 11

When It Is, and Is Not, Okay to Ask for Help

When you initially began using caregiver and PA help, it all seemed so simple. So-and-so agreed to provide the help you needed. You identified the tasks, wrote out your "wish list," and started timidly making requests. When all went well, you felt a surge of confidence and began adding tasks to the original list.

Then something strange happened. You started to feel some uneasy feedback to some of your requests. It was nothing tangible, just the vague, elusive feeling that you might have asked for something wrong. At other times, PAs would actually tell you that you had "rubbed them the wrong way." Whatever the source or reason, the message was clear: you were doing something inappropriate that was irritating your help providers.

When this happened to me, I reacted by asking my aides whether anything was wrong, but they were seldom helpful with a diagnosis. Consequently, I started trying out cause-and-effect hypotheses in attempts to correlate the PA's negative reactions and feedback to my requests for help.

Over the years I have studied these different situations that have sometimes caused friction. I have also surveyed other help recipients about their conclusions. My standards and etiquette for making requests have become increasingly refined. The result is that my aides and I both feel comfortable with my help requests.

What are the conclusions about when, how, and for what it is—or is not—okay to ask for help?

Before discussing the guidelines, let me suggest that the ultimate decisions about which guidelines will work for you must come from within you. Only you (and your conscience) can determine which of your daily needs are appropriate for requesting help from providers. Regrettably, there are no hard-and-fast formulas that can be applied to all of us, because each of us is unique.

The key to your making these personal decisions, in deciding when requesting help is or is not appropriate, is for your conscience to compare your unique set of abilities, degree of motivation, and lifestyle to your current list of help needs. You are consulting your conscience first about whether you *could* be independently performing any of the tasks or responsibilities that you have assigned to help providers. Second, you are weighing several additional factors before deciding whether you *should* be making changes. However, this is not a simple correlation between could and should—you will be evaluating some additional, personal factors as well.

Your unique set of abilities and your degree of motivation are two of several variables that you will be weighing when making these decisions regarding several topics. For example, some variables include:

- your type of disability and consequent abilities
- the type and extent of help providers available to you
- what tasks are in question, as well as where, when, and how the task occurs
- your degree of motivation in wanting to be independent
- your daily lifestyle and consequent list of routine activities.

This chapter cannot provide you with quick-and-easy, black-and-white rules to follow, but it can present a number of issues for you to consider when making your own decisions. Here are observations based on my personal experience as well as feedback from the one-on-one coaching and group classes I have taught. Over the years it has become clear to me that there are situations in which it is plainly inappropriate to ask for help, just as there are cases in which, no matter the circumstances, it is clearly appropriate. This chapter will help you discover where to draw your own line, as I have drawn mine.

Guidelines for Inappropriate Help Requests

Picture yourself in a family where each member has a set of routine chores for contributing to the smooth running of the family as a whole. Some wash and dry dishes on different nights, another takes out the garbage, another helps with the laundry, and others contribute parts of their paychecks to the family budget.

If all members but one or two were faithfully contributing, then the lazy members might feel guilty. In addition, the other members might begin to resent the lack of responsibility of the lazy, freeloading members who were not doing their share or "pulling their own weight."

Situations like this are also common in the relationships between recipients and providers of help. A former PA once related, after she resigned from her job of helping a man with severe arthritis:

> *When I interviewed for his PA job, the duties seemed to be pretty straightforward accommodations to his disability. Then, after a few days of helping him, he started asking me to do more and more of tasks that he was originally doing for himself. If his disability had*

become more severe, and his abilities more limited, then there would have been a good reason for the shift in requests. However, I think he simply found that I was a hard worker and he got lazy. When I began to resent the "extras" and asked him about the additional chores, he got defensive and angry. It was as though he was already feeling uneasy and guilty about having added the tasks. He certainly did not feel comfortable about discussing reasons why some tasks had been transferred from his list to mine.

Another woman had been married to a quadriplegic man for 15 years. Shortly after she asked him for a divorce, she told me:

Jim will always be very special in my life. I will always love him, but after 15 years of living with him, his disability finally got to me. As the years went on, he expected me to do more and more for him. It started when we initially dated with my offering to do him a few favors, a few caregiver tasks, from time to time.

What I originally meant as one-shot favors, when perhaps he was especially tired or depressed, soon became routine expectations of me. He often became angry when I failed to do a favor without his asking, or when I failed to do it when or how he preferred. The favors that he had formerly appreciated were soon taken for granted, and my performance was now being critically evaluated.

One night when he was angry, he told me that I was not meeting my responsibilities. The line had been crossed. I suddenly realized that instead of my doing occasional favors of providing physical help, in his opinion I had agreed to assume routine responsibility for these tasks. It all happened so subtly and gradually.

I had grown up with a tendency to help others and 'rescue' them. I learned from Jim that it was not appropriate for him to transfer to me—or for me to accept—the personal responsibilities for which he had previously been capable. If his disability had become worse, and made him unable to manage his responsibilities, then he could have formally asked me to assume them and I might have decided to do so. However, he was quite capable of managing his personal responsibilities, and needed only physical help. Temporary, occasional physical help—a bit of caregiver help—was all that I had agreed to provide.

In the end, I had resented him for shifting his responsibilities. I also resented myself for agreeing to assume them. In addition, he was angry at me for "failing" in my agreed tasks, and angry at himself for attempting to avoid his own obligations. I do not believe that either of us realized what had happened until it was too late to remedy things. I just hope that other couples and families will read this before this cycle happens to them.

It is very easy to misuse and abuse family caregiver or paid PA help. What initially seem like innocent requests can develop into unnecessary demands that ruin relationships and alienate caregivers. Both you and the provider feel the negative consequences of unnecessary or inappropriate requests. Although there are a wide range of requests that can lead to trouble, they fall into three main categories: tasks you could (and should) do yourself, tasks that are unnecessary, and tasks for which you ask others to assume responsibilities that you are capable of managing.

Tasks that you could, and should, be doing for yourself

One of your reasons for using minimal help is to lead an active, independent lifestyle. It is easy to become lazy and increase dependence on caregivers or PAs just because they are there.

By definition, when you start assigning tasks that you could independently do, you start becoming more dependent on the providers. Since your rehab days, your primary goal has been to maximize your independence while minimizing your dependence. When you ask for unnecessary help with independent activities, you are reversing the process and moving away from your goal.

Asking for more help than you need, and increasing your dependence on that help, is a subtle, easy trap to fall into. It is tempting to let someone else do it. In fact, the temptation can be quite similar to an addiction.

The initial habit of delegating inappropriate tasks is easy to acquire, and is partially the result of refusing to carry out one's own obligations and responsibilities. The habit can grow steadily, with the recipient expecting people around him to routinely do him more and more "favors." He then begins to feel guilty for refusing to "pull his own weight." He often slides into chronic anger or depression, and ironically aims the anger at the very providers who are helping him. Like an addiction, this is often a difficult series of habits—a difficult cycle—to correct.

There are many counseling books on addiction, codependency, and other related topics. Most of us have attempted to shift our responsibilities to someone else. It usually catches up to us in a crisis. Often an abused help provider leaves us, and we then are forced to reestablish our personal boundaries, responsibilities, self-sufficiency, and independence—and then get on with life.

Once you have listed your needs for help, look for any tasks that you could do yourself.

Tasks that are not, by nature, necessary and are actually excuses to exert control

It is also easy to create and assign to providers tasks that are simply not necessary. There are many reasons why you might do this, including an overall desire to be in control. However, the important factor is that you recognize these tendencies and try to avoid them. Following are some common character traits that get people into trouble when assigning tasks.

Compulsive control. Perhaps you are a compulsive control freak, and you cannot live through the day while knowing that there is a slight wrinkle in the left point of your shirt collar. In an extreme example, you fight the temptation to have your caregiver or PA take off your shirt and pull out the iron. Nice going. To reduce your compulsions, ask yourself, "Is the help I am about to request really important and necessary?" Start sending your shirts to the laundry, save your provider for truly essential needs, and relax the next time you are tempted to ask your provider to do something unnecessary.

Disability-related control issues. Perhaps you are not a control freak, but your disability has limited your activities and filled your lifestyle with unpredictable, sporadic, and undesirable events. In the first category, you often feel frustrated because you are unable to do many things. In the second category, examples of undesirable events include bowel and bladder accidents, bone fractures from falls, and skin breakdowns that require lengthy in-bed healings.

Overall, the disability has taken control away from you for many functions, and you miss that feeling of being in control, in charge, and having power over your body and your lifestyle. To compensate for the uncertainty and loss of control in old areas, you sometimes seek new areas that would return some stability and empowerment to your life.

The caregivers and aides who carry out your instructions are sometimes a logical target for recovering your sense of control. You are sometimes tempted to go overboard by creating unnecessary chores and detail, and by venting unnecessary anger. As a remedy, try to identify areas in your life that truly need better structure and organization, and use PA help to get those parts of your life in better order.

Chronic anger. If you are chronically angry, you may vent that anger on those around you, in part by "cracking the whip" of extreme control. As many of us have done, you should consider seeking professional help from a minister, counselor, therapist, or psychologist. Until you control and minimize your personal anger, you will prematurely lose one caregiver and PA after another. Many of us have required a year or more of weekly therapy sessions to deal with accepting our disability, as well as other anger-causing baggage from growing up. Today we are happier, and so are the longer-lasting PAs around us.

Loneliness. Problems can also develop if you are lonely and seeking companionship, or your fantasizing libido enjoys the physical attention that your PA unknowingly provides you. Consequently, you assign your provider extra, unnecessary, attention-seeking tasks, and make up false medical rationales for them.

Don't go there. Your PA, not at first knowing why, will start feeling uneasy about the made-up requests. If she senses that you are pursuing her for romantic or sexual reasons, she will usually quit. You might even be exposing yourself to a lawsuit for sexual harassment. Additionally, she could spread the word about your unwanted affections to other PAs whom you might want to hire in the future. Again, get some professional help.

Asking others to assume your responsibilities

When you initially acquired your disability, one of your first objectives was to learn to do all that you could for yourself. When you encountered old or new activities that your disability prevented, there were three choices:

- give up your interest and discontinue your performance of the task
- develop a new way of accomplishing the task, so that you could continue to do it independently
- ask for someone's help—physical assistance—in performing all or part of the task.

If most of your limitations are physical in nature, then you require physical assistance to bridge the gaps between what you cannot physically do and what you want to do. However, some folks have additional limitations that affect sight, hearing, speech, and/or their cognitive abilities to reason and remember. For them, caregivers and PAs justifiably provide additional kinds of assistance that are directly related to accommodating the specific limitations.

Another chapter discusses the sensory and cognitive impairments that often require additional help for PA hiring, training, and scheduling. If unable to manage aides independently, these help recipients—who still want to maintain maximum control and independence—can assign a personal representative or PA coordinator to act on their behalf to represent their needs. This coordinator assumes the responsibility of PA management, and can be a family caregiver or a personally employed PA. This manager, in turn, hires, trains, and schedules other hired help on behalf of the recipient. Of course, home health aide agencies are also available to serve this function.

However, for other help recipients who need only physical assistance, it is only physical assistance that they should be requesting. If you are able and willing to manage the providers and their physical help, then you should be performing all the planning and management duties. Unless you are truly unable to do so, you should not be asking your caregiver or PA to assume responsibility for:

- the coordination and management of your other PAs
- decisions about your methods of health care
- decisions about your daily activities and schedule
- remembering (without fail) each step of every task in your routine
- the supervision of whether help is provided correctly and in a quality manner.

None of your PAs should be expected to memorize all the tasks of your routine and be held accountable for remembering each one. Most of the assistance you receive will be face-to-face help, where you and an aide are working together. Typical examples include assistance with dressing, grooming, and showering.

Imagine that an aide is helping you get dressed. Two hours later, when you are working at your office desk, you discover that you are wearing mismatched socks or none at all. Is your first impulse to blame and get angry at your PA? If so, two things have happened. First, you have made the PA responsible for remembering each step of your entire routine. Second, you are denying your own, primary responsibility—especially in such a face-to-face physical situation—to have paid attention and prevented the mistake. You are blaming the PA for your failure to act responsibly toward your own needs. Indeed, if you are in a situation that enables you to act responsibly, then you are obligated to do so.

This was face-to-face help, and you were present when the aide mismatched or left out your socks, so is it fair to hold the PA responsible but not yourself? What would the PA's reaction be to your blaming her when you next see her? How would you react if you were the PA?

It is almost always inappropriate for you to shift personal responsibilities to someone else, when:

- you have the cognitive abilities to be responsible for your own needs
- you are in a physical, face-to-face (or similar) situation of receiving help that enables you to act in a responsible way.

It is easy to want PAs for more than just physical assistance. As people with disabilities, we are often chronically tired, angry, lonely, or depressed. Sometimes we even fantasize about a PA becoming a "significant other" in our life when she does not want to be. Our subconscious communication to them is, "Please take over some of my responsibilities. I need a rest, and to be cared for." For many of us this plea comes from the heart and is understandable. Just like the title of the play, *Stop the World, I Want to Get Off*, we sometimes wish we could let someone else shoulder the burden—the responsibility—for even a little while.

Is it wrong to allow someone to do a favor for you? Not at all, as long as the donor's original intent as to the nature and frequency of the favor is respected. If we appear to be tired, and a friend offers to do a favor, all is well—unless we try to unfairly extend the favor beyond the intent of the original offer. If we attempt to stretch a favor, and have the donor "take over" that responsibility, then we are covertly abusing the donor and the opportunity.

What is appropriate is that you be responsible for yourself for a lifetime, regardless of whether you are able-bodied or have a disability. It is usually wrong to shift that responsibility to anyone else, whether relative, spouse, lover, friend, or PA.

The message appropriate to the spirit of this topic is, "Do not try to assign your personal responsibilities to your PA unless your disability warrants it—instead, assign only your needs for physical help to which the PA agrees."

Deciding when it is okay to request help is not as difficult as it may seem. There are several ways to describe the needs that do qualify for requesting assistance.

Guidelines for Appropriate Help Requests

Now that we have explored when it is not okay to ask for help, and the negative consequences of doing so, here are some guidelines that are often used in deciding when it *is* okay.

It is important to remember that your lifestyle, abilities, health, and stamina often change. A physical activity that you can accomplish today might temporarily or permanently become a dependent activity tomorrow. Consequently, your need for physical assistance from others will often change.

Besides using PA help primarily for physical assistance, it is important to use assistance only for an appropriate type of activity or need. Most of these types are described in one or more of the next four categories of requests.

If you were to ask four people to describe an ocean scene, you would get four different answers. The four descriptions would each provide a different viewpoint of the same scene. For a fifth person who had never seen the ocean, providing all four viewpoints would be undoubtedly more descriptive than selecting only one. Regardless of the clarity of the four descriptions, the fifth person would still need to use imagination in combining the four versions into one composite.

In a similar way, there are many ways to describe and classify activities for which requesting help is necessary and appropriate. There are at least four viewpoints for illustrating valid requests, and there is little relationship among them. Each presents a different set of circumstances, and each provides a unique way for you to decide which of your needs are okay for requesting help.

Reasons for requests: Do your limitations justify your request for help?

There are three basic categories of help needs for you to consider: needs beyond your physical abilities, needs that would take too much time and energy (if you attempted them independently), and needs that involve health and safety issues.

Needs that are beyond your physical abilities. These are activities, or parts of activities, that are truly beyond your physical abilities. This is the primary, most straightforward reason for needing help from caregivers or PAs. Logically, does this mean that you should never, ever seek help for any task that you can perform? Not necessarily. Check out these next two types of needs.

Needs that would take too much of your time or energy (if you attempted them independently). These are activities that, because of physical limitations and not laziness, would take too long or use too much personal energy if you attempted to perform them independently.

This is the grayest, most undefinable area. There is no neat-and-tidy, black-and-white definition that can be applied, so your comfort level and conscience should guide you in this area. There are many tasks that you can perform independently. However, experience has shown that independence for some items is too costly in terms of the amount of time or energy required of you.

For example, you might be able to dress yourself each morning. Unfortunately, that independence might cost you two hours of valuable time, as well as a large portion of your day's energy. You could get dressed, but it would be 10 A.M. by the time you finished dressing yourself, and you would need a nap before facing an eight-hour day at the office. As a remedy, you use PA help, cut dressing time to 35 minutes, and arrive at the office on schedule and energetic.

The danger to your independence here lies in assigning activities to PA help because you are simply too lazy to do them for yourself. Sometimes there is a fine line between genuinely running short of the time and energy required for meeting schedules and responsibilities, and allowing laziness to tempt you to misuse or abuse help. (An in-depth discussion about misusing help in this way was presented earlier in this chapter.)

In addition to determining whether an activity is beyond your physical limitations, or takes too much time and energy, you should also ask whether the activity is safe to perform on your own.

Needs that would jeopardize your safety or health. These are activities that might cause injury or illness if you attempted to perform them independently.

The preceding example posits a situation where you might lack the sufficient time or energy for dressing or grooming in the morning. But what if dressing yourself and cooking your own breakfast routinely resulted in:

- abrasions and pressure sores on your elbows as you repeatedly maneuvered in bed
- poorly positioned support stockings that occasionally produced pressure sores on your feet or heels
- losing your balance and falling to the floor during independent attempts at bed-to-wheelchair transfers
- burns from hot saucepans or pots of boiling water as you attempt to cook?

Here, doing certain tasks without PA help would jeopardize your health or safety. When your health or safety is endangered by attempting independence, then those unassisted activities are counterproductive to independent, healthful living. After all, you would not enjoy much independence during several weeks in bed while healing a pressure sore or severe burns.

Without safety and health, there is very little independent living. If you cannot safely perform a task in a manner that preserves health, then do not allow a false sense of independence and pride fool you into refusing the help you require. Ask for help with these tasks, and know that you are justified in doing so.

Priority and timing of requests: Should you ask for help now or later?
Have you ever heard these comments from your friends, neighbors, caregivers, or PAs?

- "Anytime you need anything, you just ask and I will be glad to help you." However, when you do ask for help, it is clear that she is not entirely "glad to help you."

- "You make too many demands—I am not your slave."
- "If only you were not so needy."
- "I need time to myself when I do not feel like I am 'on duty' by waiting on you. Some of your needs could wait for a time when helping you is more convenient for me."
- "I do not have time for your unscheduled need. You should have told me in advance so I could have planned enough extra time."
- "You should not 'cry wolf' by claiming that a need for help is urgent or an emergency. You do not really need help, you simply want attention in a hurry!"
- "This was a real emergency. You should not have hesitated to ask for help at times like this. Why can't you tell the difference?"

Knowing when your request will be accepted and when it will be resented by a caregiver or PA can be confusing, frustrating, and downright depressing.

If you have live-in caregivers or PAs, you should be especially concerned about how to classify predictable and unpredictable needs, and when to ask for help. With live-in help that is continually present, there is a temptation to ask for whatever you need, whenever you need it. This means your live-in provider will soon tire of constantly being "on duty" and lacking private "time off." This can be prevented by establishing some schedule boundaries about standard on-duty times. Outside of these times, you should carefully define the types of needs that qualify for unscheduled or emergency requests.

You have probably agonized over situations like these:

- "Should I ask for help now or wait for a while?"
- "She claims that I have too many needs for help. I do not see how I can do any more for myself, and ask for any less. Maybe she should spend some time in this wheelchair. Then she might understand what it is like to have to beg for help."
- "Man, I really hate my disability and myself for having to ask for help so often. It is clear that my need for help from Suzy is soon going to ruin our romantic relationship. I hate this disability."
- "My mother has been pretty patient with my requests for help until this morning. Out of nowhere, she suddenly blew up and screamed at me, 'I cannot help you anymore. Enough is enough. You will have to find someone else. I still love you, but I cannot live in a house where you need help every five minutes. Every time I sit down to rest, you want something else.'"

Sometimes you might urgently need help, but you delay asking because you know that your aide is going to blow up in anger. You wait and wait for the right time to ask. Maybe you even start up an innocent, no-brainer conversation to get your PA into a good mood for your request. And oh, how your stomach and head can hurt with the stress! When you cannot wait any longer, you try to predict the PA's negative reaction and defuse it by introducing the request with phrases like:

- "I know you are really tired, but would you please help me with..."
- "I am really sorry to say this, but would it be okay if I asked for help with..."
- "Promise you will not get mad? Can you do me a tiny, real quick favor—p-l-e-a-s-e..."
- "You are really going to get angry, but I need help with..."
- "I promise this will be the last thing I ask for tonight..."

Here are three more viewpoints. These emphasize when it is acceptable to ask for help. There are also tips on reducing the number of special requests that are most likely to provoke resentment by reclassifying the requests from unpredictable, special requests to predictable, scheduled ones.

"Should I ask for help now, or wait for a while?" Details of the following three situations might help you answer that question in the future.

Predictable needs. Here the needs are foreseeable, well-planned, and occur routinely. The needs (and their order, frequency, and duration) can be listed in advance on your master list and schedule of needs. Caregivers and PAs rarely resent these needs, because they are expected and the provider can plan for the required time and effort. Consequently, as many of your needs as possible should be included in this routine, scheduled listing. Changes and additions should be made as much in advance as possible.

Examples of predictable needs that should be included in your "up-front" list and schedule can include:

- daily dressing, grooming, meal prep and eating
- triweekly bowel routine and shower
- biweekly laundry
- weekly shopping, cleaning your wheelchair
- routinely watering house plants
- any predictable and routine need for assistance.

Unpredictable needs. Although these valid needs are not routine, they are foreseeable, and help can be requested only near the time of the need. These should be occasional or one-shot tasks, such as:

- picking up eyeglasses or a book from the floor
- retrieving a desired, out-of-reach book
- pushing the plug to the TV back into the wall outlet
- closing the out-of-reach window shades after finding that the afternoon sun is too bright or hot
- cleaning the wheelchair after spilling soup on it, as contrasted with the weekly, routine, listed cleaning
- repairing the wheelchair after a tire suddenly goes flat, as contrasted with scheduled maintenance inspection and repair

• cleaning a spill in the refrigerator, as contrasted with the regular cleaning.

Some of these needs are urgent and some are not. A common mistake with this kind of need is to label any unforeseen need as being urgent or an emergency, and demanding immediate help. The caregiver or PA soon resents the unexpressed implication of, "I want help, I want it now, and it is your job to give me help whenever I want it because you work for me and I sign your paycheck!"

If you believe the unforeseen need is urgent or a borderline emergency, then seek help appropriately soon from any available source. (Further details are provided in the "Emergency needs" subsection.)

If the need is not urgent, but merely remedies an inconvenience or discomfort, then perhaps wait until help is next available and avoid a special request. For example, if a book falls to the floor or the TV becomes unplugged, and your PA is due to be in the area within a reasonable time, then it is common sense to wait until her next routine arrival.

While you are waiting, increase your independence by devising ways to fix future occurrences by yourself. For example, if a book is often out of reach when no assistance is available, then try to plan ahead and use setup help (see the following section for more on this type of help). Plan on which books you might need later in the day and request them before the PA leaves. If your glasses often fall onto the floor, then try to design a reaching aid to enable you to pick them up by yourself.

Watch your needs as they occur and look for any recurring tasks. Ask whether any unpredictable needs could be prevented or reduced by adding that task to your list of routinely scheduled, predictable needs.

If the need is not at all urgent, then discuss scheduling the assistance with your PA during the next time you are together. Ask to schedule help as much in advance as possible, and avoid last-minute requests whenever possible.

If you know which needs qualify for PA help and which strategy to use in asking for that help, then being assertive in making your request will be much easier for you. For example, Walter decides that he would like to have his wheelchair cleaned this week because he plans to attend his cousin's wedding on Saturday. Here is an appropriate, assertive way to request assistance for sporadic needs:

Walter: "Cheryl-Lynn, my cousin's wedding is this coming Saturday, and I would like my wheelchair cleaned before I attend the wedding. It should take about a half hour. When this week would it be convenient for you to clean it?"

Emergency needs. The third type of need is not foreseeable, can occur at any time, and requires immediate assistance or medical attention because it threatens safety, health, or property. Examples can include:

• feeling severe bowel or bladder distention

• being in the initial stages of falling out of bed

• requiring an out-of-reach medication for a sudden health concern

• smelling or seeing smoke in your environment

- hearing or seeing someone breaking into your residence
- seeing smoke coming from a motor in the wheelchair in which you are sitting.

The rule-of-thumb definition of an *emergency* is "a situation where the property, safety, or health of anyone is in immediate danger or jeopardy." If you have identified a need as being an emergency or near-emergency, then you are justified—at any time of day or night—in asking for help wherever and however you can get it.

Kinds of requests: What types of help can you request?

Here is another viewpoint of the three types of help that are available from a PA.[1] Each requires you to state your preferences about where, when, and how to provide the help you need. Generally, the more severe the limitations of a disability, the more extensive the need for help and the more detailed the preferences.

Face-to-face help. This is help provided while in the presence of a PA who accommodates you with help for some or all of a task.

Help for personal activities of daily living (ADLs) is often in this category. Preferences are usually provided here in the form of step-by-step, face-to-face instructions during each activity. Of these three types of help, your preferences for this type will be the most detailed.

When you are receiving face-to-face assistance for your ADL needs, help is usually provided by your direct instructions. These personal needs include bathing, using the toilet, grooming, dressing, and eating. Only you know best how to take care of your body, and what assistance you require to provide yourself with that care. Your preferences for receiving help for these activities are essential for your well-being. You require the most help for these activities, and you do not usually attempt to do them alone because you would be risking your health and safety.

Face-to-face tasks include:

- Tasks that are personal and involve direct help to your body. Examples include dressing and undressing, wheelchair transfers, grooming, and eating assistance.

- Tasks that require instructions or directions that are too complicated or complex for teaching a PA. The PA needs your onsite input and interaction. An example is your need to supervise a PA at your computer while he finds, modifies, and saves a specific file.

- Tasks that require you to analyze and make on-the-spot decisions about a situation, and provide directions to the PA who performs the task. Examples include assembling a newly purchased item or repairing something.

Keep those preferences logical, reasonable, and respectful of time and energy for both you and the PA, and you should hear few complaints.

---

1. Also discussed in chapter 📖 **12, "Getting It Done—Your Way!"**

Setup help. This is help provided by placing items in accessible locations, and often even positioning them, so you can later reach and use them.

Included here is the preparation for any activity that you perform independently, after the aide leaves and when help providers are not available. Examples are turning on a TV or computer, gathering books or papers into a reading area, or even setting the table for a meal that you eat on your own. Your preferences for this setup help will be the second most detailed.

If you are like most people, the bulk of your day's activity takes place after a PA leaves and you are alone. To maximize your independence, you must plan ahead to foresee where activity will take place and with what materials. Before the PA leaves, you need setup help in putting items in accessible locations and positions.

Setup help is essential for you to accomplish all that you wish while you are alone. Few situations are as frustrating as looking forward to a day's activities, and then discovering—after a morning PA has departed—that "item G" is still located on an upper shelf, out of your reach. In desperation, you grab a long stick and begin jabbing at it in attempts to knock it down to be within reach. If this is not a lucky day, a couple of fragile or spillable things will crash before you finally pull down what you were originally after!

To prevent this, you might make a habit each night of listing setup items for the following day's activities. Some standard items that you use each day will already have standard, accessible locations. Other items, that you use occasionally, must be relocated or pulled out of storage—to be within your reach—by your PA at your request.

It is important to keep especially those standard items in predictable and accessible places. First, you are physically dependent on being able to find, reach, and use those things. In addition, because your level of independent activity and function with many items is linked to their accessible location, you might even feel an emotional ease and security when frequently used items are accessibly located where they should be. In contrast, you might feel an overall discomfort and anxiety when appliances, facilities, or items that you often independently use are temporarily out of reach. For example, when the kitchen or family room is torn up for two weeks for remodeling, you are also torn up. You have briefly lost a chunk of your prized independent activity or territory. To other family members, temporarily living out of boxes is an irritating inconvenience. To you, the forced dysfunction, increased dependence on requesting help, and loss of control can be downright depressing.

Within the daily traffic routes of your home and office, there are many areas where you concentrate different kinds of activity: the bathroom sink and counter, where you wash up and do your grooming; the kitchen table, for meals and snacks; the living room table, for watching TV and reading; and a desk, where your computer, office folders, and piles of paper projects are kept.

In each area, you enjoy the freedom of working alone and on your own schedule as much as possible. If you have limited arm reach and hand grasp, you will be quite specific about what materials are to be assembled in a work area, where each should be accessibly located, and even how some must be positioned. Of the three types of help, setup help requires you to do the most advance planning of tomorrow's schedule, activities, and items. The more severe the physical limitations, including sight, the more important is each preference of location and positioning.

The following examples are typical accommodations for a spinal-cord-injured, high-level quad (tetraplegic) who has limited arm reach and no hand grasp:

- In the bathroom, at the sink and counter, your electric razor might be mounted on a special wooden stand that a therapist built. For you to shave independently, the stand must be located about 3 inches (7.5 cm) to the right of the sink. The razor must be mounted with two rubber bands, its blades pointing toward the ceiling. You shave each morning, so you instruct the PA about setting up the stand, cleaning the razor head afterward, and putting it all away.

- At the living room table, you might watch TV, read, and do homework for your college courses or career. Each morning, you instruct a PA about today's selection of reading matter and homework papers. Some items are located forward of others, for more immediate use. It is also common for the PA to follow your instructions for sorting, piling, and positioning materials. Tonight or tomorrow morning, some materials and books are returned to folders and bookshelves, while new ones are pulled out and positioned on the desk for the next day.

- Within a computer work area, the "within reach" locations of the keyboard and mouse might be especially important. The keyboard is positioned very close to the desk edge, a little left of center, and the right-side mouse is positioned at an angle and toward the right. The mouse cord should be straight, untwisted, and trail out of the way, directly over the edge of the desk. Each week, when your PA dusts the area, you try to make sure that everything is back in place or it will be inaccessible.

Remote help. Remote help is provided when you tell a PA how to accomplish a task without your being present. He might be watering houseplants in another room or running an errand across town. Here, your preferences will be mostly in the form of instructions or objectives to be carried out by the PA in your absence. When compared to face-to-face and setup help, your preferences are the least detailed—but still very significant—for this type of help.

Remote help has distinct advantages both for you and the PA. Managing a PA to provide remote help is an advanced skill. Not every recipient can do it, and not every PA can provide it. Consequently, many recipients of help assign remote tasks only when they cannot possibly be with the aide. These people assign face-to-face help 99 percent of the time. They see only disadvantages in the rare need to have a PA perform a task without them.

In contrast, PA managers who have advanced management skills use remote help as often as possible. They favor it because of its efficiency. When you can be doing something independently while your aide does a second task remotely, you are getting two tasks completed at the same time. When a PA does a remote task while you perform a second task, you save time, energy, and PA salary. In addition, when given the choice, most PAs prefer to work independently with a minimum of onsite supervision.

When assigning remote tasks, four factors will increase the chances that you can reasonably trust a PA to succeed with an assignment:

- you select which of your PAs have sufficient intelligence, common sense, and problem-solving skills to independently carry out remote task assignments

- you are able to trust that the selected aides will carry out your remote assignments, and you can be tolerant of occasional mistakes without punishing the aide

- your directions or instructions must be complete and easy to follow

- the routine steps of a task should be supplemented with "what if" comments in case your original instructions or preferences are not possible. Give the PA any extra information so he can make "Plan B" decisions without you there.

Perhaps the first hurdle is identifying which PAs have the competence to carry out instructions. It is often difficult to know when you are dealing with an efficient, conscientious person you can trust to independently meet your request, and when you are interacting with a forgetful airhead whom you must supervise and monitor to get the job done.

Your mistaken ability assessment means either using too much control and supervision, and having conscientious PAs resent you, or not sufficiently supervising less competent providers, and jeopardizing your independence, health, or safety when dependent needs are forgotten or not correctly satisfied. The latter type requires you to make your request, anticipate where the PAs might forget details, and consequently monitor them until the job is done correctly.

Not every aide is sharp enough to be able to work alone, and identifying those who are is the result of careful observation. After providing face-to-face instructions to a group of new PAs, you will soon recognize which ones are capable of working on their own. Those who need your supervision are usually comfortable working that way, whereas the sharper aides enjoy working independently.

In each crew of four or five part-time PAs, there are usually one or two who prove to have a poor memory for remembering details or an inability to plan and work efficiently. Do you fire them? Not usually. A wise PA manager merely assigns these forgetful folks the simpler, less-detailed tasks. They get a priority on face-to-face tasks of helping you that quietly permit you to keep an eye on whether all the steps of a chore are remembered and are completed in the way that your efficiency and personal safety require.

For many managers, the most difficult skill is learning to trust. To trust in PAs is to have confidence that they have a reasonable, but not infallible, ability to remember and carry out the details of an assignment. You cannot expect perfection from any PA—or even yourself. Competent people often fail to do quality work because their boss keeps interfering with supervision. If you have given clear instructions to competent PAs, then give them the chance to succeed: leave them alone and let them do their jobs.

When you first start using PA help, or during the initial training of new aides, there is a tendency to supervise everything they do to be sure it is done correctly. Then you get more experienced and smarter at this "PA stuff." You learn how to provide clear instructions to an aide, and perhaps you watch the first time the task is performed. However, you are soon comfortable to instruct, dispatch, and trust that at least some aides can carry out assignments on their own.

Directions, instructions, and comments for remote help must be especially clear, complete, and easy to follow, because you will not be there to supervise. If the steps for a task are few and especially easy, then simply run through them with each PA. However, you should consider writing or printing out the directions or instructions when:

- there are numerous steps to a task, and you want to increase the chances that none will be forgotten
- some or all of the steps or comments are very detailed
- there are specific brands, model numbers, sizes, quantities, or other specifics that are important (especially when you assign a PA to perform shopping errands). Here, you also provide "Plan B" directions and choices in case your "Plan A" preferences are not available.

You should also have written instructions as a matter of convenience to you (for example, when the same instructions will be routinely followed by a number of PAs over a number of years). To a new PA, the printed sheet provides initial training instructions; afterward, the sheet provides a convenient reference to save the PA from having to memorize the details. For example:

- Computer-printed steps to doing your laundry, with settings for the washer and dryer, can be laminated and then taped to the washer lid.
- Sticks or tongue depressors stuck into the soil of each pot, giving houseplant care instructions.

Not all of your directions and preferences will be implemented according to your original intentions. Although stating your original preferences about how you want remote help to be supplied is important, sometimes you have to settle for secondary ones because the originals are simply not possible. You will need to provide an original set of instructions and preferences, and you will usually be wise to provide a "Plan B" for when your PA runs into obstacles. If you do not provide a secondary set of instructions or preferences, then you are relinquishing this option and giving aides permission to make their own decisions.

For example, if you send a PA out to buy groceries, and one of the items is a pint of Ben and Jerry's Toffee Crunch ice cream, what is the PA to do if there is no Toffee Crunch in the market's freezer? Is it Toffee Crunch or nothing? Or is it "one pint of any of the following, listed in order of preference: Toffee Crunch, Double Fudge Brownie, Cherry Garcia, or nothing."

Thus, the process is to identify who can provide remote help, provide them with clear instructions and preferences, and then enjoy the freedom of letting them work on their own. Your time is used most efficiently when you can get two things done at the same time: the project they are working on and your own.

Locations for requests: Where can you ask for help?

There are several locations or scenarios of help that are appropriate for you to seek. The following section breaks them down into five categories: personal help, living-area help, activity help, errand help, and travel help.

Personal help. This help accommodates bodily functions and ADLs, including bathing, using the toilet, grooming, dressing, eating, and getting positioned in bed for a good night's sleep.

Similar to the face-to-face help discussed earlier, this help with personal needs is the most basic.

Living-area help. This addresses non-personal activities of kitchen, laundry, medical equipment, storage, gardening and yard work, car upkeep, and household cleaning, maintenance, and repairs (with or without you present).

Some PAs will be skilled at cleaning things; others will be inclined toward making repairs. Some needs, such as routine wheelchair cleaning, will be appropriate for PA requests, whereas others, such as the more complex repairs to a motorized wheelchair's electronic circuit board, will require outside professionals.

Here, help enables maintaining the environment that surrounds and supports your personal needs.

Activity help. This addresses educational, career, computer, financial, medical, pets, leisure, recreational, cultural, and spiritual; activities projects, meetings, appointments, conferences, and events; at home or in the community (usually with you present).

This assistance enables you to go outside the home and participate in the business, medical, and cultural communities.

Errand help. This satisfies the need for groceries and other shopping, maintenance, and repairs from the area community (with or without you present).

Similar to activity help, errands address utility needs of purchasing goods and services from the community.

Travel help. This accommodates local and distance travel, for day trips or extended overnights, for leisure or business purposes (with you present).

Travel help can be similar to activity help; however, the emphasis is on accommodating your disability for transportation and room-and-board needs. Travel help gets you there and prepares your temporary living quarters so that your PA can next provide you with personal help. Finally, activity help will enable you to participate in the events of the new locale.

Chapter 12

Getting It Done—Your Way!

When I started helping him, I often wondered why he had such specific ways of doing things, or even an exact location where he needed things placed. I had never met anyone so organized. He also seemed overly demanding about whether I arrived each morning on time for work. His day was incredibly scheduled and structured. At first, I thought he was simply a control freak who would live longer if he could just learn how to chill out!

Then, after a week or two, I was amazed at all that I had observed and learned about living with a disability—so much about his lifestyle began to make sense. Ways of doing things and exact locations were essential in order to maximize the number of things he could do alone and independently, while minimizing his dependence on others. He wanted me to be punctual in coming to work, because he was paralyzed, in bed, and unable to do anything until I did arrive. His day was structured and scheduled because he was dependent on coordinating both his own schedule and that of his PAs so he could be punctual in attending the meetings and appointments of his active lifestyle. Some of his preferences addressed ways for preventing the recurrence of illnesses and skin breakdowns, and it was understandable that these rigid preferences had to be as strongly defended as was his daily fight to stay healthy—and stay alive.

Assertively stating, explaining, and often defending your preferences with caregivers and PAs are important, and often overlooked, PA management skills. It is as important to train PAs in how to help you as it is to tell them what help you need and why. If you are unable to do so, and you give up asserting your preferences, you will most certainly lose some of your independent, active lifestyle, and perhaps threaten your health and safety.

It is not uncommon for providers to question the importance of preferences, and sometimes your lone efforts in defending and fighting for them becomes a more habitual part of your lifestyle than you had realized.

A few years ago, I was consulting with a physician about upcoming surgery and a month-long hospital stay. The doc was open to discussion, and I told him that I was concerned about my upcoming relations with the nursing staff. I was prepared to accept their instructions about my responsibilities toward my new, post-surgery concerns. However, would they be accepting of my instructions about my preferences for managing my daily disability needs? Yes, I understood my need to be flexible around the hospital setting, schedule, and staff availability, but would they be equally flexible around the unique ways that I take care of my particular disability?

After 33 years with my disability and many hospitalizations, I had learned to recognize the difference between the acute care for a temporary medical need that I must trust to the staff, and the disability-related chronic maintenance that they must entrust to me. For the acute medical needs, I gladly follow their instructions—however, for my lifelong, disability-related needs, they must follow mine.

I had heard from disabled peers and personally experienced many gruesome stories of near-fatal pressure sores and other medical horrors that develop when patients with disabilities surrender all their care to the medical staff.

Sometimes this surrender occurs because of a patient's naturally passive personality, and his consequent inability to assertively state his help needs and preferences to others. At other times, even the usually assertive patient surrenders to very aggressive medical staff because he is sick, weak, and temporarily lacks the strength required to be insistent and defensive of his routine, disability-related needs. To prevent this latter situation, it is often helpful for the patient to introduce his concerns to nursing supervisors before admission. When you employ this strategy, supervisors will usually be more willing and ready to advocate on his behalf if it becomes necessary. Their advocacy will apply to maintaining the especially high level of health care that his disability requires, as well as to defending his care preferences in the face of bedside help providers who would often resent and resist his assertive efforts.

As I used these arguments to rationalize my upcoming request to meet with the nursing supervisor in advance of my admission, the understanding doc nodded, smiled, and reminded me of the importance of my preferences in the ways help is provided to me for my disability-related needs.

> He said, "Al, you have survived over 30 years of living with a spinal cord injury, and you have led an incredibly productive and independent life. You know better than we do about how to accommodate your disability. There is no need for you to apologize about having or defending your care preferences. I admire them and your spirit. Without your advocating so strongly for yourself each day, you would have been dead a long time ago."

His comments were a real eye-opener for me. I had not realized until then how many caregivers and PAs over the years had reacted to my preferences with misunderstanding, disbelief, or even resentful anger. For decades, they had routinely questioned whether the extra steps were necessary... and perhaps I had become subconsciously concerned that I would begin to question them, also. For many years, I had been alone in fighting their resistance. Even though, deep inside, I had known all along how very important my preferences are, it was comforting to receive confirmation from my doctor.

Indeed, your preferences are absolutely essential to your continued survival with a disability. More than an able-bodied person, you are dependent on making wise choices, and even then you are often alone in your fight to defend them. Through years of difficult trial and error, you have developed your preferences by identifying what works and what does not.

This chapter is meant to assure you of the importance of those preferences, and to urge you to fight to maintain them—in getting help provided your way!

Your lifestyle makes very logical sense to you, but to others, especially your own family caregivers and paid PAs, you sometimes seem to be an inflexible person with rigid preferences. To them, your insistence on how your help is provided seems at first to point toward needless perfectionism.

It is common for the people who help you to misunderstand the importance of, or the reasons behind, your preferences. Consequently, what these people do not understand they cannot accept, and instead resent and vigorously question.

In this chapter, you will be assured that it is permitted and essential to specify how you want help to be provided.[1]

We will identify some common categories of disability-related preferences, reasons for their being essential to your independence, and strategies for explaining them to new PAs.

What are preferences, and why are they important to you?

From the first day of your disability, consciously and unconsciously, you began planning and devising new ways of doing things. The help you need bridges the gap between what you want to do and what you cannot do independently. Only you know what you want to do, how much of each activity you can and cannot do on your own, and the details of what help you need from others. In turn, the help you need from others usually carries some detailed preferences.[2]

Face-to-face help is provided when a PA works directly with you. ADL needs of dressing, grooming, transfers, bathing, and eating assistance are examples of this kind of help. Clearly, your preferences here are essential in how and in what order you want this item-by-item help provided.

---

1. In two other chapters, 📖 11, **"When It Is, and Is Not, Okay to Ask for Help,"** and 📖 13, **"Defining and Describing Your Help Needs,"** you found guidelines for listing what help you need.

2. To illustrate these preferences, let's look at the three types of help discussed in chapter 📖 11, **"When It Is, and Is Not, Okay to Ask For Help."**

Setup help is provided when a PA puts items in locations so you can later independently use them after the aide has gone. If you have limitations of reach and grasp, then you will be designating locations for items as well as specific positions for them within those locations. For example, you might ask that five specific books be pulled down from a bookshelf and located on your desk. If you have limited reach or grasp, you might additionally specify where you want this pile of books, and in what order you want them stacked, according to the order in which you plan to use them.

Remote help is provided when you instruct your aide in how to perform some tasks when you are not with the aide. Examples can include his cooking breakfast in the kitchen while you groom in the bathroom, or his selecting and buying your groceries while you are at home finishing some computer work. Clearly, your preferences about which groceries you want, which store you prefer, and when the shopping should be done are important preferences for assigning this type of help.

For additional illustrations of the variety of actual preferences you probably use everyday, think of almost any activity with which you need help. Next, think of how you would answer a new aide who asks, "What help do you need, and how would you like me to provide it?" The list of possible preferences seems to be endless.

These preferences begin to develop as soon as you create your list of needs. As you use PA help over and over, the list is routinely revised and improved. You learn what works and what does not.

The list of what help is needed is usually simple and straightforward. The items are logical and common sense in relation to the limitations of your disability. In contrast, the preferences of how you want this help provided are more subjective. They are based on your opinion of whether one method will accommodate you better than another, and why that is important to you.

You are unique. No one else has the special combination of your limitations, abilities, daily lifestyle of activities, schedule of needed help, and opinions about which types of help will accommodate you and which will not. No one else can decide how help should be provided to you, or how best to explain it. Your unique understanding of how you prefer to receive help means that *only* you can explain and teach these preferences to new PAs. Explanations and descriptions from anyone else would be secondhand, and not as accurate as those that you provide directly from the source.

Because of your disability and need for help from others, there are usually several people interacting with you at any given time. Each person comes into your life, learns your routine, provides help for a period of time, and then moves on. Each incoming PA requires training in what help you need, how you want it provided, and why these preferences are important.

Consequently, your list of needs and preferences should be taught to each new PA directly from you unless a secondary disability requires your use of a PA coordinator who acts on your behalf. There are no shortcuts.

Why PAs should understand the reasons for your preferences

By now you should be feeling comfortable about the reasons for, and importance of, your preferences. If you also take the time to explain to PAs why each preference is important, you will accomplish two things:

- the tasks and preferences will be easier for your PAs to remember, so the need to remind PAs of forgotten details will be minimized
- the extra time and effort for providing you help in specific ways will be justified, so the preferences will not seem unreasonable and the PA will keep the job longer.

Many PA managers simply tell each aide what help they need and how to provide it. When managers neglect to explain the reasons behind these preferences, they omit an essential part of training. As a result, some PAs will resent the seemingly needless, overwhelming, and unreasonable details, and sometimes the entire job of working with you.

Must you explain the reason for each and every preference? Not at all. A good guideline is to provide a brief rationale for those preferences that are especially detailed and time-consuming. In addition, keep an eye out for instances when a PA appears to be tired of and even resistant to your insistence that a task be accomplished in a specific way. Watch for the look on a PA's face that says, "My way would be so much faster and easier for me. Why are you being so stubborn and inflexible about insisting that I do this task your way? Is there a good reason, or are you instead pushing my buttons because you want to be in control?"

One approach is simply to tell each new PA that "things have to be done my way" and avoid any further explanations. The problem with this passive approach to training is that your preferences involve extra steps, time, and effort from an aide. The aide would like to provide help in the most efficient, time-saving ways possible unless the extra time is justified.

It is very common in disagreements, when the aide does not understand the preferences and sees no reason for the extra effort, for the help recipient to give up and give in. An aide sometimes has incredible bargaining power over us, especially when she is our one-and-only aide. Many of us have at some time felt, "I would rather give in about having something done, or done my way, than to lose even an undesirable PA who is getting increasingly angry."

These tense times can be minimized by explaining, as an integral part of training, why your preferences are important.

Strategies for teaching PAs what, how, and why

By nature, the work that PAs do for you involves more preferences than other jobs they have worked. You are wise to introduce this fact early, beginning with applicant interviews, continuing through training, and on into day-to-day management.

- During initial job interviews, introduce the fact that aide work has more preferences than most other jobs.

At this interview stage, you want to describe the personal nature of the work, with your physical dependence on having help provided in specific ways as the rationale for why the preferences are important. You can advise the interviewing applicants that if they are uncomfortable working with a "detail person," they would be wise to think twice before committing themselves to the job. How detailed are you? How tolerant are you when PAs routinely forget some of the details? Do you get angry, or do you keep your cool and quietly remind the aide of a forgotten step? The chance for PAs to observe the answers to questions like these is one reason for you to insist that PA applicants watch a demo of your routine before deciding whether to take the job. These are important considerations for applicants to realize before deciding whether they would enjoy working with you.

> A good teaching structure is a combination of three factors:
>   *What* (the task for which you require help)
> + *How and When* (your preferences about the delivery of help)
> + *Why* (your reason why the preference is important)
> = *Good PA training!*

Some applicants will be turned off by knowing about the exacting nature of the work, whereas others will see it as a unique learning experience. Indeed, if your applicants include college pre-med or therapy students, you can boast that working with you will provide many valuable insights about working and living with a disability.

- During the on-the-job training, use a three-part formula for teaching each element of your routine.

Demonstrate what help you need and how to provide it, with a quick explanation of why that preference is important. That way, a PA gets a complete package of information at one time. The PAs will remember more details, and will be more willing to spend their time and energy on those details, if they understand them.

Provide clear, logical, step-by-step instructions of what help you need, as well as how and when it should be provided. In addition, the cement that holds together these details is your telling the provider why each preference is important. By including why, you first give the needs credibility and importance by proving that they are necessary. Second, you make it easier for a PA to remember the details of what, how, and when.

- During later, ongoing work, provide small reminders as needed.

As you provide initial training to new PAs, there is a fine line between the stage where they are still learning and need instruction, and the stage where they have sufficiently learned the routine, prefer to independently generate their own "what's next" from memory, and actually resent your additional instruction.[3]

Avoiding unnecessary preferences

Valid, genuine preferences are essential in the help you receive; unnecessary ones are a waste of your PA's time and energy, and will be resented.

How can you tell if you might be making unnecessary requests for what help you need or how it is supplied? Watch out for two main indicators.

First, the reason for a preference should make logical sense when comparing it to accommodating the specific limitations of your disability. If a PA were to question you as to a request you are about to make, could you provide a logical explanation for its importance? If not, then the request might not be logical and valid.

Second, your expression of a preference should be a factual, objective, straight-faced instruction. Do you sometimes get emotional—showing anger, frustration, depression, or arrogance—when communicating with a PA? While facing the PA, could you deliver a rationale that justifies the preference with a straight face and a freedom from inappropriate emotions? If not, then the unavoidable emotion is usually the symptom of an unstated message. When this happens, the preference request is often a secondary way of expressing (for example) anger. "I'm really angry at this aide. I'll show her. I'll make her do such-and-such, and make her do it my way."

It is easy to get carried away with stating preferences. Some folks want to control everything they can in life; others feel an ego boost from having a PA follow their orders.

If you are getting odd looks from a PA who questions whether some preferences are necessary, ask yourself whether you are getting carried away. If you are, and the justification for some requests is getting shaky, then back off. A PA will notice hollow requests for help, and will resent them.[4]

---

3. For advice about how to make a smooth transition between the detailed instructions needed during initial training, and the occasional reminders to PAs when they forget "what's next" while providing your help, please see chapter 📖 9, **"Initial Training and Ongoing Management of Aides and PAs."**

4. For more detail about how unnecessary requests can cause resentment, and how to recognize valid and invalid requests, please see chapter 📖 11, **"When It Is, and Is Not, Okay to Ask for Help."**

Chapter 13
Defining and Describing Your Help Needs

Imagine arriving at McDonald's or Burger King to answer an ad for a cook. You meet with the manager and ask, "What will I be doing?"

The manager answers, "Gee, you...umm...just stand here and make burgers."

"But how? How do you want them made?"

"Well...you know...just cook up some patties, toss one in a bun, and add some stuff." You can bet that neither McDonald's nor Burger King trains its staff this way, and neither should you. Companies like these have formal task lists and job descriptions. Do you need to write out a formal list and schedule of your needs? That depends on your informal or formal personal style.

This chapter's objective is to prompt you to firmly identify and know, backward and forward, what help you need, as well as how and when you need it! This chapter tells you why this is important, and then gives you some options on how to assemble your list of needs and then evaluate it.

Before you hire your first PA, you should identify and then understand when and where you require help. Making this list for the first time can be tedious and time-consuming, but it serves several important purposes. Once the initial list has been completed, making later revisions is much easier (especially if it is stored on a computer).

In format, this list can be just a mental outline, a handwritten draft, or a very detailed set of neatly printed, computerized columns. Your choice will depend on your personal style and how you plan to use the information. A mental outline or handwritten laundry list is fine if you intend to discuss it with each PA. A more detailed, printed list and description are better if you wish to hand the PA— whether applicant or hired aide—a reference copy. Printed materials also can be handy for folks with communication disabilities. Those who will be using a home health aide agency can give the list to an agency supervisor.

Advantages to making your list or job description

The main advantage of making a list of routine and non-routine needs is that it assists you to identify and understand what help you need. You must know your needs, and know them well, before you can tell your aides about them.

"This is a waste of time. Why would I need to assemble a formal list of my help needs? I already know what my needs are."

In truth, your needs for help are quite extensive. Although most occur on a daily basis, others happen weekly, monthly, or even once or twice a year. If you are like most of us, you have a tendency to forget about the less frequent needs until their time arrives. It is then that you turn to your aides to add more tasks to their list. You can save yourself from having to make sporadic "add-ons" by initially creating a more complete list.

Most importantly, let's not forget an essential objective in the way you want to be, appear, communicate, and function with your help providers. Without a doubt, you want to be in control of your lifestyle and schedule. Because you have a disability and are dependent on receiving help from providers, your control includes having authority over who helps you, as well as the quality and schedule of help you receive. You should actually be in constant control of these factors, and your help providers must convinced that you have this control before they will respect your authority. There are many "wannabe" leaders who are officially in control of a situation; in actuality, though, they have insufficient operative power and are not effective in directing subordinates. Why? Because these weak supervisors do not project the appearance—they lack the outward image—of being in control, organized, and scheduled.

So, for you to be in control, you must also appear to others to be in control. When you first meet PA applicants who are considering your job, your first impression should be of someone who is clear thinking, authoritative, organized, and without any doubts knows what help is needed, as well as when, where, and how that help is to be provided. Your authoritative image will be off to a big head start if your list of help needs—in whatever format works best for you—is clear, concise, well organized, and well scheduled.

A clear list of help needs tells both PA applicants and newly hired PAs, "This person has his head together and knows what he needs. My job will be to follow his directions and provide the help."

Yes, you know your help needs, but the people who will be helping you do not. Each of these providers will need a complete list, and many will find it helpful for that list to be organized in different ways. Some providers will be working morning shifts, and will want to see the list of morning tasks. If you have been wise enough to divide your needs among several part-time aides, those aides will be examining several different combinations and schedules of duties before deciding which piece of the pie best fits their available work schedule.

To summarize, you are creating a comprehensive list of your needs so that:

- You will have an accurate, truly comprehensive view of what help needs you have, as well as when, where, and how you want the help provided.

- You will be able to personally review and evaluate the validity of asking for help with needs that occur at various times of each day, each week, each month, each season, and once or twice each year.

- You can total the weekly and monthly hours of help, and calculate and budget for these costs.

- Your first impression to PA applicants, and your ongoing impression to PA employees, will be of an authoritative person who knows what help is needed. You are clearly the boss, and the PAs' role is clearly to follow your directions and provide the help.

- Your list will make it easier to cite your needs to PA applicants or home health aide agencies, as well as to hired PAs whom you are training.

- You and PAs will be better able to visualize logical divisions of your needs among several part-time PAs.

> *Just as a building contractor requires a blueprint in order to instruct construction help, you should know your own needs before instructing PA help.*

Making your list and schedule of needs

First, clearly visualize or write out your list of help needs. In your mind, walk through the activities of a routine day from the time you wake up on a typical morning. Note each activity or group of activities. You might find it useful to visualize or write out a three-column listing that includes the following:

- A brief title or descriptor for each need or group of needs. It is not necessary to list every single step, but main headings are helpful.

- The approximate time (starting and duration) for each need. These times are merely planning guidelines, and not a rigid, minute-by-minute schedule for the PA to follow.

- A third column can show how often a need occurs, such as
  - ▸ the number of times a need occurs each day, week, month, season, year
  - ▸ morning, noon, afternoon, evening
  - ▸ each (specified day)
  - ▸ "unpredictable" (for those needs that occur without warning or occur with no predictable schedule).

Second, after you have sketched out this list, review it for the next several days as you actually ask for help. Revise the entries until they are accurate. Your list should include each predictable activity, regardless of whether it occurs each day, two or three times per week, once or twice a month, on a seasonal schedule, or even on an unpredictable frequency and schedule.

Third, review the list to decide whether all the needs are appropriate for help.[1]

A sample list and schedule of needs

You can decide how detailed you want to make your list, and whether it will be memorized and verbal, handwritten, or in computer-printed columns, like the following sample. *Figure 13-1* is a sample, partial list with illustrations of male needs for "Barry."

> *Your list should include all of your routine and non-routine needs. Do not cheat by leaving out less-attractive or unpleasant tasks.*

Barry is a C 4/5 spinal-cord-injured quadriplegic who has very limited use of arms. Although he has no motor use of fingers or wrists, he can sometimes "grasp" light-weight objects between his hands. He usually requires eating assistance, but he can independently use his motorized wheelchair and computer. For the 40 hours of weekly help that he needs, he employs five part-time aides who are recruited from both the local college and general-population communities. He is the personnel director for a utility company. He puts in long, eight- to ten-hour days at his office, to which he commutes across the city from his home.

---

1. Check out the guidelines in chapter 📖 11, "When It Is, and Is Not, Okay to Ask for Help."

Figure 13-1: **Barry's list and schedule of help needs**

Title of Need	Start When?	How Long?	How Often?
• PA arrives	6 A.M.		x7 mornings
• Takes morning medications in bed			
• Empties bladder, attaches leg bag		5 min.	
• Gets dressed w/ socks, binder, pants		5 min.	
• Transfers to wheelchair & adjusts position		10 min.	
• Washes face, brushes teeth	~6:25	10 min.	
• PA sets up electric razor and hair brush	~6:30	1 min.	
• Shaves and finishes grooming (independent)	~6:35	15 min.	
• PA does tasks while he grooms; tasks vary— empty dishwasher, start/fold laundry, water plants, start breakfast, other	~6:35	15 min.	
• PA helps him finish dressing	~6:50	10 min.	
• PA cooks breakfast, assists eating, cleans kitchen	7:00	30 min.	
• PA dresses him for outside, transfers to car	7:30	15 min.	each weekday
• PA drives him to school or work	7:45	30 min.	
• At school or work— transfers from car to wheelchair, gets inside classroom or office, gets established; good-bye	8:30	10 min.	

Figure 13-1: **Barry's list and schedule of help needs (continued)**

Title of Need	Start When?	How Long?	How Often?
• Meets PA to catheterize (or empty leg bag) in restroom (or at home)	12 noon, 3 P.M.	10 min.	Monday-Friday (or Sat, Sun)
• Meets PA for lunchroom help— Go through line, get food, carry tray to table, prepare food, assist eating	12:10	45 min.	Each weekday
(or)			
• Meets PA at home for lunch— cook, serve food, assist eating, clean kitchen	12:15	1 hour	Sat, Sun
• Meets PA, dresses for outside, transfers to car	5 P.M.	15 min.	Each weekday
• Commutes to home with driver	5:15 P.M.	30 min.	Each weekday
• At home— transfers from car to wheelchair, gets inside, gets help off with jacket; good-bye	5:45 P.M.	15 min.	Each weekday
(or)			
• Meets PA—cook dinner, serve food, assist eating, clean kitchen	6:00 P.M.	1 hour	x7 eves
• Setup help for eve activity; good-bye	7:00 P.M.	15 min.	x7 eves
• Meets eve PA— open & process mail, put away day's projects, set up next day's books-files-activity	9:00 P.M.	30 min.	x7 eves

Figure 13-1: **Barry's list and schedule of help needs (continued)**

Title of Need	Start When?	How Long?	How Often?
• Non-shower/bowel nights— grooms at sink, transfers into bed, gets undressed and positioned in bed, gets meds	9:30 P.M.	1.5 hours	x4 eves
• Bowel/shower nights— brushes teeth at sink, transfers into shower chair, does B/S routine, transfers into bed, gets positioned in bed, gets meds	8:30 P.M.	2.5 hours	x3 eves
• Grocery shop— with PA, or PA alone		2 hours 2 hours	x1 weekly x1 weekly
• Laundry— PA alone; wash, dry, fold and put away	varies	1 hour total	x1 weekly
• House cleaning	varies	1 hour	x1 weekly
• Bowel or bladder accident cleanup	varies	1 hour avg.	unpredictable
• Medical appts.— transport, assistance	varies		unpredictable
• PA cleans wheelchair while he grooms at sink		15 min.	2x monthly
• Vacations, business trips	varies varies	some same day some overnight	
• PA is called for middle-of-the-night bladder distention, trouble breathing, other	varies	varies	unpredictable, very rare 1x ea 4-6 mos

The job description and its six parts

A job description is just another way to tell help providers what you need from them. It starts with data from your list and schedule (see the first section of this chapter) and adds some supplementary detail. This detail fills the voids of a bare-bones list by answering additional questions asked by most PA applicants. Most of all, it emphasizes some important information that you want each applicant to hear and that you might otherwise not cover.

Whether or not you ever use a job description format in your interviewing, it is a good idea to be aware of its concept, structure, and details. If you decide not to use its format, you should in another way try to convey the details of its unique parts when you verbally describe your routine.

For a PA position, there are at least six standard sections to a comprehensive job description, whether it is verbally narrated from memory or written and printed as a handout.

Job title. Although this is usually called a job title, it is often also the title of the employee. It should identify the type of work to be done. Examples of titles that you might use include Nurse, Certified Nursing Assistant (CNA), Home Health Aide, Personal Care Assistant (PCA), Personal Assistant (PA), Personal Care Provider (PCP), Housekeeper, or Transportation Driver.

For more detail about the titles of providers with which you should be familiar, please see the introduction's chapter, **"Definitions of Titles and Terms Used in This Reference."**

Nature of work. This section usually consists of a paragraph or two that introduces the job applicant to the type of work to be done. Topics for these brief introductions can include:

- an introductory (brief and concise)
  description of you as the employer, and the physical limitations
  or abilities with which the PA will be working

- a brief outline of the type of work required (a more detailed list of duties
  will be provided in the upcoming section, "Duties to be Performed")

- a brief outline of the schedule of work required
  (an actual schedule of times will be provided
  in the upcoming section, "Duties to be performed").

Qualifications and qualities of employee. Here you first state whether you require the employee to have formal licensure, certification, training, or experience. You might not care whether an applicant has a license or certification, but if your salaries are funded by the government or insurance, they might require it.

If not, then the following qualifications will still be important to you. It is very important that you emphasize these following characteristics during the pre-hiring interview with applicants:

- To be dependable, by arriving for work as scheduled or by notifying you
  as early as possible when unable to work. You should run through your
  policy on recruiting replacements, such as requiring the original PA to call
  and recruit her own substitute from your other part-timers, and then to
  notify you of the change.

- To be punctual, arriving by the scheduled time or calling as early as possible when arrival will be delayed by 10 minutes or more.

- To respect you, as someone who—regardless of sickness or physical limitations—is capable of managing your PA employees, and who deserves respect and a high quality of assistance.

- To respect your confidentiality and privacy regarding your thoughts, values, beliefs, relationships, and activities ("what we discuss and you do at my house stays at my house").

- To respect your need for honesty and security, regarding your living quarters, personal possessions, and financial assets.

- To never arrive for work—or attempt to work—under the negative influence of alcohol, medications, or drugs.

- To be willing to discuss and resolve employment-related problems with you, and to provide you as much advance notice as possible—at least a full month—when resigning.[2]

Duties to be performed. This is your list and schedule of needs, outlined previously in this chapter.

Work schedule and comments. This is an overall summary statement that clarifies any policies or procedures that you want to emphasize or restate. Worthy of restating are the following:

- the need to provide an early notice of a late arrival;

- the responsibility of a PA to find her own substitute when unable to work a scheduled shift; and

- the one-month minimum advance notice for resignation, and the reason why.

Salary. This section should provide specifics regarding how the salary is computed, the rate of pay, the pay source, whether benefits are included, and the schedule that you or the third-party funding source uses for issuing paychecks.

Three sample job descriptions

Here are three examples of more formal, printed job descriptions. You should read through these if only to become familiar with the way they describe the six categories of information. You might never write up such formal descriptions, but you will want to include these details during PA interviews when you verbally describe your job and policies.

The first example illustrates a position for a transportation driver; the second and third apply to the more complex position of a personal assistant (PA).

---

2. For more detail on PA qualifications and expectations, please see chapters 📖 **22, "A Bill of Rights for You as a Help Recipient, Caregiver, or Paid Provider,"** and 📖 **25, "Your Personal Concerns as a Paid Help Provider, plus Ten Reasons Why PAs Quit and Are Fired."**

Job description No. 1

Job title: Transportation Driver

Nature of the person and work: Marge Janda, who uses motorized wheelchair mobility, works weekdays as a computer programmer at the Saratoga Access & Fitness Company. Although she owns a lift-equipped van, she does not drive and needs someone to drive her between her home and work site. The round-trip distance is 24 miles. The driver is asked to arrive at Marge's house each weekday morning, drive her to work, and drive the empty van back to her house. The driver is then on his own time during the day until the driving cycle is repeated in the late afternoon to get Marge back home.

Qualifications and qualities of employee: The transportation driver must have a valid driver's license and should have the following qualities relating to Marge and the work:

- to be dependable, by arriving for work as scheduled or by calling as much in advance as possible when unable to work
- to be punctual, in meeting the scheduled arrival time or by calling as much in advance as possible when arrival will be delayed by 10 minutes or more
- to respect Marge as someone who, regardless of sickness or physical limitations, deserves human respect and a high quality of assistance
- to respect Marge's confidentiality and privacy regarding her thoughts, values, beliefs, relationships, and activities
- to respect Marge's need for honesty and security regarding her living quarters, personal possessions, and financial assets
- to maintain a reasonably clean and neat personal appearance
- to never arrive at work—or attempt to work—under the influence of alcohol, medications, or drugs
- to be willing to discuss and resolve employment-related problems with Marge, and to provide her as much advance notice as possible (a minimum of one month) when resigning, to facilitate finding a replacement.

Duties to be performed:

- Arrive at Marge's home by 8 A.M. on each weekday morning.
- Help her with any outdoor clothing, and to get to and into the van.
- Drive her the 12 miles to work, which takes approximately 25 minutes in morning traffic.
- Return the empty van to her home driveway.
- Arrive at her home by 4:30 P.M. and drive the empty van to her job site for a 5 P.M. pickup.
- Drive Marge home.

Work schedule and comments: Assistance is needed in the morning and afternoon of each weekday that Marge works. She may make special trip requests; these will be made as much in advance as possible for the convenience of the driver. The driver is asked not to make personal side trips with the empty van unless he gets Marge's permission first. In addition, if Marge would like occasional "empty van" errands performed by the driver while she is at work, she will make these requests as much in advance as possible. The driver is asked to provide at least a two-week advance notice for vacation time and a four-week notice for resignation, to enable Marge to find replacement help.

Salary: The hourly salary is paid for the average round-trip time the driver spends on the road, from the time of arrival at the house to dropping off the empty van. These times average 8–9:30 A.M. and 4:30–6 P.M. and will be the basis for a three-hour pay period each day unless significant exceptions occur. The hourly rate is $8.50, and is paid personally by Marge. Paychecks are issued each Friday afternoon, unless requested for another time. All standard salary taxes are withheld; no benefits or paid vacation/sick time are provided.

Job description No. 2

Job title: Personal Assistant (PA), part-time

Nature of work: Suzy Rose is a college student at State University. A recent car accident caused a spinal-cord injury, and has resulted in paralysis and a loss of sensation below chest level. In addition, she has partial use of her arms and wrists. She uses a motorized wheelchair and drives a lift-equipped van. While attending SU for pre-law studies, she needs a PA who is also her campus dorm roommate. She needs assistance in the morning and at night, and is usually independent in attending on- and off-campus activities throughout the day.

Qualifications and qualities of employee: Students without prior PA experience, as well as trained and experienced aides, are welcome to apply. The following qualities are important:

- to be dependable, arriving for work as scheduled or calling as much in advance as possible when unable to work
- to be punctual, in meeting the scheduled arrival time or by calling as much in advance as possible when arrival will be delayed by 10 minutes or more
- for the PA roommate who shares Suzy's dorm room, to be always present in the room whenever Suzy is in bed, because of Suzy's inability to get out of bed independently in response to an emergency
- to respect Suzy as someone who, regardless of sickness or physical limitations, deserves human respect and a high quality of assistance
- to respect Suzy's confidentiality and privacy regarding her thoughts, values, beliefs, relationships, and activities
- to respect Suzy's need for honesty and security regarding her living quarters, personal possessions, and financial assets

- to never arrive at work—or attempt to work—under the influence of alcohol, medications, or drugs

- to be willing to discuss and resolve employment-related problems with Suzy, and to provide her as much advance notice as possible when resigning, to facilitate finding a replacement.

Duties to be performed: Suzy divides her list of needs among three part-time PAs. She holds a half-hour staff meeting with her PAs each two weeks. The PAs decide among themselves their scheduling preferences for the next two weeks, and mark their individual appointment books in addition to marking a master calendar for Suzy. If a PA cannot work a committed shift, the PA is responsible for calling the other aides and finding her own replacement, and then informing Suzy of the scheduling change.

Please see the attached, three-page list and schedule of Suzy's needs for help. This is the list that her PA staff meets each two weeks to negotiate.

Work schedule and comments: In addition to the listed duties, the PA occasionally will be asked to assist with non-routine duties. These will be requested and scheduled with the PA as much in advance as possible. Because of Suzy's continual dependence on assistance, PAs are requested to provide at least a week's advance notice of desired vacation time and a four-week notice of the need to resign. These advance notices are important for scheduling vacation fill-in help, or for recruiting replacements for resigning help.

Salary: The salary is $8.50 per hour. Suzy pays salaries from personal funds and paychecks will be issued each two weeks on Fridays.

Job description No. 3
Job title: Personal Assistant (PA), part-time
Nature of work: Tyrone Gossett, age 56, is recuperating at home from a stroke, for an indeterminate period of time after hospital discharge. He is attempting to gradually return to work during these later stages of recuperation. The left-side CVA has resulted in paralysis to the right half of his body, impaired speech, and partial incontinence of bowel and bladder. Tyrone needs several hours of daily assistance that he has chosen to divide among several part-time aides. Types of assistance include changing and cleaning of urinary incontinence devices, dressing, transfers between bed and wheelchair, grooming, showering, using the toilet, cooking, feeding, laundry, and household chores.

Qualifications and qualities of employee: Because Tyrone's aides are funded by the Dorcester County Health Department, his aides must have CNA (Certified Nursing Assistant) certification. In addition, all are expected to have the following qualities:

- to be dependable, arriving for work as scheduled or calling as much in advance as possible when unable to work

- to be punctual, in meeting the scheduled arrival time or by calling as much in advance as possible when arrival will be delayed by 10 minutes or more

- to respect Tyrone as someone who, regardless of sickness or physical limitations, deserves human respect and a high quality of assistance
- to respect Tyrone's confidentiality and privacy regarding his thoughts, values, beliefs, relationships, and activities
- to respect Tyrone's need for honesty and security regarding his living quarters, personal possessions, and financial assets
- to never arrive at work—or attempt to work—under the influence of alcohol, medications, or drugs
- to be willing to discuss and resolve employment-related problems with Tyrone, and to provide him as much advance notice as possible when resigning, to facilitate finding a replacement.

Duties to be performed: Tyrone divides his list of needs among five part-time PAs. He meets with his PAs for an hour each four to five weeks. The PAs decide among themselves their scheduling preferences for the next four to five weeks, and mark their individual appointment books in addition to marking a master calendar for Tyrone. If a PA cannot work a committed shift, she is responsible for calling the other aides, finding her own replacement, and then informing Tyrone of the scheduling change.

Please see the attached, three-page list and schedule of Tyrone's needs for help. This is the list that his PA staff meets each four to five weeks to negotiate.

Work schedule and comments: In addition to the listed duties, the PA occasionally will be asked to assist with non-routine duties. These will be requested and scheduled with the PA as much in advance as possible. Because of Tyrone's continual dependence on assistance, PAs are requested to provide at least a week's advance notice of desired vacation time and a four-week notice of intention to resign. These advance notices are important for scheduling vacation fill-in help, or for recruiting replacements for resigning help.

Salary: The starting salary is $9.00 per hour. Tyrone pays salaries from funds supplied by the Dorcester County Health Department; paychecks will be issued each two weeks on a standard day scheduled by the county.

Describing your help needs and PA job

If you are like most of us, and you are not instantly "verbally organized" like a rapid-fire radio DJ, you will find it very helpful to prepare your description before responding to applicants who inquire about working for you. The preparation will take just a few minutes, and you will make a well-organized first impression, while being less nervous and much more confident.

This may at first seem to be too easy a task to require formal preparation. However, remember the classic criticism of people who provide too little or too much detail in a description: "I asked him to tell me what time it was, and instead, he told me how to build a watch."

Over the upcoming years of PA recruiting, you will be describing selected parts of your routine hundreds of times. Some of these will be quick, phone-oriented outlines of the job; others will be more detailed descriptions for in-person interviews.

In both cases, you will want to impress each applicant that you are an intelligent and organized person who happens to have a disability. Each applicant's first impression of you is important to your image of being in control. Your description should be organized and concise. It should be comprehensive enough to fairly portray both attractive and unattractive details, and be delivered at a comfortable pace and in a pleasant tone of voice.

Avoid the tendency to quickly "ram through" your list of needs. Telephone telemarketers blitz through their sales script because they fear that a pause will give the listener the chance to say "no."

You will, indeed, be describing your routine hundreds of times; 10 to 15 times in each recruiting cycle for a new PA. To save your own time, effort, and voice, it is very wise to have two or three versions practiced for different situations.

These two different situations include the quick description and the in-depth discussion.

The 30-second quick description. Here, you provide a very brief, 15- to 30-second overview of your routine. This version is handy when you are in conversations with friends, fellow students, co-workers, neighbors, home health aide agencies, and current PAs. It is sometimes helpful to ask these folks whether they would be interested in helping you or whether they know of anyone who would.

Any more than a 15- to 30-second version would be too much for these people to remember in passing the word of your job offer to others.

Here's an example:

> *I need help seven mornings a week, from 6 to 7:30 a.m., and seven nights, from 7 to 9 or 10 p.m. I have a team of five part-time aides, usually college students, who divide this schedule of times. I have four people now, and am looking for a new fifth member. Anyone interested should call me.*

The five-minute overview. Provide a more detailed version, sometimes in two or three steps, to people who have replied to your newspaper ad, posters, or other advertising. This two- or three-step process provides bite-sized pieces of description for the caller to digest and remember.

This longer version, much like a mini job description, should address at least the following primary areas that are of interest to most applicants:

- A brief description of you—Desire for activity and independence, age, type of daily lifestyle, the general location of your residence.

- The nature of the work—Functional limitations of your disability, and the types of help you need.

- The schedule—The days and times that you need help.

- The staffing structure—How many part-time PAs help you, how they coordinate your schedule, how they provide backups for each other.

- Characteristics of the person you need—Responsible, dependable, punctual, honest, confidential.

- The salary and other appealing benefits or advantages—$8.00 per hour paid biweekly, learn about living with a disability, interesting work, their help to you will be routinely appreciated more than any other job they have had.

- The applicant's questions—To avoid sounding like a non-stop telemarketer, pause periodically in your description to ask, "Does this seem to be the type of work you are looking for? Before I go further, do you have any questions to this point?"

In addition, describing the routine in four or five steps enables the uninterested caller to bail out along the way without being forced to hear a full, five-minute script. If that happens, and she is not interested in your position, thank her and go on to the next caller. Do not try a "hard sell" to convince her to interview or take the job. Do not waste your time, no matter how desperate you are for an aide. Go on to the next prospect.

Besides being merciful to the caller who is listening, your time, effort, and voice are also saved if callers excuse themselves early. If you are responding to 10 callers at a time, you will want to spend your phone time as efficiently as possible.

For this longer description, you begin with something similar to the previous, short version, and add on.

Here is another example:

Hello, Susan. Thank you for calling about the home health aide ad. How about if I outline my situation?

I need help seven mornings a week, from 6 to 7:45, and seven nights, from 8 to either 9:30 or 10:30, depending on whether it is a shower night. I have a team of five part-time aides, usually students, who divide my schedule of needs. We all meet each four or five weeks, and everybody brings their calendar or appointment book. For a half hour, the five aides decide—among themselves—who wants which mornings and evenings. Later, if someone has committed to a morning or evening that they find they cannot work, they are responsible for calling the other aides to arrange for their own replacement. I have four people now, and am looking for a new fifth member. Each person takes on 8 to 10 hours each week. Does this sound like a time framework that appeals to you?

Okay, how about if I tell you a bit more about myself and the type of work involved? I'm 51 years old and use a motorized wheelchair each day. I'm very active, drive my own car, and work in a downtown office all day. When my morning aide arrives at 6 a.m., he or she helps me get dressed, transfer out of bed to my wheelchair, and get positioned in my wheelchair. I do some grooming at the sink on my own while they do some small chores such as laundry or watering plants. By 7:30 or 7:45, we are both finished and ready to leave the house in our separate cars.

Each night, I meet an aide at 8 for one and one-half to two and one-half hours. That's from 8 until either 9:30 or 10:30, depending on whether it is a shower night. The shower nights are Sunday, Wednesday, and Friday.

On shower nights, I meet the aide at 8 and we spend the first half hour doing clerical and housekeeping tasks. We put away files and books that I have used during the day, and put out those that I will need the next day. Dishes are put into the dishwasher, sometimes a load of laundry is started, and on Sunday and Thursday nights we water the houseplants. Next, we head for the bath and bedrooms. I first get undressed and transfer to a shower chair. The aide wheels me over the toilet, and helps me with a bowel routine that involves suppositories. Next, we wheel into the shower and I need help in showering and drying off. Finally, we wheel into the bedroom, I transfer into bed, and get positioned for the night. The non-shower nights are an hour shorter.

Does this sound like the type of work you might be interested in?

If you are still interested, I would like to schedule you to come to my house and see the longer, evening shower routine. My current aide would perform the routine while you watch. You would ask all the questions you like of the aide and me, and then go home and think about the job and commitment overnight. I would ask that you call me back the next day—one way or the other—to let me know if you are still interested.

Would you like to see the routine? Would this Sunday or Wednesday night be better? We would meet at 8 p.m. and go until 10 or 10:30. Okay, here are the directions to my house.

(You may wish to repeat the important, primary details in case the caller is a bit overwhelmed and might not remember everything.)

Thank you for calling, Susan. I'm looking forward to seeing you on Wednesday at 8 p.m. until 10 or 10:30. If you decide not to come, please be sure to call me in advance. Again, my phone number is xxx-xxxx. Do you have any questions? Okay. If I don't hear from you in advance, I'll see you on Wednesday night at 8.

All of this takes practice. To be comfortable on the phone, you might want to rehearse both routines from notes before you take the first caller who responds to your newspaper ad. When you can easily deliver the descriptions, and are pleased with the impression you will make on a stranger, then you are ready to answer phone inquiries about your PA ad in the newspaper and to conduct interviews with applicants.

Chapter 14

Say It, Ask for It, and Act—Assertively!

Have you ever heard your caregivers or PAs say any of these things about you?

- *She is so shy—if only she had the courage to speak up for what she needs.* (passive)

- *He seems afraid of asking for help and speaking up in a loud enough voice so I can hear him. It's as though he is afraid that I will yell at him or be mad at him for making his needs known.* (passive)

- *I wish she were not so demanding when she asks for help. I am not her slave.* (aggressive)

- *I like the kind of work that I do for him. I just don't like working for him—he is so abusive in the angry way he demands to have things done right away!* (aggressive)

- *He is a nice guy and I like working for him. However, occasionally, out of the blue, he gets angry and takes it out on me. It is not as much what he says, but the way he says it. His usual kindness suddenly disappears and he starts barking orders at me. I never know when Mr. Hyde, the monster, is going to appear out of nowhere and take my head off.* (aggressive or passive-aggressive)

There are four primary ways in which you can communicate with others: passive, aggressive, passive-aggressive, and assertive. Because you routinely ask for help from others, it is important that you know about the clear, direct way of assertive communication, and how to avoid the alternatives.

Using assertive statements cannot guarantee that you will be granted all the requests you make; however, it will contribute to maximizing your chances. At the same time, avoiding the other, undesirable ways of communicating will be an aid to minimizing a primary source of conflict with help providers.

It is easy to lose high-quality caregivers and PAs by stating your needs either in a passive way, and not having your needs heard or understood; or in aggressive or passive-aggressive ways, and abusing PAs with requests that are harsh, angry, sarcastic, arrogant, or demanding.

309

This chapter is about using appropriate language and mannerisms to clearly make your needs known—and keep PAs happy in the process.

> *Many of us get complaints from PAs that we are "too demanding." We often do not understand what they mean or what we can do about it—well, here are some answers!*

The four communication and interaction styles

Passive expressions and actions—To be avoided

Passive statements express (or partially express) feelings, opinions, and needs in a way that is weak, poorly understood, or inaudible. A passive style may result from several factors.

Speakers use the passive style because they lack the courage to speak up and be assertive. This shy, timid attitude is often due to fear of offending the other party and triggering negative consequences, such as an angry rejection of the request, any kind of conflict, or the PA quitting.

People choose to be passive to avoid conflict. Often, they are "gun shy" from a long history of having their requests met with the pain of interpersonal conflict and angry responses.

These people will make every attempt to avoid further emotional pain by trying to please and agree with people around them. They often assume a "victim" role of someone who expects to be emotionally, verbally, or physically abused. It is not unusual for this "victim" to weakly deliver a help request, and then to assume a defensive (sometimes almost fetal) body posture and facial expression in psychological preparation for an abusive reply.

In truly passive communication, there is seldom much outwardly expressed anger, because speakers are too afraid of the consequences. To compensate, they unfortunately bottle up and hide any personal anger. If they wish to express anger while fearing the consequences, they will usually use the passive-aggressive style, described later in this section.

When help recipients employ just one PA, and the relationship with that particular aide is breaking down, the recipients often become passive. They know that if their one-and-only aide becomes offended, the aide might suddenly quit and leave the recipient in a crisis with no available assistance. In this situation, it is also common for the PA to realize her unfair advantage. She might begin to refuse certain tasks, or play "mind games" with the recipient in making passive-aggressive, nasty, power threats.

In this scenario, the bullied and abused recipient should pull together the courage to secretly recruit and hire a replacement, and then fire the abusive PA. To avoid a recurrence of the one-aide unfair advantage, the recipient should divide his needs between at least two part-time aides.[1]

The negative effects of passive communication are felt by both the speaker and listener.

Speakers feel badly about themselves because they find that they are unable to express opinions or needs. They often feel like or accuse themselves of being wimps and lacking the courage to stand up to others and make their needs known. Consequently, they also get frustrated because their needs are not understood and go unfulfilled. They often get angry at the people who routinely ask them to repeat messages.

The listener is unfairly given much of the responsibility for interpreting what the passive speaker is mumbling. She must spend extra time and energy on figuring out what is being said and questioning the speaker. This becomes very frustrating, and she often gets angry.

Passive communication usually has the following characteristics:

- Partial, incomplete message (avoid)—
  The speaker delivers an incomplete message, hoping the recipient will *get the hint* or figure out the entire message. A caregiver or PA cannot accommodate needs that have not been clearly expressed.

  Examples
  ▸ Passive, incomplete message (avoid)—
  "Gee, the living room sure is getting dusty..."
  ▸ Assertive, complete message (preferred)—
  "The living room needs cleaning. Laura, would you please find the time before Friday to vacuum the rug and dust the furniture."

- Weak, timid, unclear, and mumbled voice (avoid)—
  The timid speaker's voice is too weak and low in volume, too low in tone, and often the words are mumbled, poorly articulated, and delivered in a hesitant speech pattern. A caregiver or PA cannot provide help to needs that she cannot hear.

  Examples
  ▸ Passive, hard-to-hear, mumbled, and swallowed words (avoid)—
  "Hea, aegen, wonna elp wif tyee meh zhoo."
  ▸ Assertive, adequate and pleasant volume, words clearly formed and projected (preferred)—
  "Hi, Meagan, would you help me with tying my shoe?"

---

1. For details about the advantages and "how-tos" of using multiple PAs, see chapter 📖 **16**, **"Dividing Your Needs, and Assigning Work Shifts, Among Several PAs."**

- Confusing, defensive, tense body language while avoiding eye contact (avoid)—
When making help requests, the shy speaker's body language and facial expression often assume a defensive and even fetal position. A PA might think she hears what is being said. However, she gets confused when the lips say one thing but the body seems to say something else. The aide's composite observations of message, voice, and body language prompt her to wonder, "*What* does he want? I do not understand what is happening here. Am I doing something to cause this, or is this entirely his problem?" Instead, the speaker's body posture should either be neutral or, better yet, illustrate, emphasize, or help convey what is being said.

  ▸ Passive, distracting body language (avoid)—
  Avoiding eye contact with the recipient of the message; routinely having a defensive, tense, or nervous body posture; using distracting facial expressions or nervous gestures

  ▸ Assertive body language that is either neutral or helps convey the message (preferred)—
  Clear, nonglaring, comfortable eye contact with message recipient; speaker's body tension is comfortable, upright, open, and not defensive; speaker's facial expressions are either neutral or (better) appropriate to the type of message and help convey the message

Aggressive expressions and actions—To be avoided

Aggressive behavior should also be avoided because it results in feelings, opinions, and needs being expressed in ways that are nasty, mean, angry, punishing, threatening, assaulting, demanding, or even hostile. Some inexperienced PA managers routinely use anger and aggression in an attempt to show power and control over help providers. Commenters about this style have noted that "rudeness is a weak person's way of exerting power and influence."

The rights and feelings of the listener are not considered. The person speaking aggressively is usually angry and thinks only about her own needs, feelings, opinions, and objectives. Goals are achieved at the expense of other people.

There are many possible reasons why someone is briefly or chronically angry. Reasons can range from temporary indigestion to long-term anger about one's childhood, current living situation, or disability. The aggressor may eventually suffer feelings of guilt and regret at having acted aggressively toward others. Regardless, he often continues aggressive behavior because his goals are realized and he feels a sense of power and control, and therefore the guilt must be overlooked. The aggressor often knows of no alternative type of behavior.

Routine, angry, and aggressive mannerisms negatively affect both the PA manager and the PA. For the aggressive speaker, being in a long-term state of anger is a lousy way to live. There is very little true joy or inner peace, and they are too often acquired by pain-relieving addictions such as alcohol, smoking, street drugs, sex and masturbation, or the abuse of medications. Sadly, the anger that is routinely vented to so many others is rarely caused by any of them—it is founded deep inside the speaker.

For the listener or victim of this aggressive behavior, the short-term response can include feelings of humiliation, embarrassment, abuse, resentment, defensiveness, or anger. She may consequently seek revenge by direct or indirect means.

> *Sometimes we make PAs mad not because of what we request, but because of the words we choose and the harsh way in which we make our demands.*

In the long term, working with someone who routinely expresses anger is a crummy way to work. These innocent caregivers or PAs rarely deserve the abuse they receive, and tend to resign after brief employments. Simply stated, people do not like to be around an abusively aggressive, angry individual—there is too much stress. As a friend, the receiver will begin avoiding contact and socializing with the aggressor; as an employee, she will begin looking for another job.

Aggressive behavior is expressed with these traits—

- Angry, threatening, four-lettered messages (avoid)—
  This is characterized by verbal assaults, name-calling, threats, or humiliating, nasty, or meanly intended remarks. Few caregivers or PAs are willing to help anyone who is routinely rude or calls them names.
  Examples
  - ▶ Aggressive message that is angry and abusive (avoid)—
    "Look, Tony, I want my breakfast cooked and I want it now. If you don't know how to cook a Johnstown omelet, you must be stupid!"
  - ▶ Assertive, clear message that respects the feelings of, and appreciates the help from, the PA (preferred)—
    "Tony, would you mind cooking my breakfast now? If you are not sure of what goes into a Johnstown omelet, I will be glad to tell you."

- Harsh, angry, loud, and disrespectful voice (avoid)—
  The voice itself conveys anger and a lack of respect. In reality, the speaker uses his voice as an assaulting weapon, much like a fist, knife, or gun. His intention is to hurt, punish, "diss," or overpower and control the listener by making his voice unpleasant. One of the most effective, quick ways of getting a PA to quit—or loving caregiver to leave—is to routinely stress them out with loud, abusive, and angry comments.
  Examples
  - ▶ Aggressively angry, loud voice (avoid)—
    "IF YOU USE INTERNET E-MAIL, THIS IS WHY 'NETIQUETTE' TELLS YOU NOT TO TYPE YOUR MESSAGES IN ALL CAPITAL LETTERS. THE RECIPIENT OFTEN FEELS THAT AN ANGRY SPEAKER IS SHOUTING."

▸ Assertively pleasant, appropriate tone of voice (preferred)—
"You can see that this clear and appropriate voice is much more comfortable to receive. Would you be more open to hearing a message from me, OR THE PERSON SHOUTING IN THE PRECEDING EXAMPLE? And it is okay to assertively show excitement, sorrow, or other emotions, JUST DO NOT YELL AT ME, okay?"

• Angry, gesturing, and crowding body language (avoid)—
The speaker uses his body to further convey the anger of his message and voice. No PA enjoys getting close to and helping an angry person.

  Examples

▸ Aggressive gestures that convey anger (avoid)—
  ▾ The speaker positions his body inappropriately close to the listener, making her feel crowded and uncomfortable
  ▾ Pointing or shaking a fist or finger (first or middle!) at the recipient, especially shaking a pointed finger at her face at close range
  ▾ Any other gestures or defiant glances that express anger or power

▸ Assertive body language that is either neutral or helps convey the message (preferred)—
  ▾ Showing respect for the listener's body space by not crowding her
  ▾ Relaxed, nonglaring, comfortable eye contact with the listener
  ▾ Body tone that is relatively relaxed and comfortable to be near
  ▾ Facial expressions are either neutral, or better yet, are appropriate to the type of message and help convey the message

Passive-aggressive expressions and actions—To be avoided

The passive-aggressive style is a hybrid. It is taking the anger of aggression and trying to hide it in innocent-looking, passive packaging. The P-A style is used by cowardly speakers who want to hide or deny to themselves or others that they are angry, nasty, or mean.

Those who make P-A remarks delight in being accused of saying or doing angry, nasty, or mean things. In defense, they enjoy making a sarcastic, defiant reply such as, *"Who, me?* How can you possibly accuse *me* of doing wrong?" At this point, their P-A style often turns into an outwardly aggressive one that accuses the other party of being the true wrongdoer. People who routinely enjoy P-A behavior also often enjoy getting into fights and arguments.

Many men communicate among themselves this way, and call it "kidding around," "busting," or "guy stuff." Discussions are very competitive. There are two ways of showing superiority over others (when someone believes that to be important). One way is simply to be better at doing something than one's peers. Another way is to routinely put down, criticize, and degrade one's peers in order to fool one's self into feeling superior. Making P-A comments about others and to others, aka "busting" or kidding someone, is common in this beer-babe-and-sports culture. It is also the cause of many ill feelings, fights, and vandalism. The sarcastic reply to someone who gets angry about "being busted on" is the classic, "What's the matter, can't you take a funny joke?" These P-A pokes are *not* good ways to communicate needs to help providers whom you cannot afford to alienate. They are not funny, but instead are mean and nasty. They do not facilitate communication, but instead impede it.

In similar ways, this undesirable behavior is a downer for both help recipients and providers, for most of the same reasons as the angry, aggressive style discussed in the preceding subsection. Consequences include an unhealthy quality of life for the PA manager and a series of premature, frequent resignations by the abused PAs.

P-A behavior is an intentionally chosen combination of passive, outward packaging that attempts to hide and excuse angry, mean, and nasty messages. Like a fish's view of a fisherman's deceptive bait, the initial impression of a P-A message is often sweet and innocent. However, as the true meaning of the message is exposed, there is a sharp, painful hook inside.

- Sarcastic, angry, barbed message (avoid)—
  The passive-aggressive message is worded for two objectives. Initially, the speaker wants to communicate a need, opinion, or information. However, as he is about to speak, he decides to use the occasion to also vent anger, exert power or control, or punish or humiliate the listener, for whatever reason. Consequently, the original message comes out with a sharply barbed spin. If the listener takes offense, as she should, the speaker often tries to rationalize and further disguise the comment—while wanting to make the listener feel unjustified and guilty for complaining—by claiming he was "just kidding." Most PAs will also take offense to this juvenile "kidding"; they much prefer the straightforward assertive approach.

  ▸ Sarcastic, insulting, and yet sugarcoated anger (avoid)—
    "Gee, the kitchen sure is dirty. Sure would be nice if somebody would do something about it someday. Oh, ah, I was just kidding, Mike."

  ▸ Assertive, clear, direct, and complete (preferred)—
    "The kitchen needs cleaning. Mike, would you please put the dishes in the dishwasher and clean the counters."

- Sugarcoated, angry voice (avoid)—
  You have heard it thousands of times: the sarcastic, insulting message that a bozo delivers with a sugar-syrup twang—like adding "accent to injury." The actual message would have been a straight stab in your gut, but the vocal inflections additionally twist the knife. A double-edged comment like this would be justified cause for a PA to drop everything and walk out your front door.

  Examples

  ▸ The P-A voice is often not predominately angry, but usually has a sarcastic, defiant, arrogant, and stick-it-to-you tone (avoid)—
    *"Hmm, 15 minutes late for your work shift, Jim. It is **so** nice of you to spare me the time this evening to **show up**. I hope this is not **too** much of a sacrifice from your useless leisure time. Ah yes, guess I am lucky that today is payday or maybe I would not **see you at all!** See if you can arrive on time tomorrow."*

  ▸ The assertive voice is open, honest, comfortable-sounding, and without a hidden, sarcastic hook inside (preferred)—

"Hi, Jim. It is good to see you. Hey, guy, I know the traffic is heavy out there and causes delays, but when you are delayed I end up delayed in meeting my schedule. Would you mind leaving your house just a few minutes earlier? It would make a big difference to me, in turn, to get to my meeting on time. I really appreciate your extra effort."

- Defiant, arrogant, and angry body language (avoid)—
  Body language adds to the negative effects of P-A behavior. Once more, passive-aggressive communication will anger and drive away the help providers on whom you are dependent.
  - ▶ The P-A speaker uses angry gestures and defiant glances that are a bit more subtle and disguised than outwardly aggressive ones. This person has two objectives: to express anger or control, and to convey a factual message.
  - ▶ The sole objective of the assertive speaker is to communicate, and her honest body language is comfortable, appropriate, and respectful. If you respect her, she will probably return the gesture with the help you require.

Assertive expressions and actions—To be adopted and routinely used

Of these four styles of communicating, assertiveness is the only desirable one.

The assertive speaker uses communication that is clear, direct, complete, honest, and comfortable. His sole objective is to communicate, and there is no hidden intent to imply anger. If the speaker is indeed angry, he is direct about expressing it, without hidden agendas of being mean or nasty.

Listeners have no need to interpret the message being delivered and no need to defend themselves against abuse, threats, punishments, or other negative feelings of fear and anxiety. The two parties can disagree, but there is a constant level of respect for the rights, feelings, problems, and concerns of each other.

> *Your PAs will appreciate clear, direct, pleasant, assertive requests, and not angry demands.*

When assertiveness is used for requesting help, the message content as well as the speaker's voice and body language are all coordinated and reinforce each other. The style is comfortable for both speaker and listener. The listener feels no fatigue or anxiety from wondering whether there is a hidden message in addition to—or different from—what is being said. All the messages are up front and conveyed by the verbal statements.

Using assertive statements does not guarantee that you get what you request; however, you will feel satisfaction that your request, feelings, and opinions are clearly expressed and heard. Of the four styles, assertiveness will maximize your chances of having needs fulfilled. In return, if the PA is also assertive and cannot fulfill a need, you will clearly know the reason why and whether an alternate plan might be possible.

Assertive behavior lessens the chance of conflict between two people, but it cannot always prevent it. After all, it is opposing ideas and values that cause conflict, and not always the way in which they are expressed. When both parties are assertive—and avoid the other three undesirable styles—bargaining negotiations and alternate proposals can be comfortably discussed. This additional discussion is usually not possible if either party is passive, aggressive, or passive-aggressive.

Finally, when both help recipient and provider are assertive, the relationship enjoys a maximum comfort level. This is not to say that disagreements will not occur; however, they will seldom occur around communication issues. Routine assertive behavior minimizes the chances of frustrations, depression, anxiety, and even psychosomatic disorders (stress-related head and stomach aches) that come with the other three communication styles. Consequently, PAs seldom resign because of "bad-attitude communications"—you keep good PAs longer!

- Clear, complete, logical, easily understood, and polite message that serves your purposes while respecting the PA's feelings—
  When an aide hears and sees angry communication coming her way, she psychologically shuts down to minimize the pain of insult. Consequently, she often cannot—or chooses not—to hear the fact or opinion in the message. In contrast, when you speak assertively without anger, she opens up to the comfortable style—and message. As the saying goes, "she hears you."
  - ‣ Complete and easily understood
  - ‣ All necessary details are included
  - ‣ The order of details is clear and logical
  - ‣ The message—especially if a request for help—includes polite expressions of respect and appreciation, such as *please* and *thank you*
  - ‣ If a need for help, the message is often phrased as a polite *request*, instead of an *order or demand*
- Voice is clearly articulated with comfortable volume and tone—
  Again, the comfortable and clear voice reinforces the assertive message.
  - ‣ Clearly articulated words that are not mumbled
  - ‣ A comfortable volume level and tone
- Body language of appropriate gestures and respectful closeness to listener—
  The speaker's respectful and appropriate body language further confirm what the assertive message and voice are conveying.
  - ‣ Gestures and facial expressions that reinforce and emphasize—and avoid distracting from—the message

▸ A physical closeness to the listener that respects her need for personal territory, and avoids crowding or violating
▸ Relaxed, nonglaring, comfortable eye contact with the message recipient
▸ Relaxed and comfortable body tension

Make Requests for Help, Not Demands or Orders

So, you have adopted the habit of being assertive, and avoiding the other three styles. Congrats! Being clearly, directly, and respectfully assertive with caregivers and PAs will earn you an overall acceptance for most of your help needs.

However, you might still occasionally rub a PA the wrong way while stating a few needs. There is one more rule of thumb for stating needs: Make *requests* or *polite statements* for help, rather than issuing *orders* or *demands*.

Now your reaction to this might be, "Give me a break! What do I look like, a drill sergeant? Of course I make requests and I am polite, that is common sense." What might seem to you to be a request might be heard, perceived, and interpreted by a caregiver or PA as something else.

To *request* is "to ask for, especially, formally or politely." To *order* or *demand* assumes that one has the authority to command, and consequently the expectation that the act will be done. As help recipients, we do not have that kind of authority, and should not be making that assumption.

The fine-line difference between the two styles is sometimes in the choice of words, and at other times in the tone of voice used. Consider the different interpretations that a PA can make when you simply emphasize different words in different ways—

- *"Would you please tie my shoe?"*
- *"Would YOU please tie my shoe?"*
- *"Would you PLEASE tie my shoe?"*

It is likely that the first two statements would be accepted as *requests*. The third, however, introduces a hint of stress and anger—and thus the potential to irritate a help provider.

If this happens once during an otherwise smooth evening routine, the PA will probably ignore and forget it. Let it happen five times in the same work shift, and the aide will probably assume you are not in a good mood this evening. If you are "not in a good mood" for a straight week of evening routines, the provider will typically become irritated.

Inherent in a *request* is the PA's unspoken interpretation that you technically respect her right to refuse to perform a task. Technically, she indeed does have this task-by-task right of refusal, and her sense of dignity and importance wants that right to be acknowledged. The need for acknowledgment does not require you to beg—it asks merely that you avoid ignoring it or running your wheelchair over it!

To ignore her need for respect is to imply to her that she is not important to you, that her help is not important to you, and that she and her help are such small change that they can be *taken for granted*.

Most people who have been in any kind of a relationship—parental, romantic, job-related, or with a PA—have probably accused or been accused of *taking for granted* the other party. Indeed, this is a "phrase that pays" in most relationships. It literally means "to assume without question, to treat with careless indifference." The bottom line here is that everyone likes to feel important, and few people like to feel that they or their work is not.

This chapter has been about using appropriate language and mannerisms to clearly make your needs known and keep PAs happy in the process. The two-part package that you want to use is

- to use assertive communication, and avoid passive, aggressive, and passive-aggressive styles
- to make requests or polite statements, and avoid demands or orders—or anything that resembles them.

Your *requests* should sound like questions. Good requests begin with polite lead-ins, such as

- *"Would you mind doing…"*
- *"Would you please do…?"*

As an alternative, *statements of need* are fine as long as they are polite, show respect, and avoid any chance that the PA can feel "dissed." The magic word that you first learned as a kid is still the most important for moving helpers to fulfill your needs:

- *"Please…"*

And regardless of whether you express your need with a polite request or statement, at least one-in-ten fulfilled requests should be acknowledged by, you guessed it:

- *"Thank you."*

Your author has taken many informal surveys over the years to determine the most effective ways of asking for help and still keeping aides happy. Scores of responding PAs have confirmed over and over the powerful importance of routinely saying *please* and *thank you*—your mom and kindergarten teacher still rule!

As the saying goes, "If it sounds, looks, feels, and smells like a polite request (or demand or order), then it probably is one." Your caregiver or PA has the only opinion that counts.

It is a good idea to make eye contact with a help provider each time you make a request. After all, a request usually prompts a brief answer or acknowledgment. As you look at your aide while she responds, watch for any facial reaction that indicates any questioning or irritation, and follow up as necessary. If she is interpreting your requests as anything else, consider revising your delivery. Occasionally fine-tuning your style is a small price to pay for showing your providers that you value and respect them and want to keep them as long as possible.

Examples

Here are five examples of the four communication styles. In each of the five examples, the *assertive* style also illustrates the appropriate use of *requests* or *polite statements* for asking for help.

As a refresher, first please remember:

- Passive expressions and actions—To be avoided
  - ▶ Partial, incomplete message
  - ▶ Weak, timid, unclear, and mumbled voice
  - ▶ Confusing, defensive, tense body language while avoiding eye contact
- Aggressive expressions and actions—To be avoided
  - ▶ Angry, threatening, obscene or foul messages
  - ▶ Harsh, angry, loud, and disrespectful voice
  - ▶ Angry, gesturing, and crowding body language
- Passive-aggressive expressions and actions—To be avoided
  - ▶ Sarcastic, angry, barbed message
  - ▶ Sugarcoated, angry voice
  - ▶ Defiant, arrogant, angry body language
- Assertive expressions and actions—To be adopted and routinely used
  - ▶ Clear, complete, logical, easily understood, and polite message that serves your purposes while respecting the PA's feelings
  - ▶ Voice is clearly articulated with comfortable volume and tone
  - ▶ Body language of appropriate gestures and respectful closeness to listener

Examples

①   Passive: *"My wheelchair is pretty dirty. I hope nobody notices at the Friday meeting."*

Aggressive: *"This chair is getting dirty again. I thought we said you would clean it each week. Let's get it done before Friday or there won't be any Friday paycheck!"*

Passive-aggressive: *"My chair is filthy. Somebody around here is not doing her job. You don't suppose you might have time this year to get around to it, eh?"*

Assertive: *"Judy, I have a business meeting on Friday morning.*
Would you mind cleaning my wheelchair by this Thursday night?"

②   Passive: *"Gee, my shoe is untied."*

Aggressive: *"Hey, tie that shoe up, will ya?"*

Passive-aggressive: *"It is nice to see that your own shoes are so neatly tied. It is obvious that you have the skill. Would you mind terribly applying the benefit of all that expertise to my shoe, also?"*

Assertive: *"Steve, my shoe is untied. Would you tie it for me?"*

③ Passive: *"Could you spend some time in the kitchen?"*

Aggressive: *"The kitchen is a pigsty. If you take any pride in the way this place looks, would you take three minutes and stow the dishes?"*

Passive-aggressive: *"I don't know why these dishes can't be put away. They've been here all morning."*

Assertive: *"Gillie, before we leave for the shopping mall, would you please put the dishes away?"*

④ Passive: *"I have had a stomach ache all day. Maybe I should use the bathroom sometime."*

Aggressive: *"I have not asked for your help all afternoon, so I doubt that it will kill you to help me use the bathroom. It is the least you can do for me, and if you put it off much longer you will also have a laundry to do."*

Passive-aggressive: *"I don't know what time you were hoping to leave tonight, but at 8 o'clock I will need help for an hour in using the bathroom."*

Assertive: *"Cheryl-Lyn, I think I had better use the bathroom before going to bed tonight. Would you mind helping me?"*

⑤ Passive: *"My pants sure are looking sloppy lately."*

Aggressive: *"When I leave for work, I look like a slob because of the lack of caring that you put into this job. Let's be sure those pant cuffs are straight or you and I will have a lit tle talk. Understand?"*

Passive-aggressive: *"If I am not interrupting you, and if this is a convenient time, and if you do not mind, and if your back is not hurting, would you mind giving me just one lousy minute to pull down and even my pant cuffs? I don't think that is too much for me to ask, or do you?"*

Assertive: *"Rose, I have noticed the last few mornings that my pant cuffs have been uneven. If you do not mind, would you try to remember to check them each morning to be sure that they are the same height?"*

Part V

Strategies for Being a Good Manager

Part V

Strategies for Being a Good Manager

The four chapters of Part IV provided pointers on defining and describing your help needs. Some chapters offered tips in deciding whether all those listed needs were valid for help requests. In addition, they assured you that your preferences in how help is provided are essential to your independence and health, despite the negative reactions that you might receive from PAs. Finally, Part IV wrapped up by encouraging you to state your needs assertively, and avoid weakly passive or abusively aggressive communication.

Part V presents some golden strategies for your becoming a first-class manager. The first chapter is packed with time-proven, experience-driven, solid-gold management strategies. You will find methods that have been collected from your author as well as dozens of other experienced PA managers. You will be coached away from being a stressful, demanding boss who must crack a whip to make PAs work, and instead, toward being an efficient, effective, and appreciative facilitator for whom aides want to work. PAs will usually enjoy working with you, and will often work beyond the date of their original commitment.

If there were a list of the top ten PA management tips of all time, near the top would be that of dividing your needs among as many part-time PAs as possible. Gone are the crises that arise when a one-and-only PA tires of working for you and starts acting as though he were indispensable. When you put all your help needs in just one PA basket, that sole provider has enormous power over you. This power can be used to unfair advantage, if the provider is so inclined. You should also remember that it costs no more to employ four aides as it does just one, for the same total of hours. Additional advantages to using several aides are outlined, as well as the steps for assigning work shifts to your aides.

You can be the nicest help recipient of all time, but still experience an unnecessarily frequent turnover in aides if your residence is not reasonably clean. Additional PA turnoffs include poorly planned work areas where supplies are not well organized, are not well stocked, or otherwise waste a PA's time and energy. The chapter on work areas and maintaining adequate supplies offers tips that make your residence a desirable place to work. After reading these tips on keeping a clean and efficient place, none of your PAs will have a reason to say "This job stinks!"

The people on whom you most rely and trust are those who too often let you down. They might be 20 minutes late in arriving to get you up in the morning, or they may completely fail to show up until you repeatedly call to wake them up. Other providers seem to be so stable and secure when they promise a work commitment of the next 12 months. You hire them and relax, trusting that your staff is firmly in place—until two weeks later when they give you a seven-day advance notice before resigning. Your year-after-year survival depends on how well you cope with and react to these frequent and sporadic failures of PAs toward their commitments. Although you cannot always depend on your help providers, you will be able to depend on the advice in this chapter.

After brushing up on the strategies of first-class managers found in Part V, it will be time to check into Part VI. The topic here is money. You will find comprehensive lists on what it costs to nail down each new help provider, from placing your newspaper ad through training the applicant whom you select and hire. Additionally, there are three primary ways to pay your aides: a cash salary; a non-cash salary of exchanging room and board to live-in aides for an equivalent, fair value of their monthly help; and a combination of cash and non-cash perks. But how do you calculate all this? The methodology presented in Part VI is impressively simple. Finally, a list of IRS publications will assist PA employers who live in the United States with a basic understanding of their tax obligations, as well as potential money-saving deductions.

Part VI *The Costs of Your Personally Employed PAs*

Chapter 15

Your Qualities and Strategies as a Good PA Manager

You have probably worked at jobs where you either hated a boss who was demanding and stressful, or liked one who was caring, friendly, and appreciative. You soon quit the unpleasant job (or wanted to!), and you stayed longer and work harder at the positive one. You will probably have fond memories of the supportive boss and job for your lifetime.

So what is the point? When you manage your own PAs, you are the employer. And your working environment can make the job one that your providers enjoy and want to keep for a long time, or one that they dislike and from which they will resign as soon as a better job comes along. To make sure you are in the first category, consider some of these issues:

- Which kind of PA employer do you want to be?

- How would you like to be remembered by a former aide ten years from now?

- Have there been times when several of your hard-working, quality aides have quietly resigned after a few weeks, and provided you with merely a nondescript, generic reason for leaving?

- Would you like to provide a more favorable work environment so current PAs would enjoy their work and stay longer?

- When you and a current PA are interviewing new prospects, and the prospect speaks alone with the current PA, do you have any concern about whether the current aide is expressing cautions and reservations instead of recommending your job?

- If one of your current aides who now knows you and your work had a second chance, would she still apply for your job, or would she look elsewhere?

If these topics concern you, then this chapter has some hot guidelines for you!

Please note that this chapter provides valuable guidelines that apply equally to using unpaid family caregivers, personally employed PAs, or agency-supplied aides. There will be many references to managing a business of employees, but these principles are just as important for volunteer family caregivers as for salaried workers. Paid or not, these people provide help for your needs. Paid or not, they prefer a boss and work environment where they enjoy their work and are appreciated.

In this section, you will find simplified, but very important, versions of some primary strategies used by all good managers (not used by all managers, but all good ones). Good help is hard to find, and if you ignore these strategies you will fail time after time to keep good help for very long. If you ignore these strategies, good help will not want to stay with you—I guarantee it!

First, let's define some management concepts.

Your objectives as a PA manager

Many books have been written, and many university courses and seminars taught, on various theories of management. These theories have been studied by top corporate executives as well as small-business owners. Executives often manage hundreds of employees in multi-billion-dollar industries, while folks with disabilities quietly manage one, five, or twenty people. Regardless of the operation's size, everyone who employs and manages people should learn the basic strategies of being a good manager.

Your objectives as a PA manager begin with comparing the qualities that you want in providers with the qualities they want in their work environment. Your aim is for a win-win situation where everyone is satisfied. When one party succeeds in getting its wish list, it is more willing to accommodate the other party.

Qualities that you prefer in the PAs who help you

Let's begin by listing what you prefer in the PAs who help you.

- Providers are dependable in arriving for work, or provide advance notice when they know they will be unable to arrive on schedule or at all.

- They are reasonably clean and professional in personal hygiene, clothing, language, or habits.

- They never jeopardize your safety or health by:
  - ▸ performing a poor quality of work
  - ▸ not observing the safe procedural methods that you request
  - ▸ becoming physically or verbally abusive
  - ▸ working while smoking or under the influence of drugs, medications, or alcohol.

- They are physically, cognitively, or emotionally able to perform the duties, and reasonably fast and efficient while working.

- They are trustworthy with your work time, possessions, finances, medications, or food. In addition, they are honest with fellow PA employees, routinely completing assigned duties and not leaving them for completion by the PA who has the following work shift.

- They rarely have a bad attitude, or fail to assertively communicate in a clear, direct, and pleasant manner. In addition, the aide is neither weakly passive nor abusively aggressive when discussing standard needs, special needs, changes in duties or schedule, opinions, preferences, or feelings.
- They agree to perform their work duties according to the schedule, methods, and amount of salary which you require and to which they originally agreed.
- They respect your rights and your need for confidentiality and privacy with regard to your personal preferences, opinions, feelings, problems, values, beliefs, relationships, and activities.
- They have an appropriate attitude toward people with disabilities and a respect for you. They see you as an individual who, regardless of physical sickness or impairments, has a mind that is fully capable of knowing personal needs, making decisions, and managing the physical assistance that your body requires.
- They respect your right to be in control and to make decisions regarding:
  ‣ the selection and number of employed PAs
  ‣ the choice and schedule of specific duties to be performed
  ‣ the preferred methods for fulfilling those duties
  ‣ the quality and dependability of help that you need.
- They always complete their work efficiently. *Efficient* can be defined as "providing a high quality and quantity of work for the lowest cost." If you are using a paid PA, costs to you include the time and effort that you spend performing your duties as a manager plus the salary you pay. Costs to the caregiver or PA include mostly the time and effort that they spend giving you assistance.

Qualities that PAs prefer in their work environment
Now let's look at what PAs prefer in a supervisor and job site.

- PAs are clearly told, from the beginning, about the nature of the work, list of tasks, and schedule that are expected of them.
- The methods and step-by-step order for performing duties are logical, and do not waste the PA's time and effort.
- Their work areas are clean, well organized, and sufficiently supplied.
- When more than one PA is employed, their supervisor is respectful and fair by:
  ‣ not favoring one provider over another
  ‣ not tolerating one PA who routinely leaves unfinished duties for the next PA to complete
  ‣ not tolerating the poor performance and habits of uncaring aides with bad attitudes, while unfairly expecting different standards from other, quality aides
  ‣ not speaking unfavorably about one PA to the others

> not shaming, harshly reprimanding, or otherwise embarrassing one aide in the presence of others

> not initiating, tolerating, or contributing to gossip, favoritism, unfair advantages, inequitable salaries, or other injustices.

• Their supervisor is reasonably happy, and lacks the anger, depression, and bad attitude that some other people with disabilities routinely display.

• Their supervisor can be trusted, and is never dishonest regarding the PA's possessions, time worked, or salary owed. He never has hidden expectations of the PA such as unstated duties, extra work hours, sexual favors, or loans of money or possessions.

• Their supervisor is never abusive, unreasonable, or stress-inducing in demanding that duties be performed that are inappropriate because:

> the help recipient could easily perform certain duties himself, and should not be requesting PA help

> certain tasks are not appropriate for the PA to perform

> there are too many duties for a specific period of work time (or not enough aides to do the work), and the duties must be performed with unnecessary speed or urgency

> the duties are to be performed in ways that are detailed and exacting without a good reason

> the duties are being performed under unnecessarily tight, stressful control and supervision.

• Their supervisor is understanding and tolerant of their honest mistakes, occasionally forgetting details, being unable to physically perform certain duties, or needing occasional sick or personal time from duties.

• Their supervisor respects the aide's personal life, rights, time, and other concerns by recognizing that job responsibilities and schedules cannot take priority over the aide's personal life.

• PAs receive the clear, honest, and assertive communication that makes their job easier and less stressful. They dislike passive, aggressive, and passive-aggressive styles.

• They are paid a sufficient salary that is generously supplemented by your routine expressions of appreciation for their help.

Traditions to avoid and alternative approaches

Traditional bosses tend to be concerned with meeting their own needs. They tend to believe that their only obligation toward employees is to provide a weekly paycheck, and at as low a salary rate as possible. To many bosses, employees are like machines: plug them into the weekly payroll office and expect that they will do what they are told without further attention.

In their self-serving value system, some bosses believe that employees should feel fortunate to have their jobs and can be replaced if they begin to feel otherwise. There is nothing unique or important about each PA, because a replacement could do the job equally well.

These inexperienced, inflexible bosses use the same stressful, uncaring, production-oriented strategies that their father or mother used. They believe they must maintain an image of authority, power, and tight control. They seldom provide workers with routine personal caring and appreciation, because they fear losing their authority image.

These bosses rarely acknowledge any of their own personal faults, because they will not listen to—and are defensive about—any criticism. Their beliefs, values, and methods are not to be questioned. To quote the title of a book by Rush Limbaugh, they enjoy lecturing to others about The Way Things Ought to Be, and the way employees should conduct themselves.

> *The "caring, appreciative management approach" results in PAs who routinely work hard for you because they want to, not because you try to force them to.*

Would you enjoy working for this type of manager? Is this the kind of PA manager you want to be? Probably not, and yet each of us has occasionally managed PAs with this value system. When that has happened, we got some quite negative feedback from aides as they resigned.

From now on, you can be the high-quality manager that PAs want to work for. Let's look at *Figure 15-1*'s comparison between two PA management approaches: the stressful, demanding PA boss and the caring, appreciative PA manager.

Figure 15-1: **Two Management Approaches**

Stressful, demanding PA bosses	Caring, appreciative PA managers
Dislike their disability, and consequently resent their dependence on PA help	Have reasonably accepted their disability, and are comfortable with their dependence on PA help
Resent the PAs whom they must hire for help	Enjoy working with the PAs whom they hire
Have chronic personal anger, stress, and depression about their disability and other issues, and often vent these feelings on the PAs who help them	Have accepted the negative emotions related to their disability, and are reasonably happy around their PAs
See themselves as bosses who must tightly supervise and control the PAs, because they cannot otherwise be trusted to do quality work	See themselves as managers or coordinators who can provide initial instructions to PAs, and then trust PAs to do a good job. They provide ongoing supervision and control only when needed
Believe they must maintain an image of authority, and the only way they know to prompt respect is to demand it	Want to have an image of caring and friendship—to receive respect from PAs, managers must earn it by first respecting the PAs
View PAs as pawns who are paid to help them, and have little interest in the PAs' petty, personal interests and concerns	View PAs as interesting people who have feelings and concerns, and enjoy discussing topics that are important to each of them
Are seldom willing to occasionally modify their schedule when PAs have special needs—after all, they pay PAs to be flexible around their schedule	Are willing to be reasonably flexible about modifying their schedule when PAs have special needs—just as PAs do around the manager's needs
Tell PAs what their needs are, and expect them to satisfy those needs—that is what PAs are paid to do	Make requests and polite statements to PAs about their needs for help, and then express appreciation for PA efforts
Rarely express appreciation to PAs for their help—their paycheck is more than they deserve	Routinely express appreciation in addition to monetary salary—managers try to provide a sincere "thank you" for at least 1 in 10 tasks

Two primary management styles are discussed here. The stressful, demanding bosses know no other way of management. They tend to be rude and rule over PAs with an iron fist to force them to work hard and fast. In contrast, the caring, appreciative managers provide a reasonably pleasant, trusting work environment where providers want to provide a high quality of help. They respect their PAs, and the PAs respect them in return.

The stressful, demanding boss

The erroneous and traditional way of "motivating" a donkey that is hitched to a cart is to hit or whip the animal to keep it moving. Bosses who adopt this traditional style feel that they are powerful and in command by conditioning the animal to perform tasks in order to avoid pain. Punishment occurs whenever the animal does not perform as instructed. When the animal jumps from a sense of fear, the trainers falsely believe that they have earned power, control, and respect. Neither donkeys nor PAs respect or like working for these employers.

Rudeness has been defined by smart managers as "a weak person's way of showing power." This approach is loaded with disadvantages to both bosses and PAs. The PAs resent the bosses as much as the work they are performing under constant stress. Knowing this, the bosses find it necessary—and very time-consuming and tiring—to spend most of their time tightly supervising ("riding herd on") the people who help them.

Rude communicators favor passive-aggressive and aggressive styles to get their point across. To rude bosses, aggressive statements are paths to power and control; to the workers on the receiving end, aggression is the torn-up road to tension headaches and the fantasy of quitting.

A final disadvantage of this approach is that PAs feel very little loyalty to or respect for their bosses, and thus give very little notice of their upcoming departure. There is little reason to respect or care about someone who, in turn, has seldom respected or cared about you!

> *Good managers do not force or command employee respect; instead, they earn it by first respecting employees.*

The caring, appreciative manager

The second approach is loaded with advantages for both managers and PAs. Here, you do not force the aides to work for you. Instead, you provide a pleasant working environment so they decide on their own that they want to work for—and please—you.

In a pleasant working environment, you first respect the PAs, and in turn they respect you. When you provide a nice place to work, your help arrives to find that work is easier; their duties are clearly defined and reasonable in nature, and the work area is efficiently laid out and well equipped.

The time and effort that you spend in supervision is cut to a minimum. The quality and quantity of work are much higher than can ever be realized under the other approach, because you and the providers are working together. PAs tend to keep their jobs longer, even in the sight of other jobs that pay slightly more, because they like the work they are doing. When PAs have been respected and do decide to quit, they are more inclined to give generous advance notice in return for the respect they have received. They often offer to briefly work beyond their quitting date if you are having problems finding replacements.

A mutual respect between you and PAs is a key ingredient of this approach.

Respect is "showing regard, consideration, and caring for another." Between you and PAs, it means that if you care about what is important to your PAs, they will usually care about what is important to you. Each of you benefits in this win-win situation.

"I really enjoy working for him, because he cares about me, he appreciates my work, and he is not afraid to routinely tell me so." Or, as Lea, a valued PA, once told me about the importance of respect from an employer, "I really enjoy working here, because I feel that what I am doing is important. On top of that, I personally feel important because Skip cares about me as a person. I get appreciation for my work and respect for being me. If occasionally he needs something extra done, or my time goes over, I do not mind because I like helping him—often, I actually do not think of it as being work."

By now, you are probably saying, "Okay, you have convinced me to break down and show respect to my PAs, and probably get the same in return from them. Where do I start?"

Review the comparisons in *Figure 15-1*. Avoid the nine factors in the "boss" column, and adopt the nine factors in the "manager" chart.

The three boomerang courtesies

In summary, here are the three most important boomerang courtesies to remember. Give these courtesies to your PAs, and they will almost always be returned to you!

First, *your caring attitude* toward each PA ensures that PAs will care about you. Mutual caring is the foundation for maintaining a friendly and pleasant working environment.

Caring must be a sincere attitude and consistent habit. It should not be the plastic management strategy that you have seen from others. Your ability to naturally and sincerely care about others is possible only if you first care about yourself. If you are chronically angry or depressed about yourself—your disability or other long-term baggage—you will find it impossible to sincerely care about others.

It is true. If you cannot like, respect, and love yourself for who you are, then you cannot genuinely feel these emotions toward others. If you are overflowing with anger, depression, or other personal emotions, get help. Until you do, you might not be able to give a damn about anyone else's concerns. What is more, the anger and depression that are inside of you will ooze out in what you say to your aides. Few PAs want to work in a stressful environment, and you will encounter frequent resignations.

If your caring about others is sincere, you will find many ways to express it daily. During the initial interview with PA applicants, your questions about their personal interests will come naturally. Your interest will not be a strained gimmick or "noble thing to do," but will come from a genuine interest in learning more about each applicant. As PAs arrive for work each day, you will be asking about updates on their activities. You will find yourself remembering their birthdays or upcoming college graduations, and maybe even sending a card or pint of ice cream. And they will start doing the same for you!

Second, *your routine expressions of appreciation* for PAs and the work they do ensure that they will appreciate you and the help you need. Mutual appreciation reinforces your commitment to them and their commitment to you.

Remember that routinely expressing appreciation is often more powerful in pleasing a PA than the weekly paycheck (although the paycheck is still essential). Appreciation makes PAs feel personally important and tells them that they are doing a good job. (Further comments on the importance of routinely expressing appreciation are found in the next section.) The powerful effect of expressing appreciation is for your aide to hear and feel, "Thank you for what you have done— you and your work are really important to me."

Third, *your consistent respect for the PA's rights* ensures that your rights always will be respected as well. Your respect for the personal rights of each PA is basic to a solid employee-employer relationship.[1]

The importance of expressing appreciation

For unsalaried, family caregivers, constant, sincere appreciation is as vital to their health as the oxygen they breathe. For salaried PAs, it is actually more important than (although it cannot replace!) their paycheck.

Anyone who provides you with help expects routine "payment" in the form of appreciation, and it does not cost you anything! To *appreciate* "is to recognize someone's services by outwardly expressing gratitude." *Gratitude* speaks of "being thankful for the benefit of comforts received or discomforts relieved."

Appreciation is a very powerful force. It is so powerful an incentive that several huge volunteer agencies with very dedicated members throughout the world pay no formal salaries to the majority of their workers. Examples include the American Red Cross, the Peace Corps, hospital auxiliaries, school PTAs, and scores of clubs and groups in every community. These are volunteer agencies that have designed and implemented highly sophisticated programs for expressing appreciation to volunteers who are willing to work very long hours and years for free. These programs include certificates, pins, award banquets, media releases, and a whole hierarchy of ranked titles that the volunteers earn by routinely donating their services.

---

1. For more detail on the natural rights that each of us expects—and appreciates from others— please see the lists of employee and employer rights in chapter 📖 22, "A Bill of Rights for You as a Help Recipient, Caregiver, or Paid Provider."

The end objective of these recognition strategies is merely to say, "Thank you for what you have done—you and your work are really important." That may seem syrupy and corny, but workers often lose interest in even high-salaried careers unless they regularly receive appreciation for their work.

A worker's need to receive appreciation, and the employer's responsibility to provide it, are not inversely based on the monetary salary paid to the worker. Many managers mistakenly believe that by providing a worker with a decent salary, the worker is being shown sufficient appreciation. In contrast, unpaid volunteers, min-imum-wage workers, and even six-figure corporate executives all want to feel the figurative pat on the back that comes from routine appreciation.

Many traditional bosses, who believe that they must keep a rein of tight super-vision and power over employees, refuse to outwardly express sincere apprecia-tion. Some believe that to express appreciation is to show dependence on employ-ees, to invite the worker to become uncomfortably close, and therefore to lose the boss's sense of supervisory power and respect.

Today's more modern employers are taking deliberate steps away from that outdated approach. These modern managers who express appreciation find that they do not lose "face." To the contrary, by respecting employees the managers earn increased power and respect.

As a PA manager, you are wise to benefit from the experience of big business. In addition to the salaries you pay PAs, express appreciation to PAs who deserve it.

> *There are four main elements to powerful expressions of appreciation.*

According to most psychologists, one of the most effective, powerful incentives for both learning and remembering tasks, as well as for correcting bad habits and main-taining good ones, is to "positively reinforce" desired behavior. If a puppy hears the evening newspaper being delivered, gets the paper, and brings it in—and you would like this to happen each evening—then the most effective way to reinforce the behavior is to praise him at the time you receive the newspaper.

This strategy might sound hackneyed, but it remains the most effective answer to the frequent question, "How do I train and maintain good habits in PAs?"

There are four factors that will make your expressions of appreciation especially effective.

- First, express appreciation only when you sincerely mean it. If you do not feel appreciative, get into the habit.

   If you do not routinely feel appreciative of a PA's help to you, ask yourself "why not?" You should realize either that the PA is doing a good job and deserves some kudos, or that she is doing a poor job and should be corrected.

If she deserves your routine gratitude and you "feel funny" about expressing it, then discipline yourself to "feel good" and make it a habit. Get your feet wet by expressing an appreciation, and then observe the recipient's reaction. That smile, facial blush, and maybe even an expressed "thank you" should tell you something. You have not lost any of your authority, but instead have enhanced it. The recipient likes you a tiny bit more now than she did ten seconds ago. However, beware. If you adopt a habit of routinely expressing these things, you could be looking at a very favorable change in your whole image!

Do not insult your PA by expressing insincere, cold, plastic appreciation—it is worthless and often sarcastic. If you need to develop an appreciative mindset, think about how impossible your life would be without her help. At each time that you know you should express appreciation, but cannot, play that tape in your head, "What my life would be like without her help." You will probably be grateful for the task that she has just done well; tell her about your sincere feelings, now! Repeatedly play your "head tape" until you naturally feel the appreciation and can easily verbalize it. As further reinforcement, start to notice her favorable reaction to your expressions.

• Second, when you express appreciation, be sure your message is clearly delivered and understood.

Speak assertively with sufficient volume, speak clearly (avoid mumbling), and use a tone of voice that shows the warm sincerity behind your expression. When you are about to speak, lift up your chin and eyebrows, smile, and make good eye contact by looking at the PA.

Looking at an aide when you address him is a powerful way of making sure he is listening and understands your message. The strategy usually assures him full attention and ensures that he will remember your message. Appreciation that the PA does not hear, does not understand, or does not think is sincere is wasted.

This body language has the basic, powerful elements of any clear, direct, assertive communication.[2]

• Third, each effective expression of appreciation should convey at least two messages: what you appreciate and why you appreciate it.

The most effective expressions of appreciation have this one-two knockout message:

▸ "Earl, I really appreciate the way you clean my glasses—they really make a difference when I have to study for several hours."

▸ "Kathy, I like the way you hang up the towels after my shower—that is the only way they will dry out."

---

2. For more details on and strategies for being assertive, please see chapter 📖 14, "Say It, Ask for It, and Act—Assertively!"

▸ "Fran, I am grateful for your calling ahead tonight to tell me you would be 20 minutes late—I would have been concerned when you were late, and I was able to finish some work that I had to get done for a meeting tomorrow."

▸ "Kim, thank you for helping me with the interview of the PA applicants. Have you ever considered being an instructor? You have an especially clear way of explaining difficult concepts, and creating examples. You are really skilled at it."

▸ "Dave, I want to thank you for all of the help you've given me this past year—it is a relief to be able to depend on your help."

• Fourth and final, vary how and how often you express appreciation. Patting your PAs on the back should become a routine habit.

Although there is no set formula for your expressions, you might remember the Psychology 101 adage that random positive reinforcement is more effective than patterned reinforcement. By *random*, we mean "with no recognizable pattern or schedule." In everyday terms, this is why a romantic mate especially enjoys getting flowers and an "I love you" for no special reason.

If your two-hour evening routine has 86 tasks, should you express 86 compliments? No, that would be overkill. Is it enough to save your thank yous for one, really assertive and sincere, eyeball-to-eyeball expression as a PA says good night at her shift's end? Perhaps.

DeGraff's Appreciation Rule of Thumb for his personal PAs is that roughly "1 in 10" tasks gets some sort of thank-you. Roughly and random means sometimes 1 in 5 and other times 1 in 15. One night, when my current PA and I were interviewing some applicants, I heard my current PA mention to an applicant, "I don't know exactly why, but I usually feel really good after I finish one of his routines."

In addition to random frequency, deliver a variety of expressions or reasons why you appreciate the task:

• "I appreciate... because... "

• "Thank you (thanks) for... it is really important because... "

• "You really do a great job of... and that makes it easier for me to... "

• "Nice going... that will make my day a lot easier... "

• "I am especially grateful for the way you... and let me tell you why... "

• "You are one of the best... that I have seen in a long time."

• "You are becoming a real pro at... look at how clean that is... "

• "Where did you learn to do such a great job of (to be so good at)... "

• "I am really grateful that you did... as a result, I was able to do... "

• "Nice job... "

• "You take a lot of pride in the way you do... "

• "It has been a long time since anyone has done that good a job of... "

• "You are great... "

Among those random times, there are four especially good ones. Be sure not to miss out on these opportunities.

On arrival. Greet every PA arrival with a smile and hello. You are really glad to see him, and that he has arrived on time. Provide special appreciation if you know that he overcame a difficulty to arrive (bad weather, illness, Monday morning or Saturday night). "All right, there he is, right on time—wow, am I glad to see that you made it here despite all that rain!" In the PA biz, if you are consistently glad to see your aides arrive—and say so—they will tend to look forward to coming to work. Conversely, if you are a consistent whiner and complainer, most PAs will soon begin to frown as they come through your door.

Want to test it? Select two of your PAs for an experiment. Give "A" a glad greeting for each of seven mornings, and give "B" a depressed greeting on seven evenings (or whatever works). On the eighth day, before you say anything, check out the facial expression of each aide on arrival. Which is smiling and looking forward to seeing you, and which is looking at the floor and not really wanting to be there?

During training. Use appreciation during training both to reinforce the first sign of a good habit, and to boost the self-esteem of a new PA who needs a boost.

Randomly reinforce work details that are done well by a new PA who is learning your routine, or by a current PA who is trying to correct bad habits. In addition, watch for new PAs who are doing a good job and who need a little extra support. To maintain morale during your initial training instructions, emphasize what she is doing right, instead of commenting only when she does something incorrectly. If a new aide looks overwhelmed by all the task details, give her extra energy with extra appreciation.

"Gee, Gordie, you learn quickly. You have been doing a great job in keeping the kitchen clean—it looks great!"

"Hey, Jamie, are you okay? This routine has a lot of details for a first night. But you know what? Tomorrow night will be easier, and the next night easier yet. Remember how confusing it was the first time you went through all the steps to drive a car? After a few times, you no longer had to think about them. The same will happen here, I promise. Together, you and I can clobber this routine."

Bad days and boredom. Everyone has a bad day, and we all respond better to a sympathetic show of support. And sometimes the routine can get people down. Show gratitude when a PA gets bored or feels taken for granted.

"Gillie, please remember how grateful I am for your help. I doubt there are many other jobs where you would be appreciated as much as you are here."

On departure. Close out every PA's end-of-shift departure with gratitude and enthusiasm for the next time you will see him.

Remember how important it is to greet each PA arrival with a smile? Well, the same importance applies to each departure. As an aide walks out to her car to go home, do you want her to think about how tired she is, or how good she feels because you just told her how much you appreciated her work and how much you are looking forward to seeing her next time?

"Barry, thanks so much for your help tonight. It means a lot. Have a great weekend and I will look forward to seeing you on Monday night."

Perhaps the power of routinely expressing appreciation is best summed up by what Joan, one of my PAs, once told me. She had left my employ and moved with her husband across the country. Two years later she called me for an employment reference. I readily agreed. As we were ending our phone call she said, "You know, I really miss working for you. You are one of the few employers I have ever had who cared about me, made me feel important, and appreciated my work."

It does not get much better than that!

Chapter 16

Dividing Your Needs, and Assigning Work Shifts, Among Several PAs

Has either—or both—of these scenarios happened to you yet?

Scenario #1. You have been employing Fran as your only PA. The woman does a fantastic job, and everything has been running smoothly for a couple of years. She is very healthy, never gets a cold, and thoroughly knows your routine. However, this afternoon she called you, very apologetic, and announced that she had broken her leg while doing farm chores for her folks. She will not be able to help you for several weeks.

Politely, you wish her well and hang up the phone. You are in shock.

For two years, she has been your only PA. How will you get into bed tonight? Everything was so perfect. You never imagined anything would happen to this smooth routine, nor have you even wanted to consider the possibility.

Sure, you fantasized once about having the luxury of two or three aides. But who could afford them? Also, you have only 20 hours of needs each week. There just would not be enough work for two or three people. And imagine all the headaches of scheduling, keeping track of work hours, and calculating paychecks. For more aides, you would have to multiply the effort you now spend managing just Fran by two or three! Besides, she takes so much pride in her work, she would probably be insulted and get mad if you brought in anyone else.

If only you had even one backup PA, you (or Fran) could call the other to do a sudden fill-in. You would not have to train him, since he would have been routinely working with you and Fran. But, given your situation, how could that have been possible for you? So much for being naive in believing that Fran was invincible. Your nightmare has come true. At eight o'clock tonight, just five quick hours from now, Fran will not be coming through your front door to help you into bed!

Scenario #2. You and Steve have shared an apartment in downtown Denver for almost a year. When you first moved to the city, the two of you met at a bar. He needed a place to live and you needed a live-in aide. He learned the routine quickly, and within a week you had developed a romantic relationship. As a couple, you shared so many current activities as well as dreams about the future. Each of you would do anything for the other, and this included the unquestioned PA help of every kind that Steve provided for you.

341

You were unable to imagine that anything could happen either to the relationship or to his PA help. Indeed, it seemed inconceivable that anything could interrupt the help, because the other relationship was so strong. You have trusted Steve without reservation, even to the point of a steadily growing financial loan to him while he has been out of work. However, what's a few hundred dollars and his borrowing your credit card when you consider all of the free help you have received?

All went so well until about three weeks ago, when you got the flu and needed extra help—and time—from Steve. Small disagreements and arguments turned into bigger ones. Then, last week, it subtly became obvious that he was not as available for assistance as he had been. You got the hint, and brought in another friend to do some errands and housecleaning for which Steve was "no longer available."

So, the romantic relationship had suddenly disappeared, and you began to doubt that you will ever again see your finances or credit card. However, most importantly, your one-and-only live-in aide has begun curtailing, one by one, the PA tasks that he has heretofore been willing to perform. In addition, his personality and attitude toward you are fluctuating faster than the stock market. Each afternoon, when he arrives at the apartment, you drop what you are doing to check his facial expression and mood. Your quickly growing experience has taught you that his hourly mood and attitude toward you are pretty reliable indicators of whether he will abruptly agree or refuse to provide PA help.

You hate living this way. What incredible power he now has over your lifestyle! Your daily schedule of when you get help out of bed, when—or if—your meals are available, and when you are assisted back into bed was so regular, constant, and dependable for months, until just ten days ago. You have lost your appetite, because your stomach hurts each time Steve opens the apartment door. He now controls the quality of your life, and he obviously enjoys his newfound power.

You have no idea how to get out of this nightmare. If only you had a second or third aide, you could fire and evict him, using the other PAs both to enforce your decision and to seamlessly provide transition help. After you get out of this, it will be "one-and-only, live-in PA—no way!"

The importance of dividing your needs

In my three-plus decades of managing PAs, I have found few other strategies as important as this one. This single strategy answers so many questions and prevents so many problems—that once routinely happened—from ever happening again.

If you are truly dependent on help from others, then

- you probably have enough weekly hours of needs to divide between at least two aides

- you should not even consider placing all of your needs with, and becoming totally dependent upon, just one aide

- you should divide your weekly needs among as many part-time PAs as is practical for you and them.

As an example, I am a C 5/6 quad (tetra) and have always personally employed and managed my PAs. I need about 30 hours of weekly help. Wherever I have lived, I have recruited and hired from a local college campus and maintained a staff of about five PAs at all times. Each works an average of six hours a week, two mornings and one evening or one morning and two evenings. Once each month, we have a staff meeting and, with calendars in hand, the PAs select their assignments for the next four weeks. After these formal, face-to-face schedule commitments are made, if an aide then encounters a personal emergency and cannot work a shift, she is responsible for calling her four colleagues and finding her own replacement. The original aide informs me of the change, and notes the change on my master calendar that reflects all assignments.

It costs me the same to address my 30 weekly hours of help whether I use one or five people. When I employed just one aide at a time, and that one aide was suddenly unable to work, I was forced to call friends and neighbors for favors. At other times, a sole PA sometimes knew that he had an unfair advantage over me, and an occasional aide abused it. My personal schedule was often dictated by his preferences. I experienced many kinds of abuse. Now, with a constant staff of five, I am always in control of my schedule, quality of help, and possessions. With four instant backups at all times, I could easily fire an undesirable. However, because of a well-designed recruiting and screening procedure, I have fired less than a handful of people in all of these years. I sleep soundly, knowing that I am sure to get up on schedule each morning.

Employing more than one PA seems impossible!

There are several reasons why employing at least two PAs may seem impossible for you. You may be concerned about increased costs, or spiraling management responsibilities, or declining privacy. But careful consideration will show that, whatever the concerns, they are far outweighed by the advantages of having additional help when you need it. Here are some common reasons why you may think you cannot hire more than one PA, and then the arguments in favor of doing just that!

Enough hours. You may think you do not have enough weekly hours of help needs, so there would probably not be enough work for two or more people.

In truth, the majority of people who are interested in doing PA work either cannot or do not want to work full time. Most will consider only part-time work of 20, 10, 5, or even fewer weekly hours. It is true that most part-timers have a weekly minimum and maximum of hours in mind that will fit into their schedule. When you are answering phone inquiries about your PA newspaper ad, the first caller might require "at least 20 hours" to balance his budget and make your job "worth his time." If this is a much bigger block than the five hours you are offering, do not give up. Thank the first caller, save his name and number just in case, and take the next.

An old adage says that for every item that is up for sale, there is at least one buyer. The same is true for your PA jobs. It is especially true if you market to college students.

If you are truly dependent on help from others, then you probably have enough weekly hours to divide between at least two aides. How many PAs should you hire? Check out the discussion later in this chapter within the section called "Tips for recruiting, scheduling, and managing multiple PAs."

Affordability. You can barely afford to hire one PA, and cannot imagine affording more.

Just as it costs you no more to keep your car's gas tank constantly full than to keep it one-quarter full, it costs you no more to employ five PAs than it does one PA, for the same total of hours.

For example, if you have 30 weekly hours of needs and pay an hourly salary of $8, the weekly salaries will cost you around $240. The cost is the same regardless of whether you employ one, three, or five aides, and divide the total hours among them. However, as discussed later, it will cost you slightly more in advertising because you will be placing ads more often.

Management. You have trouble managing and scheduling one PA, and cannot imagine the extra time, effort, and paperwork.

There was a movie in the 1950s, when families were into raising lots of children, called *Cheaper by the Dozen*. The premise of this wry comedy was that once parents have learned about raising (and managing) one child, they might as well have more. Once they had learned and tooled the formulas and strategies for the first child, additional ones would not require that much extra effort. There were also a number of situations where the parents actually assigned some of the parental management duties to the older children. The idea was that some of the children could be taught and made responsible for their own management tasks.

In reality, "PA parenthood" can be managed the same way. If you can manage one PA, you can manage three, four, or five, and you can use some of the aides to help you with the duties.

These economies of scale are common. In printing, the per-copy price becomes cheaper as you have more copies made. The per-copy cost of paper is a constant, rising uniformly as more copies are printed. However, once a printing press is set up, the ink flow is adjusted, and the paper stack is located correctly, the per-copy labor cost drops sharply for higher quantities. As printers say, "Once we have everything set up and running smoothly, extra copies get cheaper because you are paying mostly for me to stand here and keep my finger pressed on the operating button for another 30 seconds."

Once you have formulated your PA management strategies and have employed a few sole PAs, one after the other, you might as well "keep your finger on the button" and employ more than one. Managing several part-timers, beyond the initial recruiting, hiring, and training, is really not that much extra work. In fact, later in this discussion you will find ways of having the PAs manage themselves. Examples include making them responsible for deciding their own schedules and recording assignments on your master calendar, recruiting their own replacements, and helping you with salary calculations and check writing.

Insulting the current PA. You are concerned about insulting or making angry your current PA or family caregiver by hiring additional ones.

In the world of business, decisions must be made that keep the business strong and improve it. Two sayings come to mind that address the fact that in any business, periodic decisions must be made and new directions taken regardless of their popularity with all employees. First, in the direct simplicity of the baseball legend, Yogi Berra, "Business is business"; in a John Wayne style, "You do what you have to do."

Your ongoing, day-after-day, life-sustaining, salary-paying need for PA help is most definitely a business. You must periodically make business decisions around what has not worked, what can be done to resolve the problems, and what you need to change. And then you proceed to make those changes.

It is a fact that more than 50 percent of family caregivers who help us are overworked and chronically tired, and are experiencing some degree of depression. This does not mean that they love us any less or that they do not want to help us. It does mean that our caregivers usually need some supplemental help and a rest. It is also very common that they feel guilty about telling us their needs, and often deny their need for additional, outside providers.

It is often up to us to watch for symptoms of their ongoing fatigue, and out of our love for them, for us to volunteer—and often insist—to find them some relief or replacement. The decision to hire some outside help and divide needs among more people is one to be made with a rational head, not an emotional heart. This is business—we do what we have to do. The decision to hire more help is not a sign of a failing family or romantic relationship. Instead, it is a way of preventing a relationship from becoming strained and preventing failure from happening.[1]

Location. You live in a rural area, had difficulty finding your current PA, and cannot imagine being able to recruit others.

If you live in a sparsely populated area, it is easy to imagine that your current PA is the last one in existence. What's more, you might be overpaying your current PA and requesting that she help only with pleasant tasks, because of fear that you might otherwise lose her. There are even days when you fear that you might go without help after she ultimately leaves and cannot be replaced.

It is very likely that your current aide will someday resign. Few PAs work forever. If your need for help is ongoing, then you will have to recruit her replacement sooner or later. If you recruit the "replacement" now, while you still have the original aide, then you will benefit from two part-timers. When one does resign, you will feel less stress because there will be no potential gap in your coverage.

---

1. For more details about the concerns of recipients, caregivers, and paid providers, please see the chapters:
📖 23 "Your Personal Concerns as a Help Recipient"
📖 24 "Your Personal Concerns as a Family Caregiver"
📖 25 "Your Personal Concerns as a Paid Help Provider, plus
  "Ten Reasons Why PAs Quit and Are Fired"

It is not uncommon to think of a current aide as the "one and only" who is available, especially if you have not hired many aides. However, as your need for help will outlive the current PA, and you will eventually have to replace her, why not hire that second aide now and benefit from two concurrent ones?

Privacy. You value your privacy, have adjusted to one outside PA, and cannot imagine being invaded by more.

Chances are that you use only one PA at a time, so whether you employ one or five PAs, you will still not be "invaded" by more than one at a time. When you divide your needs among two or more part-timers, you will have more than one person with whom to become acquainted and in whom to trust.

If you are concerned about personal security and stability, you will find comfort in having your dependent needs entrusted to more than just one aide. If you like the secure feeling of being able to trust that your needs will be continuously fulfilled, with minimal chances for no-show gaps, you will enjoy employing two or more providers and not putting all your needs into one "PA basket."

Now that you have addressed some of the more negative reasons for dividing your needs among more than one PA, it's time to consider the large number of positive reasons for pursuing additional help. These can range from maintaining more control to preventing PA burnout, but they all provide tremendous benefits.

Control. You are in control by having instant substitutes and backups for sudden PA sick times, vacations, no-shows, resignations, or firings.

Perhaps the major advantage in employing several, concurrent PAs can be stated in one word: *empowerment.* When you are dependent on just one aide, that person can have incredible power over you. For most respectful relationships, this is not an issue. However, it is not uncommon for a sole PA to take advantage of his or her monopoly.

If an "only" aide is so inclined, he knows that without him, you are in trouble. Without him, you might not be able to get into or out of bed, use the bathroom, or get your meals. This unscrupulous person knows that you fear suddenly losing him, and that you probably want to keep him happy. He knows that you probably will not, and cannot, object if he:

- wants to refuse to do some of your less desirable tasks
- wants to modify your schedule to better fit his sleep pattern
- wants too often to arrive late or leave early
- wants to sample your liquor cabinet or narcotic medications
- wants to routinely feed himself from your refrigerator
- wants the help of your wallet in giving himself a pay raise
- wants to borrow your wheelchair-accessible van to help a friend move a heavy kitchen stove
- wants sexual favors
- wants to suddenly take vacation time
- wants to slack off in the quality of help he provides.

In short, he knows that he cannot easily be replaced. He can choose to take control of you, your lifestyle, and your possessions. He can choose to create your worst nightmare, if he is your only aide.

In contrast, when you spread your needs among several PAs, you have several assurances that your needs will be met—your way. Wall Street financial investors have proven for decades that the cardinal guideline for maximum security and stability is to diversify where one invests. Only foolish investors and inexperienced Las Vegas gamblers trust all their money to just one chance to win. If that one chance fails, they lose everything.

Consequently, why should you trust all of your life-sustaining needs to just one aide? When you have several PAs and one breaks a leg, wants time off for a ski weekend, wants to resign, or has to be fired, you have instant, well-trained backups and replacements.

When several aides are helping you, only you are in control—and that is a very stable, secure, and powerful way to live.

Time and stress. You have more time and less stress for recruiting, hiring, and training new PAs.

The period of time between a PA announcing her resignation and having in place a new, trained, and trustworthy replacement can be both lengthy and stressful. Will you be successful in finding a high-quality replacement, and finding one before the current aide must leave?

Most of that uncertainty is minimized when you have the support of one or more continuing PAs to bridge the recruiting gap. There is no chance that you will temporarily not be able to get into bed if the PA vacancy is not filled in time. If the departing aide must leave before the new one is in place, each of the continuing PAs simply takes on a few extra hours to meet your needs.

Talents. You have a variety of people and talents to accommodate your variety of schedule, routine tasks, and special projects.

If you have physical limitations and are dependent on physical help from others, you probably also have many types of needs. At the most basic level, you might need help for ADLs, which may include getting dressed and undressed, transferring between bed and wheelchair, performing bowel and shower routines, and perhaps assistance with food preparation and eating.

However, you undoubtedly need help in areas beyond these very basics:

- watering and repotting houseplants
- vacuuming the carpet and dusting furniture
- cleaning and making minor repairs to the wheelchair
- cooking special dishes
- weeding the garden
- cleaning the barbecue
- wiring new speakers to your stereo

- replacing a light bulb in the front porch lamp
- washing the car
- hanging a new picture on the wall
- selecting the best produce, meat, fish, or bread at the market.

All of the people you interview and hire should have the ability to help you with ADLs. For additional types of needs, you may discover some PAs who are "jacks of all trades," naturally skilled at almost anything. However, most people are skilled in some areas and not good at others.

Most of these additional tasks are best done by people with somewhat specialized skills. There are some people who are skilled at cleaning things, and others who "do not do windows." Some folks are mechanically inclined and have a talent for fixing things, whereas others can't use a screwdriver.

Asking someone to do something at which he is clumsy or about which he is unknowledgeable can be futile, counterproductive, and downright frustrating. If the task is completed at all, it will probably require your constant supervision and instruction, take twice the necessary time, and not be done well anyway. In contrast, assigning the same task to someone who has the required skill means that she can do the job alone, in half the time, and it will be done well.

When you have three PAs helping, you often have three times the skills available when compared to employing just one person. Each of the PAs routinely helps with the everyday, basic ADLs. However, when it comes to special projects, you can match each task to a PA who shines in that area.

Attractiveness. Your PA job is more manageable, and thus more attractive, to applicants.

Your recruiting is easier when the job is more attractive to applicants. It is more attractive when the work, time commitment, and responsibilities are not borne by one person, but instead are divided among several co-workers. In addition, dividing tasks means you can better accommodate each PA's personal schedule.

Your needs don't usually all occur in one convenient package of time, on one day, and in just one location. Usually needs occur morning and night, on as many as seven days each week (including every weekend). Perhaps there is also a variety of locations, such as home, job site, college campus, and community. If this is your lifestyle, you will have a problem finding a single person to cover all of that variety. (More than one PA over the years has told me, "I cannot keep up with your on-the-go daily lifestyle—I am resigning in order to get some rest.") In contrast, if you divide your needs into manageable portions like blocks of time, days, and locations, then hiring and keeping good PAs will be easier.

When initially describing the position to responders reached by your newspaper ad, be sure to explain the advantages of your multi-PA staff, including the availability of substitutes. These features are very attractive to prospects, and you will be establishing your policies early.

Burnout. You will be reducing the incidence of PA burnout and keeping PAs longer.

Burnout from overwork is much more common when you load all your needs onto the shoulders of just one provider. In contrast, when each member of a PA team shares the work and time commitments, each load is lighter. Burnout is reduced, PAs are happier and stay longer, and you recruit, hire, and train less often.

Financial investors have long known about the safeguards in diversifying. They would never consider gambling all of their money in just one fund. Especially if you personally employ, you should not gamble all of your needs on just one PA.

In an overall sense, one family caregiver or PA working alone has no opportunity for time off from the work, and no relief from the feeling of being constantly on duty for assistance to a very dependent individual. Help providers need time off for at least two reasons: to provide a real break from the constant responsibility of the work (and the feeling of your dependence on them), and to provide them with the chance to pursue their own interests of career, education, or leisure activities.[2]

Scheduling. You have several people—and not just you—scrutinizing your schedule and supply of continuous help, and there is less chance of a no-show gap for a shift.

Later in this chapter, you will find details about scheduling and assigning tasks among several PAs, with an emphasis on sharing these responsibilities with the PAs. For example, instead of you assigning tasks to PAs, have them select and negotiate your schedule among themselves. Arrange a staff meeting with you every four or five weeks where the aides can meet and work together in selecting and assigning work shifts. Later, if a PA is unable to work a self-assigned shift, she is responsible for calling her colleagues to recruit her own replacement, and for notifying you of the change. If she cannot recruit a substitute, then she cannot take the time off. In this way, the PAs assist you with your responsibility for maintaining continuous coverage. Indeed, all of you work as a group to avoid no-show gaps.

Variety. You enjoy and benefit from a variety of people, cultures, conversations, and problem-solving ideas.

Your interaction with PAs is an important and unavoidable part of your daily lifestyle. If you resent the required intrusions into your privacy, then you can cope with them by viewing the interactions as simply work-related sessions for which you receive help and the people who provide it receive paychecks.

In contrast, if you enjoy socially interacting with the PAs, then life for each of you can become richer and fuller in addition to the help you receive. If this is your viewpoint, and you look forward to seeing each aide, then employing more than one will multiply the ideas, cultures, and problem-solving abilities that you encounter.

---

2. For more detail about family caregiver burnout, please see chapter 📖 24, "Your Personal Concerns as a Family Caregiver."

The primary disadvantage to dividing your needs

The only significant drawback to dividing your needs among several PAs is the more frequent cycle of recruiting, hiring, and training, along with the associated cost. However, for those of us who have reaped the numerous advantages of multiple PAs, this single disadvantage is relatively minor.

Tips for recruiting, scheduling, and managing multiple PAs

"Okay, you have convinced me to divide my needs among as many PAs—resources—as possible. What should I know about setting up this PA personnel office of mine?"

There are some key strategies that make it easier to recruit, schedule, assign, and manage multiple PAs, and to get the most out of them. These tips are repeated in other appropriate areas of this reference book.

How many PAs should you hire?

Hire as many as the market allows. For your interests, the more PAs you concurrently employ, the better your needs will be served.

Some PAs will want to maximize the weekly number of hours they work, so as to maximize salary; others will limit the hours they can work by limitations in personal schedule. If you are employing college students, experience has shown that students carrying a heavy course load often find six to eight weekly hours of work quite attractive. If you are advertising to the general, non-student community, you will usually encounter people wanting more hours.

Examine your list of routine, weekly needs for help and total the average number of hours. Start by trying to offer each PA six to eight weekly hours, so divide your total weekly hours by six to determine how many aides to hire. For example, if you have about 30 weekly hours of needs, you will initially be trying to hire 5 PAs for about 6 hours each.

How do you know if six weekly hours will be attractive to the people in your area? There are two factors that will help you decide:

- When placing your newspaper ad, cite "six hours average per week" and monitor the responses. If this attracts enough responses, and you can hire enough people, then you have the formula that works. If there are not enough responses, change the ad to eight hours and try again. Keep repeating this trial-and-error procedure until your offer matches the work load needs of the PA prospects.

- When you are speaking with applicants, or after you have hired, ask for additional feedback advice. This is market research. Ask about what wording in your ad attracted them and what they think about the number of weekly hours.

Advertising and recruiting

Experience has shown that it is usually wise to include the average number of weekly hours per aide in your newspaper ad. Including these kinds of specifications in your ad will attract responses from the people who meet the profile you want. This will reduce the number of unqualified callers who ring your phone.

Here is an example of a PA newspaper ad that cites the average number of weekly hours.[3] This can be a very attractive, bite-sized work load for college students or anyone with an otherwise busy schedule:

> **$9 for Help to Man with Disability**
> Get experience working with a disability. Cool, active guy who uses wheelchair needs help with living activities, 6-8 hrs weekly. Just 10 min from campus (car required), routine easy to learn. Needed now. Call Skip today & lv message, 555-3721.

Training

There are three steps to training new providers.[4] Schedule the new people:

- to watch a current PA perform each part of your routine
- to complete the routine once or twice while a current PA stands by
- to finish their training by working with you, and receiving your occasional reminders and lots of patience.

If you employ more than one part-time PA, be careful in selecting which one to use as an example, both during early interviews and demonstrations and during post-hiring demonstrations and training. Choose a current aide who has the personal qualities and work habits closest to those that you want the new PA to adopt. The new PAs will tend to model what they see.

As the current aide demonstrates the routine, her primary role is to narrate what she is doing and how she is doing it. These are the parts that she knows best, and she can explain as she provides you help. Your role should include explaining why you prefer that tasks be done in certain ways.

Nine steps to facilitating staff meetings and assigning tasks

This is the beginning of the heavy-duty advantages of employing several PAs. You have them negotiate and self-assign their own scheduling, and consequently be more firmly committed to it.

❶ The foundation for the PA's clear understanding of policies is the routine staff meeting. Once every four or five weeks, hold an hour-long scheduling meeting and ask each PA to bring an appointment book or calendar. To minimize the need for after-meeting shift changes, advise PAs to carefully check their personal schedules before the meeting. With just a few minutes of cautious planning, they can avoid committing to work shifts that already have conflicts.

---

3. Additional ad examples are outlined in chapter 📖 8, "Where and How to Advertise for Your Own PAs."

4. These training steps are outlined in chapter 📖 9, "Initial Training and Ongoing Management of Aides and PAs."

❷ At the meeting, first be sure that everyone has been introduced and that each PA has a complete, up-to-date list of the crew's phone numbers. You will want all members to be well acquainted, comfortable, and well connected with each other.

❸ Next, make any staff announcements and ask for any concerns that any PAs would like to discuss. This is a golden opportunity to address any concerns, complaints, gossip, or job dissatisfactions that have been left up in the air since the last meeting. If these are left unaddressed, they can often cause discontent and departures. This is also a great time to do your market research about whether everyone likes the weekly number of work hours, and to inquire about other suggestions for improving your system.

❹ Next, if a meeting includes new recruits, you might remind everyone about the routine, weekly schedule of needs that they will be accommodating. For example:

- each morning, 6 to 8 A.M.
- each bowel and shower evening, Sun-Wed-Fri, 8 to 10:30 P.M.
- each simple evening, Mon-Tues-Thur-Sat, 8 to 10 P.M.

In addition, remind the group about the two ways to view each PA's weekly work load. One is to take the weekly total of hours and divide by the number of PAs. For example, if you have about 30 weekly hours of need, and there are 5 aides, then each aide will be committing to about 6 weekly hours.

A second viewpoint helps PAs decide how many weekly shifts each PA should average. Here, you divide the total number of weekly shifts by the number of PAs. For example, if there is a morning and evening shift each day, 7 days per week, the total is 14 shifts per week. Divided by perhaps five PAs in your group, that comes close to three shifts for each PA, each week. Translated further, that means that each aide will be aiming each week for two mornings and an evening, or one morning and two evenings.

❺ Also announce the dates and times of any special projects or appointments with which you will need extra help within this upcoming four- or five-week period.

I would like you all to note some special requests that I have for these upcoming weeks:

Friday, May 11, is my birthday. I would like to get up at the usual time, but my family is having a party for me and I would like to postpone the evening until 11 p.m. That Wednesday would ordinarily be a bowel/shower night. Due to my request for a later bedtime, let's change the bowel/shower nights that week from Sunday-Wednesday-Friday to Sunday-Tuesday-Friday.

On Monday, May 14, I would like to do some shopping down in Dallas. Is anyone available for a five-hour period to give me a ride, help with shopping, have a nice dinner on me, and give me a ride back?

6 Ask the PAs to decide among themselves which shifts each wants. Then sit back and watch the negotiating, stepping in only if questions or problems arise.

PA crews have been known to use several different ways in making their self-assignments. The crew will soon decide for itself which it prefers.

Some groups prefer consistency in making PA-shift selections. For example, one PA might ask simply to take all of the Tuesday mornings, Thursday evenings, and every other Saturday morning. Another might prefer each Sunday and Wednesday morning, and each Tuesday evening.

Other ways of consistently making PA-shift selections include:

- Time of day—morning needs to one PA, evening needs to another.

- Days of the week—M-W-F needs to one PA, T-Th needs to another.

- Weekends—weekend needs to one PA, or to different PAs on different weekends of a rotating monthly schedule.

- Location—home needs to one PA, work or school needs to another.

- Types of work—divide different types of needs among different part-time PAs who have various skills and interests, such as medical assistance, household cleaning, mechanical repairs of mobility equipment and household furnishings, yard work, and transportation.

- Amount of work—divide your total schedule of needs into bite-sized blocks of time.

Other groups dislike this consistent approach and opt for variety. The following, more democratic approach is preferred especially within larger groups and when some PAs are less assertive than their more motivated counterparts.

These groups often prefer to have each person take a round-robin turn in having first choice for a selected week. For example, if the aides are sitting in a circle and Sam is somehow selected to go first, he gets first pick of his share of the mornings and evenings for the first week. To finish that week, each aide takes turns in committing to the remaining shifts. For the second week, if Suzy is sitting next to Sam, then she begins by taking her preferences of the second week's shifts. When Suzy has finished committing to her preferences (and share) of the second week, the rest of the crew takes turns finishing off the week. The third week begins with the third PA, and so on.

7 Supply the negotiating PAs with a master calendar for you, and ask for a volunteer to mark it with all the shift commitments as each day is negotiated. In the end, you will have each calendar day marked with one PA's initials for each shift of each day. For example, if you have two shifts each day, there will be two sets of PA initials within the box for each calendar day: one at the top of each day's box, identifying the morning PA, and one at each box bottom, identifying each night PA (see *Figure 16-1*).

The individual PAs probably will not keep a comprehensive master calendar like yours. However, each will be marking his or her own calendar or appointment book with personal commitments.

Figure 16-1: **Sample master calendar**

This example of a month-long master calendar shows the handwritten initials for morning and evening work shifts for five part-time PAs who have scheduled four to five weeks in advance.

M	T	W	TH	F	S	SU
MAY	**1**	**2**	**3**	**4**	**5**	**6**
	JH	FS	PR	PR	FS	JH
	FS	PR	ME	ME	JH	ME
7	**8**	**9**	**10**	**11**	**12**	**13**
KK	PR	ME	ME	FS	PR	PR
JH	JH	KC	JH	KC	SB	ME
14	**15**	**16**	**17**	**18**	**19**	**20**
PR	PR	ME	PR	FS	SB	PR
FS	JH	FS	FS	JH	FS	KC
21	**22**	**23**	**24**	**25**	**26**	**27**
SB	PR	ME	PR	FS	SB	FS
ME	JH	KC	KC	KC	JH	PR
28	**29**	**30**	**31**			
JH	PR	ME	PR			
ME	JH	KC	KC			

❽ Within a half hour, all your needs will be scheduled by the PAs' choice. When all shifts are taken, ask everyone to check their individual calendars while you call out each day's commitments from the master calendar that someone has created for you. This is a very important step to catch any discrepancies:

- "Sunday, May 6—Janis has the morning, Megan the evening."
- "Monday, the 7th—Kim has the A.M., Janis the P.M."

In an upcoming subsection, "The master calendar," you will see the importance of this master calendar as a graphic reference for both you and your staff.

❾ Before the meeting adjourns, make sure you accomplish two things.

First, have the PAs schedule the next staff meeting (for five weeks from now, if you are scheduling five weeks at a time). This date and time should be marked on individual calendars and your master.

Second, remind everyone of your "sub and backup" policy. If a PA cannot (or does not want to) work a committed calendar shift, she is responsible for finding her own substitute and for notifying you in advance of the change. She has a complete listing of all PA names and phone numbers, and she calls her teammates to ask for a willing sub for her shift. In return, *during that same phone call*, she negotiates an exchange of taking a shift for the willing substitute. If she cannot recruit a substitute, then she cannot take the time off. No one should ever call you to announce, "I can't work my shift tomorrow night—I hope you find someone to fill in. Bye."

Also emphasize that the "sub and backup" policy should be used sparingly. For complete details about using this policy, please see the following subsection, "Ready access to substitutes and backups."

The master calendar

In Step ❼ , while PAs selected their shifts, you or someone else marked a master calendar for you. After the meeting, your master calendar should be conspicuously posted at your residence for easy and routine reference by both you and each shift's aide. The two favorite posting locations include a central traffic area, like the kitchen fridge, especially if this is near the counter where the aides complete their time sheets at the end of each shift. Or, you might prefer your bedroom wall, where you can quickly reference it from bed if a PA fails to appear for a shift and you want to know who to call.

Your master calendar is the only comprehensive record of everyone's commitments, and is important for three reasons.

First, toward the end of the scheduling meeting, it is quite important that you call out the assignments marked on your master, while PAs check their own appointment books. At each meeting, while you recite the month's series of day-by-day shift assignments, at least one or two PAs will usually catch discrepancies between your master calendar and their appointment books. In addition, as the aides listen to you and scan their appointment books, it is common that they will suddenly remember previous commitments or other reasons to speak up now and make last-minute changes. Now is the time to find problems, instead of later in the month when no one appears for a work shift.

Second, the master serves as a handy daily reference for your needs. As you head for bed each night, make a habit of always noting who is scheduled to get you up in the morning. This is important if the morning arrives and the scheduled aide does not—you will know who needs a wake-up call from your bedside phone. In addition, it is common for your aides to call you several times each month when they want to check the accuracy of their own appointment books. Your master calendar is the authoritative reference that settles all disputes.

Third, it serves as your way of reminding PAs of their upcoming shifts. At the very end of each work shift, just before you say good-bye to the departing aide, make a firm habit of asking him, "Okay, when do I get to see you next?" Make sure that he personally checks your calendar, instead of your telling him about his next shift. When you force the aide to check your calendar, he dedicates a few seconds of his time and attention to researching his next shift date. In this way, he is much more prone to pay attention and remember the date. In contrast, if you were to tell him the date, he would tend to passively agree with whatever you said. In addition, you are providing one more chance for PAs to find discrepancies between their calendars and yours.

The master calendar is a very simple strategy, but very effective. In each situation, you are assured that the departing aide knows when next to show up for work. It is yet another way of preventing no-shows from happening.

Ready access to substitutes and backups

Your substitute and backup policy is one of the real beauties of having several PAs. You should never have no-show gaps in work shifts due to accidental oversight, illness, or lack of desire to work.

As outlined previously, if a PA cannot—or does not want to—work a shift, she is responsible for finding her own substitute and for notifying you in advance of the change. She has a complete listing of all PA names and phone numbers, and she calls her teammates to ask for a willing substitute for her shift. In return, *during that same phone call,* she should negotiate an exchange of assuming a shift for tonight's willing substitute.

If she cannot recruit a substitute, then she cannot take the time off. This is one of the policies that you clearly state from the beginning, as early as the pre-hiring interview stage.

The group, at a staff meeting, should decide for itself what reasons are valid or justified for calling teammates to request a substitute or backup. Some PA groups will decide to be very strict—emergencies only. Most groups will be flexible around concerns that are common to their culture.

Most will accept requests for more liberal reasons when made several days in advance, but often only emergency reasons are acceptable for last-minute requests. For example, college students might be willing to consider and negotiate a shift exchange for an unexpected, hot ski weekend if made in advance, but not if requested the night before.

Almost any group-made policy is acceptable, as long as the group agrees to it, it is not abused, and your help needs are continually staffed without no-shows. It is important for you to realize that valid reasons for aides might not be the ones that make sense to you. Their valid reasons will reflect their specific concerns, whether the PAs are college students, blue-collar factory workers, soccer moms, moonlighting home health aides, retired folks, or a combination. This is a time for you to let democracy reign. There is no reason to get caught in the middle unless PA complaints indicate that the group's decisions are not working.

The self-assigning of work shifts and the substitute and backup policy work well when:

- Your PAs understand both your policy and their responsibilities from the early stages, beginning when you answer inquiries from newspaper ads, during pre-hiring interviews, and again at staff meetings.

- Your PA staff meetings require the PAs to select and calendar their own work shifts for four or five weeks in advance.

- Your staff meetings require the PA group to create its own list of reasons that are valid for requesting substitutes and backups, and then periodically to review and comment on whether the system is working well.

- You are routinely notified, by the requesting PA, of a substitution she has arranged.

- The substitute system is used sparingly and not abused.

- A requesting PA schedules her debt repayment in the same phone call as her request, and the granting PA cooperates by offering repayment dates.

- You keep your ears and eyes open to individual PA complaints, as well as group discontent, and you promptly address these concerns until solutions are implemented.

The system fails, and creates resentment among PAs—and no-shows for you—when:

- You weakly propose the substitute and backup policy late, after each PA is hired. It is unfair for PAs to not know the rules, or for you to change the rules after PAs are hired.

- You attempt to create and mandate the calendar schedule of work shifts as well as the rules that define your reasons for valid substitutes and backups. Your schedule and rules will probably not work for their concerns, and your staff will resent and ignore them (making you angry and creating a struggle for control).

- PAs who have arranged for a substitute do not notify you about the changes.

- The sub system is used several times each week, and the calendar work shifts become meaningless and ignored. If the integrity of the original schedule is repeatedly compromised, you will begin to experience no-shows.

- The PAs do not promptly repay their sub and backup debts, and the granting PAs become resentful and quit.

- You hear of individual or group discontent, but ignore the problems and allow them to cause low morale and unnecessary resignations.

A key strategy to making requests of other PAs, and increasing the chances for success, is for the requesting PAs to repay their debts in the same phone call, and for the second PA to cooperate in proposing some exchange dates. This on-the-spot debt repayment is very effective in preventing the granting PA from feeling taken advantage of.

Overall, this policy is a great remedy to one of the all-time, classic problems in employing aides: finding substitutes for PA sick-outs and personal crises, often in a hurry. When the policy is respected, it works really well. I have taught this procedure to my own PAs and used it successfully for more than 20 years. I have heard of no better system from the many PA users I have interviewed and coached.

Assertive and complete communications

When you and your PAs need to communicate with each other, clear, direct communication is essential. The most common reason for two-ways between aides to take place is for one to want another to substitute for one of her shifts. In turn, the usual reason for communication failure is when the original PA calls a substitute, finds her not at home, and simply leaves her request-message with a roommate or voice mail.

The caller assumes that the sub will both receive the request message and be willing to fulfill the work-shift void. When these assumptions are wrong, then too often neither PA thinks he has one of your shifts. Consequently, no one arrives to help you and you are forced to contact an available aide for immediate help.

For each new group of PAs, run through these precautions. When PAs are trying to communicate about your schedule, you have a right to ask that each PA who leaves a message for another does the following:

- Leaves a clear and complete message—what is requested, why, when, and what phone number to call to respond.
- Leaves her phone number (for convenience) and asks for a response.
- At no time assumes anything—that the second PA has received the request or agreed to fulfill it.
- Notifies you, the recipient of help, of the exchange only after actually hearing—and not assuming—agreement from the second PA.

Your overall control

The emphasis of these strategies is for you to make these policies, guidelines, and procedures, and (as much as possible) for the PAs make their own subsequent operational decisions. This strategy helps keep them happy and saves you a lot of go-between negotiating.

The emphasis of this book is for you to work in harmony with the people who help you. You respect their ability to make certain decisions within your policy guidelines, and they respect you in return. It is important to realize that your degree of control is not compromised by having PAs make decisions that you have selected. You have not surrendered authority to them. By putting them in an advisory capacity, you—the manager—still retain the right to make all final decisions. However, you override their decisions only when you obviously must, and not arbitrarily to demonstrate your authority.

While they do their deciding, your management role is only to facilitate and guide the process, as long as it goes smoothly. If the process stops working, and the PAs stop making decisions (or stop making good ones!), you have veto power. At any point of their face-to-face negotiating, you have the continuous power to interject advice or to terminate their decision process and supply your own. This is rarely necessary or appropriate ("if it ain't broke, don't fix it"), but it is always your option.

Take care, however, when exercising this absolute authority. If you abuse it, and simply substitute your decisions for those made by your PAs, they will soon see their "scheduling authority" as a sham and place all the burden on you. The role of the PAs in this process should be respected. Maintain your role as the facilitator as much as possible. Your efforts and theirs should be directed toward working together, as a team, to produce the help you need each day.

Chapter 17
Setting Up Efficient Work Areas and Maintaining Adequate Supplies

When you set up your personal computer at home or office, you instinctively begin gathering the printer paper, pens, pencils, scratch paper, wastebasket, lighting, and other items that you will be using near the computer. You pay a lot of attention to locating the computer, monitor, keyboard, mouse, and printer on a desk that is an ideal height and easy to approach. Lighting is important so you can see well. Perhaps you bring in a radio or stereo to make work more pleasant. You probably also arrange a supply storage area that is close by. In addition, you keep an eye on your supplies and periodically restock so you have everything necessary for work.

You probably do all this without consciously thinking about it. Why is it important? The reason for all of this gathering, locating, and coordinating is to save you time and energy. You want to make your own work easy.

You would not want to work very long for a boss who insisted that your computer stuff be scattered in out-of-the-way and hard-to-reach locations in two or three different rooms. You would be wasting time and energy, and you would be considerably less efficient and less productive.

Keep these factors in mind when setting up work spaces for your family caregivers and hired providers. They have limited time and energy for helping you, so more efficient work flows mean they will enjoy their work more and perhaps stay with you longer.

"Working with Phil? Yes, he has a really nice place to work, and even though I help him with a lot of detailed needs, somehow the work is not difficult or tiring."

A clean and pleasant work area

Few of us would like to live in an area that smells of urine, bowel, or dirty laundry; has trash overflowing from garbage cans and wastebaskets; has sticky and dirty kitchen counters, tabletops, and bathroom sinks and toilets; has cockroaches or other crawling pests; or is dark and musty smelling from dirty windows and dusty, drawn shades.

Likewise, few PAs want to routinely work in such an area, either.

A clean and pleasant living area for you, and work area for the PA, does not have to be sterile. Routinely keeping the area clean is not overly time-consuming, either. It should include some of the following features:

- Not even the slightest trace of smell or odor from urine, bowel, dirty laundry, mold, mildew, or dirty kitchen.

- All trash, wastepaper, or food garbage kept in wastebaskets or covered trash cans that are kept clean and lined with a plastic bag.

- Clean kitchen counter tops, stove areas, and refrigerator interiors. Spoiled food anywhere in the kitchen or refrigerator/freezer areas should be promptly disposed of. After all, if you can no longer eat it, why save it? Throw it out.

- Bathroom sinks, toilets, bath/shower, floors, and mirrors should be cleaned at least once a week.

- Bed linens should be changed and all laundry done either promptly after "accidents" or at least once a week.

- The overall living area should be dusted, vacuumed or mopped, and aired out regularly.

- Personal living items should be reasonably organized and neatly stored, as opposed to living among piles of junk throughout various rooms.

Although it remains your responsibility to provide the PA and yourself with a clean and pleasant area, the actual work might be beyond your own physical abilities. If so, it is then your responsibility to instruct PAs in methods and a routine schedule for keeping the areas clean. In addition, you are responsible for stocking an adequate variety and quantity of cleaning supplies so that PAs can do their work. Tips on keeping adequate stocks of supplies, and not running out, are provided later in this chapter.

> *Providing an efficient and pleasant place to work is important to PAs having enough time and energy to meet all your needs, and to keeping good providers happy with their jobs.*

An efficient layout for each work area

Picture yourself with the job of making hamburgers at a fast-food restaurant. Your main work area is a cooking grill and an adjacent table for putting together and wrapping the burgers. Each meat patty is taken from a freezer and cooked on the grill. Then it is placed on a bun and given ketchup, mustard, onions, and two pickle slices before the top bun is put into place. You then wrap each burger in paper and place it on a chute where it travels to the customer serving area.

This is really a simple process and should take very little effort. However, suppose each of the ingredients is kept in a different part of the kitchen. You fry (or flame broil!) each patty, walk ten feet to where the buns are piled, walk three feet in the other direction for the ketchup container, reach under the counter for the mustard, and go to the refrigerator for the onions and pickles.

After making just your third hamburger, you would probably turn to your boss and say, "Hold it, why can't I organize all of these items around the grill within my reach? This current system is a waste of my energy and time, and therefore wastes a lot of the hourly salary you are paying me." In the back of your mind you are also telling yourself, "This setup doesn't make sense and it's difficult to work in. If my boss refuses to make it more efficient, then I'll quit and work somewhere else where the work is easier to perform."

Fast-food restaurants and all other businesses carefully plan and lay out their various work areas to make them as efficient as possible for employees. So should you for PAs.

The advantages of efficient work areas for PAs include saving their energy and time. The PAs can perform their duties much more easily with far less frustration, and therefore you will tend to keep good PAs longer. Not only do you keep good PAs longer, you get more duties performed during the time the meter is running.

Steps to planning efficient work areas include the following:

- Identify each work area, or separate location, where the PA performs a specific set of duties for you: bedside, dressing area, bathroom, kitchen, eating area, etc.

- For each area, first think about the set of duties to be performed. Then think about the equipment, medical supplies, articles of your clothing, or food that the PA needs in that area. For example, at your bedside work area in the morning the PA might help you get dressed. This might require your urinary leg bag, socks, abdominal binder, pants, and belt. Try to locate these items within a reasonable distance of the bedside.

- Design standard locations within the PA's reach for storing the equipment, supplies, and clothes within each work area: for example, a shelf, drawer, closet, cabinet, pantry, or footlocker.

- Routinely encourage the PA to keep an organized arrangement of these supplies within each storage area, and to return items to their storage places promptly after each time the duties are performed.

A sufficient inventory of supplies

Many of us are quite dependent on a daily or routine use of prescription medications, over-the-counter medical supplies, and specially prescribed medical appliances and equipment. In addition to these personal supplies for our own needs, other types of supplies are required by our family caregivers and PAs. Examples include cleaning supplies, laundry soap, and tools for repairing medical equipment.

Whether an item is used by you or the provider, exhausting the supply of an item can result in either a considerable inconvenience or occasionally a health- or life-threatening circumstance. Here are some proven strategies for minimizing the chances of running out of important supplies.

There is little reason to completely run out of most items. All that is required is some organization, a periodic check on supply levels, and some advance ordering of new supplies. There is no additional cost to keeping adequate levels of supplies. It costs no more to keep a car's gas tank at least half full than it does to allow the tank to reach "empty" before each filling. The overall cost is exactly the same, since the same amount of gas or medical supplies is used in either case, so why risk running out?

Keeping an adequate inventory of supplies depends on being able to periodically compare the current quantity of each item that you have stored with the quantity needed during the time it takes to reorder.

To avoid running out of a medication or other supply, compare—

Your supply of an item
(e.g., you currently have a three-week supply)

- How long it takes to reorder and receive this item
(e.g., two weeks)

= How long before you should reorder
(e.g., you should reorder one week from now!)

For example, if you find that you have a three-week supply of a medication left, and you believe that it will take two weeks to order and receive a new quantity of that medication, then you have about one week before you should reorder that item.

How long does it take to receive a reordered item? Different items require different times. Some items are always readily available from the shelves of the local pharmacy. Others might require funding approval and a physician's prescription before the actual order can be placed. To safeguard yourself, allow extra time for unexpected delays that can include:

- a physician's unavailability during her vacation
- the physician's secretary forgetting to promptly mail you the prescription
- the pharmacist forgetting to promptly order the item
- the medical supply company's inability to promptly send the order to the pharmacist
- a UPS or other courier strike that delays delivery between the manufacturer and the pharmacy
- Medicaid's backup of paperwork, which results in an extra two-week delay in approval for funding
- a three-day holiday for everyone during this time.

How easily you can make this periodic comparison of "how much I have" with "how much do I need to get me through reordering" depends on two factors: the location and organization of the stored supplies.

First, you alone are always responsible for keeping an adequate supply of each item. Therefore, the physical storage location of your supplies should be within your personal level of sight (or touch, in the case of a significant sight impairment). In living areas with limited storage space, where not everything can be located at your level of sight or touch, store the least frequently used items where a PA can easily check quantities for you upon request.

Second, the arrangement of items within these storage areas should be well organized. A reasonably neat arrangement of items enables you to do two things: to quickly count up the actual quantities of items for inventory purposes, and to quickly locate a specific item whenever it is needed in a hurry. In addition, good organization means that you can easily describe the location of needed items to a PA who can retrieve them for you.

This arrangement of stored supplies should take into consideration the following points.

Store each type of item together, so that you can determine how many containers of the same item are stocked ahead. For example, store all bottles of medical adhesive together in one section, and all boxes of bandages together in another section.

When storing each type of item together, use reasonably neat rows or sections within a drawer, box, closet, or footlocker. This will make counting stock much easier than if similar containers are merely tossed into a pile in the back of the closet.

Use the entire contents of one container of an item before opening a new container. It is much easier to take inventory if all containers of an item, such as pills, are known to be full except for the one presently being used.

In using each container completely before proceeding to the next, it is wise to use the oldest stock first. To make "rotating the stock" easier, many folks write the purchase date on the caps of supplies on the day the purchase is made and the container is stored. Finding the next oldest container when you need it is made easy.

To make reordering items easy, keep a computer listing of all the facts you require to reorder each type of supply. List the name of the item, the manufacturer, model number, size, and name and phone number of the local store where the item is available. You may wish to include the length of time typically necessary for reordering the item. For example, "Urocare urinary leg bag, 1 liter size, # 9032, $52.89 from Wyman's Drug Store, 853-6969; reorder time is usually 2 weeks."

When requesting prescriptions for ongoing medications from your physician, ask the doctor if each prescription can be written for a two-or three-month's quantity with each refill, and that each prescription be refillable several times. This strategy can save you extra trips to the pharmacy and to your doctor. If your insurance company allows it, you might consider getting a two-or three-month supply of a prescription at one time.

The medical supply and equipment business is constantly making improvements in their products. Keep your eyes open at pharmacies and medical supply stores for new or improved supplies that appear on store shelves and in catalogs.

Preventing theft

You have many possessions that are either attractive or valuable. You will want to reduce the chances for loss by routinely practicing two or three strategies.

Attractive items are those that people like to "borrow" because they are fun or useful. Included here are music CDs and tapes, tools, food, books, calculators, and a variety of other electronics. The strategy here is to be somewhat organized, so you will promptly notice if something is missing, and to be aware around light-fingered people who enjoy one-way borrowing. These friends and PAs have no intention of stealing anything, but they think nothing of borrowing something and honestly forgetting to return it.

Your valuables can get you involved with hard-core thieves. For our disability population, high-theft items are most often money, prescription medications, certain kinds of medical equipment and supplies, jewelry, electronics, silver and gold, and even postage stamps.

If you live in a high-crime neighborhood and have valuable possessions, or if your agency or personal aides make you uncomfortable, you might encounter con artists who will attempt some form of theft. Certain kinds of prescription medications deserve your constant attention: narcotics, tranquilizers and sedatives, and stimulants. There is good reason *never* to include your last name or street address in a PA advertisement, because there are crooks and addicts (besides the nicer people who apply for your PA job) who will then target you and your place for a break-in or personal-visit theft.

You should carefully guard physician-signed prescriptions before they are filled, while they are being filled, and afterward when the bottled pills are in your medicine cabinet. If aides do errands and script refills for you, select those people carefully and have them deliver the bottled pills to you the same day they get the script refilled.

It is seldom a good practice to discuss what medications you are taking, because you will seldom know which of your PAs or their friends might have special interests in your collection. Some people will be interested in tapping your supplies because they are personally addicted, and others will want to sell your meds to addicts.

During research and writing on this book, I saw a *Newsweek* article stating that certain narcotic pain relievers have a street value of $1 per milligram. That means your pill bottle with a 30-day supply of 40-milligram oxycontin that is taken four times daily (120 tabs) can be worth $4800.00! The article also cites cases of addicted realtors who would rob the medicine cabinets of clients while holding "open house" showings of their homes. Undoubtedly, there are also health aide addicts and cons who feel no guilt about their routine med thefts from help recipients.

If you have any of these "hot" medications in your medicine cabinet (you need not worry about laxative thieves!), and you are unsure about the honesty of your aides or friends, first consider dividing each month's supply into two containers: one stays in your medicine cabinet and the other gets stowed in a secret place that you can independently access. If there is a maximum half-month's supply available to outsiders, then that's all they can steal at one time. Also, if they do steal a few pills each time (hoping you will not notice), you will have a better chance of noticing a small theft from a half-month's supply than from a full one.

> *It is your responsibility, not the caregiver's or PA's, to keep adequate levels of supplies to prevent running out of items.*

In addition, some people keep any attractive meds (plus a couple of laxatives as decoys) stored in pill bottles that have the descriptive prescription label hidden under masking tape.[1] By writing an unrelated alpha letter on the masking tape, they can tell their PAs, "I need one of the 'B' pills and two of the 'G' tablets."

If you will be storing unfilled prescriptions, cash, blank bank checks, or other valuables, consider getting a small-business safe. Get the kind that requires a key or key and combination. Any lockable area to which PAs will have periodic access with your permission should be locked with a key that you keep with you, and not locked with only a combination or combination lock. With a key lock, the PA has access only when you momentarily give her the key; be sure she promptly returns it to you. If you give a PA the numbered combination to a lock, the PA can then access the lock whenever she wishes, perhaps without your knowledge.

Prescribed medical equipment

You are probably dependent upon specialized, expensive medical equipment for your mobility, vital body functions, and otherwise staying active and preventing illness or poor health. It is very important to keep an adequate stock of repair supplies and tools. This enables you or a provider:

- to perform preventive maintenance that prevents many breakdowns from occurring
- to perform actual repairs when the inevitable breakdowns do occur.

---

1. If you do this, be sure the prescription label is first protected by a layer of clear desk or shipping tape before you cover everything with opaque masking tape. This allows you or medical authorities to confirm a bottle's contents by peeling off the masking tape without harming the original label.

You often check out the weather forecast. If you have not heard the forecast, you still pay attention to nature's early warning signs, such as dark clouds or thunder. If you are outside, you take these warning signs seriously and run for cover early. Preventive maintenance toward your important medical equipment is similar to watching the weather, and just as wise. Breakdowns in your equipment are certain to happen, but your preventive maintenance can provide you with big advantages.

Routinely taking care of your equipment, and having advance repairs made, will prevent some needless breakdowns that would occur from neglect. At other times, paying attention to warning signs of an upcoming breakdown again enables you to plan for an early repair before a breakdown actually happens.

These warning signs can include equipment squeaking or making a strange noise, operating slowly or with difficulty, giving off a strange smell or odor, or flashing or beeping of an equipment's formal warning system. These warning signs are telling you of upcoming problems. Be tuned into early warnings, be grateful for them, don't ignore them, and take appropriate action to promptly remedy the problem before the equipment dies completely.

If you purposely ignore all early warning signs, and the equipment suddenly dies, then you may have to do without it for a while so parts can be ordered and repairs made. In contrast, if you are alert to early warnings, you can often prevent a breakdown by being early to book repair appointments and order replacement parts.

As you first acquire a new piece of medical equipment, do some research in advance to find a shop where it can be repaired. Are parts readily available, or must they usually be ordered? Is loaner equipment available while parts are being ordered and repairs made? What preapproval paperwork and time are required by any funding source you use?

Some equipment exams and repairs can be made by you, possibly with help from a caregiver or PA who follows your instructions. Avoiding the need for professional repair help by doing it yourself whenever possible means a quicker repair without many of the delays and paperwork headaches mentioned earlier.

> *Most sudden equipment breakdowns can be avoided by routine, preventive maintenance.*

Become very familiar with each piece of medical equipment you use. Learn how to spot early warning signs of upcoming breakdowns and act quickly to fix any problem. Learn how to make basic repairs yourself, even if you have no physical ability to perform them. If you need physical assistance, then you can instruct an available help provider, step-by-step, in making those repairs. Do not expect a typical PA, who does not use your medical equipment, to know how to repair it. That's your responsibility.

To make these repairs, be sure you also have an adequate supply of tools. Keep them in a key-locked tool box so that no one "borrows" them.

Have some of these basic tools at home, and purchase good-quality ones:

- a set of screwdrivers (several sizes, regular and Phillips head)
- a pair of pliers
- a set of combination wrenches
- adjustable wrenches (one large, one small)
- Allen wrenches (one set on a ring or in a jack knife-type casing)
- two tire irons
- a bicycle pump (with a built-in pressure gauge).

One set of good-quality tools, such as those frequently on sale at Sears, is considerably less expensive than buying two or three sets of cheap tools that must be replaced with each tool that bends or breaks. I know; I learned this lesson the expensive way!

One final word on prescribed medical equipment. Each piece of medical equipment you regularly use will eventually wear out, no matter how well you maintain it. Learn to recognize, in advance, when a piece of equipment is about to wear out, and order a replacement.

How much in advance? A rule of thumb on replacing major, funded equipment says "at least twice as long as you think necessary to acquire the funding approval, to place the equipment order, to receive the new item, and to have the shop adjust it to your particular needs."

There are three primary ways to estimate the order and delivery time on a piece of equipment:

- Get a time estimate from each party involved in the ordering process with regard to how long their individual involvement will take (physician, therapist, funding source, pharmacist, medical store, etc.).
- Ask a friend who has ordered and received similar equipment about his or her experience with the length of the entire process.
- Provide your own estimate of time based on your experience in ordering and receiving similar equipment.

> *When you use medical equipment, watch and listen for warning signs that a part is wearing out—and get it fixed before it breaks down.*

If your current wheelchair will soon need replacing, and you believe it will take three months to receive a new one, then speak up and start the replacement process at least six months before you expect the old wheelchair to become unusable.

After you receive your new wheelchair and you are sure it is working smoothly, give strong consideration to getting the old chair repaired for ready use as a backup to your new one. The objective is not to replace each old part until the old chair looks like a new one, but instead to repair or replace the few parts that are most worn out and most likely to break down. Consequently, the older wheelchair can be used for brief periods of time when the new chair must be away, either for periodic preventive maintenance or for unexpected repairs.

> *When you receive new equipment, have the basic functions of the old equipment repaired right away. You will then have a readily available backup if your new equipment needs time-consuming repair.*

The older wheelchair can also be used as your "travel chair" when traveling by air. All airline carriers have a well-earned reputation for being rough and frequently breaking medical equipment. If your travel chair is damaged, your better chair will be waiting for you at home and ready to use. Your travel chair can be repaired at airline expense, without timely inconvenience to you, and be ready for the next airplane trip you take.

Chapter 18
Coping with and Reacting to PA Failures

Regardless of whether your paid aides come from an agency or personal recruiting, many will disappoint you with broken promises of many kinds.

It's a fact: The people upon whom you most depend each day will too often let you down.

Given that you realize the "certain" things in your life include death, taxes, and the eventual resignation or firing of each paid PA, why do you inescapably feel let down each time you are disappointed? Is your anger or depression caused simply by an employee leaving, or are there additional, less obvious reasons for your feeling the way you do? Why do so many recurring, predictable departures usually come as a surprise? Your ability to cope with these emotional events, as well as logically respond to the realities, is a learned skill—and a very important one.

As with any topic in this reference, you could gradually learn the skill through years of trial and error, or you can get a mega head start by investing a few minutes with this chapter. This chapter introduces the most common ways for PAs to fail in meeting their responsibilities and your expectations. In addition, it reviews your typical feelings when failures occur, and then offers some experience-proven strategies for fixing the current problem and reducing the chance that an aide will fail again in the future.

As you review the list of common ways that aides fail to deliver on their commitments, you might notice a very obvious omission: PAs who fail to work for the entire duration of their job commitment by quitting well before the promised date. This is one for the "Failure Hall of Fame."[1]

---

1. It deserves special attention, and gets it in chapter 📖 10, "Recognizing and Resolving Your PA Problems, or Parting Ways."

Don't you hate it when they do that?!

PAs can pick some of the worst times to let you down. In addition, their wide variety of disappointments often come one after another, without offering you much recovery time. While some superstitions claim that unfortunate events and deaths come in groups of three, there have been times when I have been convinced that disappointments from PAs seem to come in groups of ten!

To introduce this chapter, let's investigate a scenario that is regrettably common during the recruiting, screening, and hiring process.

Some promising applicants answer your newspaper ad for a new PA. Each of the four has answered the ad by leaving a well-organized, articulate message on your answering machine. Each respondent seems warm, caring, well-grounded, and experienced. You need only two new PAs at this time, but experience has shown that you will need more applicants than you have positions; some will drop out along the way. You trust that these are great prospects and you should have no trouble ending up with two good aides.

You always feel anxious and uneasy when it is time to hire someone new. Will you find anyone as good and reliable as Susan and Jason, who are leaving you after two years of being your best aides ever?

You call back each of the four prospects to explain the routine and all are eager to meet with you for the group interview and demo session. As you wrap up the initial "scheduling calls," you stress the importance of calling you in advance, should the applicants foresee being late or decide not to come to the appointment. All promise to do so, and assure you that they will be on time for the meeting.

On the night of the meeting, one applicant simply fails to show up.

The remaining three applicants arrive on time, observe the routine, and are very enthusiastic about working for you. At the end of the session, you ask them to carefully consider the responsibility of the position. You ask them to call you sometime the next day to let you know whether they are still interested in the job. When you check your voice mail at the end of the next day, two applicants have left messages that they would like to be hired. You never hear from the third again.

So, out of the four original candidates, the remaining two ask to be hired and agree to at least the nine-month commitment that you have proposed. Furthermore, they firmly agree to give a one-month minimum advance notice when they eventually have to resign after that nine-month commitment has been completed.

These new PAs are eager to learn your routine, and begin providing you with high-quality, dependable work. You slowly begin to trust them. After three short weeks, one appears uneasy as her evening shift is ending. She approaches you, looks down at her feet, and mumbles that she must quit at the end of the week. She has found a higher paying job, and her new employer insists that she begin immediately. She is very sorry, and is also sure you will understand. She states that she has no choice in the matter, and wishes you luck in quickly replacing her.

You have one new PA remaining. Since you are now short one of the two PAs you originally needed, you begin recruiting again. Can you trust the remaining PA? How could the others be so irresponsible? What caused this chain of premature resignations and other disappointments? Are you at fault, is your job too demanding, or are these people simply members of an untrustworthy generation?

PA failures like these are common to the disability lifestyle; this scenario is not an exaggeration. Your able-bodied (A-B) peers might be disappointed or frustrated when a friend fails to meet them for a restaurant meal, for the joint review of a business proposal, or for a round of golf. In contrast, the emotions you feel around a PA failing to meet the commitments are often more intense.

Why? For your A-B peers, a friend not appearing for lunch has little effect except for some missed conversation and camaraderie. Consequently, they feel mainly disappointment and maybe a little annoyance. For you, with your disability-mandated dependence on physical assistance, a PA's failure to appear for providing help might mean that you cannot get out of bed, eat lunch, or shower and get back into bed. Consequently, your emotional reaction often includes anger, depression, and a feeling of helplessness.

The next sections address very common situations where a PA fails to honor a commitment made to you. For each topic, a failure is described, your typical emotions are discussed, and advice is offered on how to remedy the effects of the current failure as well as on how to reduce the chances of a recurrence.

What to do when your PA—

- Fails to keep an appointment for your job interview and demo, or to call you in advance to cancel?

Ironically, an applicant who fails to show for an interview and demo, or to call back with her job decision, is doing you a favor.

You should expect that 25 to sometimes 100 percent of the applicants who answer your PA ad will not make it all the way through to the final hiring. Not every applicant has the qualifications to be your aide, and not everyone is truly interested in doing so. It is far better to identify weak candidates now, during a screening step, than to have one fail to appear on a work morning to help you out of bed.[2]

The key here is to not take personally the PA's failure to keep—or call to cancel—an interview appointment. The PA's failure is due to his inability, lack of responsibility, or a set of personal values that differ from yours. The applicant's inability to meet many responsibilities and appointments has affected his relations with probably hundreds of people over the years; you are just one person in a long line.

When an applicant fails in a situation like this, you probably had no influence and cannot consider yourself to be a cause. In addition, the candidate is rejecting an employment situation, not you personally.

---

2. In chapter 📖 7, "Ten Steps to Getting All or Some of Your Help from Personally Employed Aides," describes an eight-part screening procedure that is designed to weed out undesirable candidates.

In a final piece of advice, your interviewing and screening steps will frequently screen out 75 percent or more of applicants. This does not indicate that an interview and screening process is being too selective in screening out too many candidates. Instead, it indicates that the process is doing an excellent job of what it was carefully designed and field-tested to do. At times like these, you should guard against any impulse to short-circuit the process and bypass some of the screening steps, so more candidates will seem to qualify for hiring. The unfortunate consequences of hiring poor-quality candidates today will usually haunt you later.

Here is another approach to understanding the importance of a good screening process. Imagine that you are an apple farmer who grows apples, and then sells both apples and cider at the local market. After the apples are picked by farm hands and trucked to the processing center, you expect that a certain percentage of the entire crop will be unsuitable for sale. There is a variety of reasons, including apples with worms, bruised and rotten apples, and those that are too small. But why must this occur? Why can't all of the apples qualify to be sold at the market?

Your father told you long ago that there is no logical reason for many phenomena in life. As a farmer, you initially got angry that so much of your time was spent in picking out bad apples. However, after a few harvest cycles, you finally accepted the fact that bad apples are always part of your harvest. Nature puts them in every farmer's orchard, through no fault of even the best and most experienced farmers.

Just as all apple farmers screen their apple harvest for undesirable apples, you, as a help recipient and PA manager, must also screen your PA applicants for those who are undesirable.

Much like the farmer's observations about apple crops, you can be certain that there is a percentage of the general population, and therefore of the people who initially answer your PA ad, that cannot or should not perform the work you need. Your hiring process has two objectives: First, you want to filter out the applicants who should not work for you; *then* you can decide which of the rest you want to hire. PA applicants who fail to keep their appointments with you are actually helping you to accomplish your first objective.

The wide range of reasons why applicants fail to honor their own commitments—and also should not work for you—include the following:

- not being comfortable with the very personal nature of helping someone with physically intimate needs

- not being dependable, punctual, honest, trustworthy, or responsible about commitments

- not having appropriate reasons for wanting the job you offer

- not having sufficient time, energy, health, physical strength, or intelligence to perform your job.

Some of these undesirable job applicants are aware that they should not apply for your job, but will apply anyway while attempting to conceal their undesirable traits. For example, alcohol or drug abusers will often be undependable in meeting the routine schedule of any job. They know this, and have been fired from several other positions for it. When they interview with you, they will be very clever at hiding their addiction and its effects on responsible performance of your job.

Therefore, your objective now toward these people is to be a detective in uncovering their bad traits and refusing to hire them. Additionally, if you identify seriously bad traits after hiring, your role then is to promptly fire them.

Indeed, these applicants are usually very good at hiding the truth. Wouldn't it be great to know of a screening procedure that would usually expose them before they might otherwise be hired? You are in luck, because this reference's carefully designed ten-step chapter (chapter 7) for personally employing aides, includes eight screening opportunities.

Whereas some knowing applicants try to conceal their bad traits, others applying for your job do not sufficiently understand the level of commitment required for the position. This is especially true for one of your best sources of applicants—college students—although the trait can also appear in others. It is very common for students or other applicants to simply not be sufficiently aware of their own personal limitations. Too often, they become overextended for their available time, energy, or health. They impulsively agree to committing to a neat job like yours and then realize, after a month of adding your job to their full-time studies or other commitments, that they cannot do it all.

Your objective here is to know their potential limitations better than they do. During their interview with you, find out what you can about their other workloads: the number and schedule of semester classes, time committed to family or children, other jobs, level of recreational and leisure activities, and their degree of health. If you begin to suspect that some applicants are already stretched to the max, tactfully ask them if it is wise for them to consider adding your job. Tell them that you admire their high level of activity, but when they are weighing their decision about accepting your job, you would like them to be careful about not taking on too much. (As the film comedian, W.C. Fields, once said, "Isn't it a shame to waste youthful energy and optimism on children!") Thus, sometimes your interviewing, screening, and hiring experience will enable you to counsel a job applicant to be cautious about becoming overextended. You are making this suggestion because you care about both them and the validity of their commitment to your job. The ten-step procedure also details the interview opportunities for discussing these concerns with applicants.

So, what do you do when a job applicant fails to show up for your job interview, and even fails to call you in advance to cancel? Initially (the first few times) you might be disappointed and angry. However, with experience, you can then be grateful that your well-designed and structured procedure has accomplished its screening objective.

Forget about the failed, poor-quality applicants, and concentrate on the others. Out of applicants? Get your PA ad back into tomorrow's newspaper or Internet bulletin board, and start again. Experience will prove that these failures are a regrettable but foreseeable step to finding the upcoming, excellent PAs who will be glad to hear about your job. Yes, you will find some!

What to do when your PA—

- Fails to call you back with her decision of accepting or declining your PA position?

Again, the screening procedure that you are using has done its job, as you just saw when an unworthy applicant failed to keep her appointment for your interview and demo. For this additional concern as well, your well-designed screening process is meant to filter out those who either do not have a serious interest in the job, or are not dependable in honoring appointments and other commitments.

Following another part of this reference's interview and screening steps, you meet with a candidate for an interview and demonstration of your routine. As the meeting wraps up, you ask her to go home and carefully weigh the job commitment in light of her other responsibilities and schedule. She is asked to call you back sometime the next day to indicate whether she is still interested in the job.

You can plan that about 25 percent of all applicants, regardless of their enthusiasm during the interview and demo, will never call you back.

If you are desperate to hire an aide, you might be tempted to track down the applicant to beg her to take the job. In another instance, you might be angry enough to call her just to vent your feelings. In either case, you will almost always be wasting time and energy that would be better invested in recruiting the next (quality!) candidates.

There are, however, a few rare cases when it seems essential to call someone back after she has failed to call you. Indeed, there may be desperate times when you will have to hire an undesirable applicant in order to get into bed that same night. Your *modus operandi* is to call her back, sugarcoat the less attractive details of your routine, and otherwise "sell" or "con" her into helping you for at least a few days.

Most old-timers have had to temp-hire on rare occasions. In truth, we are being deceptive in very cautiously hiring an undesirable PA for temporary survival, while quietly recruiting a trustworthy, long-term replacement. This can be dangerous, but we do what we must to endure our short-term nightmare at Maslow's lowest stage of survival.

For the majority of other recruiting times, however, it is wise simply to hear the applicant's message when she *fails*—in reality, she *purposely decides not*—to call you with her decision. Statistically, of the applicants who will be calling back, 19 out of every 20 will call the day after the interview, as you requested. About 1 in 20 will take an extra day. Half of all callers will decline your job, but half will accept!

If you haven't heard from an interviewed applicant by the third day, there is little chance that she has simply forgotten to call you and needs a reminder call from you. "Oh, Lou, thanks for calling me back to get my decision. My, my, I must have forgotten all about having applied for your job! Ah, sorry, I just can't fit it into my schedule right now. But if you ever need a temporary fill-in, be sure to call me. You know you can count on me—I will be so very glad to help. Bye."

It is very common for someone who feels guilty or uneasy about declining your job, or resigning from it, to offer to fill in "anytime you are in a bind." If you find yourself in that situation in the future, rarely will any of those Good Samaritans be available. They have made that offer primarily to ease their own conscience; they feel better if they believe you will be grateful rather than angry.

Cross them off your list, and respond to the next one who saw your newspaper ad.

What to do when your PA—

- Ultimately fails to accept your job after interviewing and consistently showing interest in the job?

Sometimes a PA will not accept your job offer even after interviewing and consistently showing interest in the position. The frustration felt when this happens is very similar to being in the final stages of reeling in a trophy fish, and then watching it slip off the hook as you lean over the side of the boat to net it.

Here, a quality applicant, who was punctual for the interview, enthusiastic while watching the demo, and faithful in calling back, is now about to deliver her decision. Much like the glistening fish that is finally at the edge of your boat after a 20-minute fight, this ideal aide is almost within your grasp.

As promised, she calls you with her decision about the job and says, "Hi, Jerry, this is Margie calling back as you asked!"

At your end of the phone, you remember that Margie interviewed with you last night. She was ideal. Wonderful personality, raised near your hometown, and even likes your kind of movies and music. She was so comfortable with helping you that she jumped in to help with the demo of your routine. What a great fit. You are so glad to hear from her.

"I really enjoyed meeting you, the experience appears to be ideal for supplementing my OT studies at the campus, and the hours fit nicely into my schedule. However... "

Ding dong. Hold everything. News flash. What is with this "however" stuff? Something is wrong here. There should be no need for any "howevers" in this acceptance speech. Margie, please do not tell me you said "however."

"—my boyfriend has just started an espresso shop here in town and I've decided to be his first waitress. Isn't that romantic? He is so nice, he said he would name his latest peppermint cappuccino after me! A chance like this doesn't happen very often. I'm sure you understand."

At your end of the phone line you silently smile, wish her a happy latte, and hang up. Then you scream in frustration.

In my experience, I have heard a wide variety of reasons for last-minute declines. Some are humorous, and some very sad. Regardless of the reason, my initial reaction is still, too often, "Why couldn't this reason have occurred to you earlier in this long, tiring process?"

Too often in life, we struggle to find the logic for a happening that inherently has none. As the legendary TV news anchorman, Walter Cronkite, would say in closing each night's broadcast, "And that's the way it is." So, when one of your star candidates jumps off the hook at the last minute, smile, scream, and then put fresh bait on your hook and cast out for the next one!

What to do when your PA—

- Fails to appear for a work shift?

When you are initially meeting and interviewing PA applicants, part of your standard presentation should be to clearly state your list of expectations. Your list should include the need for your aides to be rock-solidly dependable, responsible, honest, confidential, and punctual. Prospective PAs should know that if they expect to be even five minutes late for any shift, they should call you in as much in advance as possible. If they cannot work a shift, they will be responsible for calling your other part-timers to arrange their own coverage and exchange. That way, you are not caught in the middle.[3]

If you sleep alone in your residence, and are unable to answer the phone while in bed, at least get an answering machine that lets you monitor incoming messages. Keep the volume cranked up so you can hear incoming, live messages from bed. In this way, a morning PA calling in can tell you, "Mariah, this is Colin. It's 5:45 and my car won't start. If I will be any later than 6:15, I will call you again with an update." You hear the message and take comfort in knowing that the scheduled PA is on top of things.

Emotional reactions. It helps for PAs to realize, from the beginning, why it is so important to keep you updated. Instead of telling them why, you can give them the experience by conducting a quick role-play at your initial staff meeting. Ask them to imagine that they are lying in bed, paralyzed below the chest, alone in their house, and unable to get out of bed by themselves. An aide is scheduled to arrive at 6 A.M. and has a long track record of faithfully arriving at your front door precisely at six o'clock. It gets to be 6:05, 6:10, 6:15, and 6:20. Ask the applicants, "What emotions would you be feeling while watching the clock and listening to the silence throughout your house?"

Some answers include:

- Worry and fear that if the aide does not show, I might be left alone in bed all day without water, food, or medications.

---

3. For details about why and how to use two or more part-time aides, please see chapter 📖 **16,** **"Dividing Your Needs, and Assigning Work Shifts, Among Several PAs."**

- Concern about the welfare of your PA. She might have been in an accident of some kind, because this failure to arrive on time is very unlike her. I hope that she is okay, for her sake and mine.

- Anger at your PA, if she could have prevented this. Anger at myself, for not having had the courage to replace her when this happened once before.

- Anger that this scary situation is happening, and perhaps at a god and my disability for forcing me to be in such a helpless state.

- Concern about how I will get out of bed. Also embarrassment about cold-calling my other PAs, relatives, neighbors, or friends at 6:15 in the morning, waking each, explaining the urgent situation, and begging someone to help me get out of bed.

- Commitment that somehow I will devise a system to prevent this from ever happening again!

The conscientious PAs will feel a bit of what you would feel and have a first-hand respect for arriving to work on time. However, what would you do at 6:20 A.M. in this situation?

Wow, a nightmare that none of us wants to think will happen. However, if you live alone, it both can—and probably will—happen. If it does, you will be extremely glad that you started taking planning steps now to get through it more easily.

Most important is that you keep your head together. Try to prevent emotions from taking over. Begin right away to think about your alternatives and start working through them.

Four common reasons for a no-show. When a PA fails to appear for a work shift, there are four primary possibilities.

First, she is faithfully on her way to your place, and has been delayed by a dead car battery, car accident, or traffic ticket. She will eventually be there or call you to explain. Wait until she is 15 minutes late, then proceed to the next step of calling to wake her.

Second, she has overslept and needs a wake-up phone call(s) from you. Once you wake her, she will rush to get to you and arrive full of apologies.

Third, she has completely forgotten about her work shift, and might or might not be at her residence. Depending on what you know about her lifestyle, you have a 50–50 chance of reaching her by phone if this is the situation.

Fourth, she has suddenly decided to quit working for you and this is an example of her passive-aggressive communication style. In this rare instance, she would probably be expecting you to call. She would not answer, so there is no sense in phoning her.

For the usually conscientious PA, the odds are highly in favor of one of the two initial situations. If she has been dependable and punctual until this morning, concentrate on the first two items in this list.

Options for action. What do you do as you lie in bed wondering? First, assume that she is merely delayed, and wait 15 minutes before doing anything. Indeed, in the vast majority of times when PAs do not arrive on time, they are en route and will arrive less than 15 minutes late.

If she arrives late, greet her with concern and a reminder of the importance of punctuality. Try to avoid unproductive anger. If you greet her with anger, you will probably be subconsciously attempting to punish her to discourage her "from ever doing it again." It is far more effective to greet her with concern that she is okay. She will probably react with guilt, and feel far worse about being late. After all, think how well guilt from your mother worked for many years!

"Oh good, Katie, there you are. It is quarter after and I was worried that something was wrong—I was just about to call you (or did call you). Katie, if you will be late in the future, and near a phone, please remember to call me as early as possible so I will know what is happening."

At the point when your PA is 15 minutes late, do not wait any longer. Start calling her. With luck, she either is still on her way or has merely overslept.

There is always the possibility that you will not be able to reach her. You have two choices: staying in bed all day (or out of bed all night), or calling someone else to help you. If you will be calling a fill-in PA, you had better start very soon—your other aides are now getting out of bed and might very soon be heading out for the day. You might have to make several calls before your sunrise recruiting is successful.

If you live alone, it is essential to sleep within reach of a phone and phone numbers. A trip to Radio Shack each six months will keep you up-to-date with the latest hardware technology. A speed-dialer will enable you to store a long list of numbers, and dial any by pushing one button. A speaker phone allows hands-free dialing, answering, and conversing. In addition, today's voice-recognition phones perform all functions, including finding and dialing any stored number, from your voice commands. Perhaps the simplest way to providing an in-bed phone, for people who are able to hold a phone and manually use a keypad, is to go wireless, with either a cordless phone or a cellular phone.

If you lack a speed-dialer or voice-recognition phone, then you would be wise to sleep next to a regular phone and a list of phone numbers. The phone numbers in bed with you can be in the low-tech format of a handwritten sheet, or a higher-tech computer printout. If printed, use large, bold characters that are more easily seen in pre-dawn bedroom light. The numbers should include a variety of people whom you can call for a variety of urgent reasons, including this morning's no-show if the scheduled PA cannot be reached.

Your bedside list of phone numbers could include:

- your complete list of current PAs
- a couple of former, recent PAs who could be called
  if current aides cannot be reached
- family caregivers, or appropriate relatives or friends
- emergency numbers, although 911 should do the trick
- three or four next-door neighbors, who could arrive much faster than more distant PAs, in case of fire or an emergency medical crisis. None know your routine, but they can carry out urgent instructions.

If your speed-dialer phone has a limited memory, these are the people to prioritize for one-button calling.

> *To cite a real-life example of the importance of a bedside phone, I was lying in bed alone one morning at four o'clock. I was awakened suddenly by a pounding headache from rapidly increasing blood pressure. My urinary night-drainage jug had filled, my bladder was distending, and my BP was skyrocketing. I knew that I needed to relieve the urinary pressure within the next three minutes, or the increasing blood pressure would cause a stroke.*

> *There was no time for 911. I shot a glance at the buttons on the speaker-phone that I keep next to me in bed. As a quadriplegic with no use of fingers, I doubted that I could quickly remember and manually knuckle-dial any neighbor's number. I looked at the stored, one-button numbers in my phone's memory speed dialer. The handwritten list began with "Sally and Greg," my back-to-back neighbors. Desperate for help, I punched "speaker," got a dial tone, punched their button, and heard the speed-dialer rip through their seven digits.*

> *I did not want to waste any precious time having to repeat my message to sleepy people, so I concentrated on speaking slowly and very clearly, "Sally, this is Skip. I have an emergency. I do not need 911, but I do need your help right away for a medical problem that you can do alone. Can you come over now? My back door is unlocked."*

> *Within two minutes Sally was at my bedside, following my concise instructions for disconnecting my catheter and letting its pressure drain out.*

That morning, my speed-dialer and neighbor most definitely saved my life. I urge you to prepare yourself for these kinds of emergencies—today.

An answering machine is also very useful. You might well consider buying your own machine instead of subscribing to a phone company service. Your own digital machine will enable you to monitor live messages from callers. You will be able to hear messages from PAs, even though the phone might be out of reach. Phone-company services do not usually permit live monitoring of incoming calls.

Now back to the missing PA. If you reach her answering machine, carefully structure your message. If your aide has overslept, it is likely that you will repeatedly reach her answering machine until she wakes up. Leave an "emergency" message during your first call (yes, this is truly an emergency). Remember, your voice and tone should convey concern, not anger.

First, identify who you are calling, state your name and number, and then state "this is an emergency." Sometimes her roommate will hear your message before she does, and will help you to reach her. State a brief but complete message. State the time, for several obvious reasons. Ask her to call you right away, before she does anything—if she heads for your place, you will want to know that fact.

"Hello, Sherry, this is Joel at 555-7967. Sherry, it's 6:15, you haven't yet arrived, and I am getting concerned. I hope everything is okay. Please call me right away before you do anything. I am waiting for your call. Thank you."

Next, hang up and call five more times, pausing about 15 seconds between calls in case she tries to call you. Let her phone ring each time until the machine picks up. If she is sleeping or in the shower, your repeated calls will get her attention and tell her that the call is urgent. She should eventually check for a message that explains what is going on.

If she has a phone-company voice mail, she will hear her phone ring four or five times before your message is recorded. However, she will not hear your live message while it is being recorded. Therefore, there is no point in leaving additional, duplicate messages—besides the first one—when you make the additional calls.

If you believe she has her own answering machine, then she might be able to hear your live, incoming message after the phone stops ringing. In this case, talk to her each time by leaving a message each time. If you are angry, try to avoid the temptation of showing it or panic; instead, the tone of your voice should show your ongoing concern for each of you.

If you reach her, ask her to come as soon as she can. If you are angry, you are wise to control it; showing it now could be counterproductive. Stay cool until after she arrives and gets you out of bed. She will probably arrive in a gush of apologies. Stay cool, smile, and if necessary tell her that you prefer to discuss the matter later. This is an excellent time to quietly plan what to eventually tell her, and how to say it.

If you suspect that her upcoming behavior might be negative, be sure that this morning's routine is completely finished before you initiate discussion of the matter. Her reaction to whatever you say might be totally unpredictable. If you suspect a negative conversation is coming, prepare accordingly, just in case. If it is remotely possible that she might throw a tantrum and walk out, be sure that she has first met all of your needs for assistance.

Whether she is sure to be calm, mature, and supportive or angry, unpredictable, and abusive, her late arrival for work is a serious matter to you, and you want to minimize the chances that it will ever happen again. Appropriately, address your concerns in a discussion that is somewhat formal and serious. This is not a topic to talk about while she has her head buried in the refrigerator, with a stereo or TV blasting, and her mind preoccupied in cooking your breakfast.

Communicate with your PA first by setting the stage, and then listening to her concerns before delivering your own. When you are ready to discuss the situation, invite her to go first: "Kim, what happened this morning?"

Studies have shown that people most want two things from communication: to be heard and to be understood. Studies also show that many people are unwilling to hear and understand the other person's message until they believe their own has been received.

Now it is your turn to speak. However, before saying anything, weigh a number of factors in deciding about her future. Before you speak, decide what your end message will be, and be concise in delivery. Avoid a five-minute rambling and venting of your emotions.

Decision: Keep or fire the aide? Before speaking, you should decide between two basic choices: Do you want to keep this aide or fire her?

As the saying goes, "Good help is hard to find." As discussed in another chapter, each of your hired aides has cost you a considerable amount of time, physical and emotional energy, and advertising costs. Each time an aide leaves, through resignation or termination, a lot of time and money walks out the door. More important is the loss of one of your most valued assets: dependable, trustworthy, and trained help for your dependent needs.

There is no question that a PA who has seriously bad, incorrigible habits must be fired. Ignoring untrustworthy employees can further cost you your possessions, the resignation of other PAs, or even your health or life.

However, if you are careful while hiring, there will rarely be a need for a firing. Indeed, a well-designed hiring process, such as the ten-step procedures found in this reference, includes steps that will screen out the majority of undesirable applicants before they are actually hired.

This is not to say that carefully screened PAs are flawless. Everyone has bad habits, but those that truly merit firing a PA should be both serious and not correctable. In more than three decades of hiring and managing more than 350 of my own PAs, I can count on one hand those I have been forced to fire.

"If in doubt—don't," is an adage that should be applied to nearly all of your impulses to fire someone. Most of these impulses occur during short, temporary, and emotional crises. If you give yourself the benefit of taking a hour-long walk, getting a good night's sleep, or talking with a friend over a cup of coffee, most emotional impulses to fire a PA will cool down to an objective evaluation of differences in opinion or style.

So, returning to the question of whether to fire a PA who didn't appear on time this morning for work, ask yourself the following questions. If the majority are answered with "yes," then firing this otherwise high-quality aide might be a regrettable mistake.

- Has this aide consistently been a mature, stable, and level-headed person whose behavior is generally logical, rational, and within predictable paradigms of common sense?

- If it were possible to clone the qualities of a select few aides and duplicate their rare qualities in others, would you want to clone the qualities of this aide?

- Has this aide been consistently providing you with quality help?

- Has she had a good attitude toward you, respecting both you and your possessions?

- Was there an excusable reason, truly beyond her fault or control, for her failure to appear on time?

- Was today's failure a sharp departure from her usually dependable and punctual style; is this the first time this has happened?

- Does she seem to sincerely regret today's failure, and be serious about taking steps to avoid a recurrence?

- If you have decided to keep her, does she need a punishing reprimand, or just your very serious request that she avoid any chance of a recurrence?

In contrast, carefully consider firing her if:

- She consistently has been an immature, unstable, and unbalanced person whose behavior is generally unpredictable and not grounded in common sense.
- She has not previously provided you with quality help.
- She has proven herself not to be responsible, dependable, or punctual.
- She has often had a bad attitude in not respecting you or your possessions.
- She does not have a good reason for this morning's failure, and does not seem to care.
- She does not seem to care about her failure's negative consequences for you.
- She does not seem eager to immediately take steps to prevent a recurrence.
- She has often shown some of the other negative traits listed in another chapter.[4]

In addition to carefully weighing the factual answers that she states, use your intuition—gut reaction—to identify any hidden messages. If she is favorably answering your questions, does your sixth sense tell you she is being honest and sincere, or is she trying to snow you? While she answers your questions, watch for body-language contradictions to what she is saying:

- While she is talking to you, is she making good eye contact with your eyes, or is she mostly looking off to one side?
- Is her tone of voice warm, apologetic, and a bit nervous (consistent with the sincerity of apologies), or is she instead somewhat arrogant in trying to hide the anger that she actually feels toward you?
- Is your overall impression that she is sincerely sorry about her failure, or is she instead struggling through anger and impatience to tell you whatever you want to hear?

Is she being both truthful and sincere? Do you believe what she is saying, and is what she says also what she seems to feel?

If you keep the PA, decide also on your instruction to her for preventing a recurrence. If you want to fire her, first plan very carefully for her replacement.

An aide may state that she made a mistake, is very sorry, and will do her best to prevent it from happening again. If you believe her, then tell her that you are concerned that it never happen again, and let it go. If she is truly sorry, then there is no need to reprimand or punish her; she will already have done that to herself.

---

4. Please see chapter 📖 25 "Your Personal Concerns as a Paid Help Provider, plus Ten Reasons Why PAs Quit and Are Fired."

Perhaps the most frequent question inside you right now is, "How many serious failures should I allow her? How many times will I forgive her for being late, requiring me to phone her with wake-up calls, stealing my possessions, or continuing other bad traits? Due to the risk to my possessions, health, or life if she fails me again, should I allow the possibility of another occurrence, or fire her?"

In the PA ball game, just two strikes should make an out. If she fails a second time to show up, then she truly can't be trusted. She must be replaced. For even more serious problems, such as stealing, there should not be even a second chance. At the first occurrence, you should decide immediately to fire her, and actually do so as soon as circumstances permit.

In summary, the PA who overslept this morning, but who has otherwise been dependable, probably requires merely a firm request not to oversleep again. Remind her that if she foresees being delayed in the future, she should call you as much in advance as possible. Statistically, she will probably not mess up again. However, if she fails to show up a second time, and this second no-show has serious negative consequences for you, then her continued employment should be in serious jeopardy. After a second no-show, additional promises to reform are probably meaningless.[5]

What to do when your PA—

- Fails to be honest by lying to you or stealing your money or possessions?

We are accustomed to the traits of a disease or virus. Either can suddenly appear without prior notice. Either spreads quickly if ignored. Either can quickly do irreparable damage if not immediately treated. Either has the potential to completely consume your health and your financial resources.

A PA's lying or stealing is, indeed, a disease or virus. Each requires your immediate attention and reaction. Neither can be ignored. An aide who lies or steals once will do so again and again, and will try better next time to prevent you from finding out about it. As discussed in the previous section, serious lying or stealing is a one-time strikeout in the PA ball game.

Lying or stealing is almost always serious, regardless of whether the actual value of today's lie or theft was relatively small. It will happen again, and a second lie or theft is rarely smaller than the first!

You would be wise to consider promptly taking three types of action:

---

5. For more details on whether to fire, and how to do it wisely, see chapter 📖 10, "**Recognizing and Resolving Your PA Problems, or Parting Ways.**"

- If you have caught an aide lying or stealing, call him on it. Tell him you cannot tolerate that behavior, and that he is not to do it again (even though he will). He is hoping that you will not discover his deception, or that you will be afraid to confront him. When he knows that you know, and you are deliberately not addressing it, he will assume that you lack the strength and courage to be assertive. He is winning this hand of poker, enjoying his victory, and looking for another opportunity to bully you. While he is feeling stronger each day that his victory remains unchallenged, you are probably feeling increasingly sad that you have wimped out. Show him your strength, and reclaim your rightful control of the help recipient-provider relationship.

- You may decide to fire him today, but you may want to delay the actual firing until you have a replacement. If he is your sole aide or you are otherwise dependent on him, begin advertising today for a replacement—without the PA's knowledge. This is tricky, but it can be done. As soon as you have hired and scheduled a replacement, fire the dishonest aide while telling him that he is being replaced because of his lying or stealing that occurred on Tuesday.

- After firing him, take precautions to avoid additional theft. If necessary, have a locksmith change your locks on the day of firing. The alternative, collecting your keys from him, might be meaningless if he has made copies. If he is angry about being fired, he might now have a new motive objective for additional stealing—revenge.

What to do when your PA—

- Fails to be the type of traveling companion-aide that you expected

When you use personally employed PAs, you will commonly find that these folks are willing to travel without an hourly salary, as long as transportation, room, and food expenses are paid.[6]

As your author, I have traveled from coast to coast many times and seldom paid a salary to the PA who traveled with me. If my travel is financially sponsored, I am very forthright about my need to include the airfare, room, and board for my aide. If my travel is personal, I build the extra expense into my vacation budget, save receipts, and deduct my out-of-pocket PA expenses on my taxes as a medical or business item.

Because I usually personally employ my PAs from local college students, I have little trouble finding travel companions when I need them. I employ four to six part-timers, and within two or three phone calls I usually hear an enthusiastic "Y-E-S" in response to my request. "Hetty, I want to fly to San Francisco on the 11th, attend a three-day conference, and sample some great restaurants. I need someone to travel with me and do PA stuff, all expenses paid except personal spending money. Are you interested?"

---

6. For additional notes and cautions about traveling with PAs, please see chapter 📖 4, "Settings Where You Use Help."

Selecting and accommodating your travel providers. There are some cautions about being on the road, totally dependent on your companion, and a thousand miles from any of your backup aides:

- Select your travel PA very carefully, choosing someone who is stable, mature, flexible, and drug-free. Regardless of how well you plan a trip, problems and crises are very common. Airlines routinely damage wheelchairs, hotel rooms are often not as accessible as they claim to be, and a medical need will occasionally send you or your PA to the local ER. Most of all, travel can make even the nicest people tired, cranky, and a little crazy. Select a companion who has "staying power" to be there, and be innovative, when you need her to be.

- Plan on a sole travel PA to need either relief help or time off each three to four days. On long trips, take either two aides or a lot of patience. Whether you are at home or flying friendly skies, PA work is still work—it is not a vacation. It is a fact that X amount of help with your routine ADL needs at home will probably require 2X or more of help while traveling and camping out in hotel rooms. In addition to your usual ADL needs, you are traveling!

> *Plan on a sole travel PA to need either relief or time off each three to four days—travel long trips with either two aides or a lot of patience!*

If you are traveling several days with a one-and-only family caregiver or hired aide, you are wise to routinely schedule PA "R&R" time. You might be psyched for traveling eight progressive destinations in eight days, but few aides would survive. Ideally, plan for a half-day when a caregiver or aide has off-duty time to sleep, take a long walk, or spend downtime—alone. If you can travel with a caregiver and an aide, or two aides, suggest that they alternate duty days. If you are traveling with two or more providers, and they will be alternating days or duties, have them negotiate the work schedule among themselves.

Before leaving home, discuss your PA's probable need for private time. Some PAs depend on a daily fitness routine, and will need formal exercise during travel days. Once on the road, watch and listen to her for signs of chronic fatigue, and respect them. Let her routinely recharge.

- If you are traveling with hired aides, and are offering to pay travel expenses in lieu of salary, make sure that the financial terms are well understood in advance. Does there seem to be an expectation for cash spending money, or have you formally discussed all the terms?

- Although assistance with very personal needs will come from your family caregiver or PA, be prepared to accept—and manage—supplemental help from strangers. Hotel staff, airline and cruise ship personnel, and passersby often offer, or can be summoned to provide, valued help. Give your personal travel aide a welcomed break, and ask an airport skycap to carry the luggage!

Roadside concerns of your help providers. Suppose you have heeded all these cautions. What problems can occur that would cause a crisis? Let us count the ways!

- Sudden illness or need for medical help for you or a provider

   Yes, this is a vacation and these things are not supposed to happen. However, they frequently do. Assess the medical situation to determine whether a restful day by the hotel pool will do the trick, or whether an emergency-room visit is warranted. If you are staying at a hotel or motel and need resources, call the front desk for advice in coordinating anything from a pharmacy location to having them arrange an ambulance pickup.

- Fatigue

   Travel is tiring. As discussed earlier, a common problem during adventures is simply overdoing it. The remedy is usually twofold. First, take an extra half day or day to rest. If you are staying at a hotel or resort, and have people who need rest and others who need activity, there is usually a variety of resort facility choices.

   Second, after your "roadies" have rested, call for a discussion on whether the remainder of the outing should be down-paced. Develop a game plan that integrates more rest into the remaining schedule so crises can be avoided. The toughest part of this planning is often to get members of the travel party to assertively state their needs, and be flexible around the needs of others.

- Tempers flare up, arguments escalate, and communication breaks down

   Let's go for broke, and discuss a worst-case scenario that might happen while you are on the road. You are on a road trip with a one-and-only PA who suddenly loses her composure and has an emotional breakdown. Here is another real-life, golden experience from your author.

   A few years ago, I felt the urge to spend a few days at the ocean. Since I personally employ my PAs from a nearby college campus, I asked my 20-something PAs for a willing travel companion. Only one of my five part-timers was available. I was well aware of the risks of hitting a high-paced highway trip for several days with just one caregiver or PA. It is a classic prescription for help provider burnout, as I was soon to be reminded.

Chelsea was a 22-year-old, free-spirit college student who had been working smoothly for several months as part of my PA team at home. She was sharp, enthusiastic, and we headed west in my mini van with some great CD tunes. After three days on the road, we pulled into our San Francisco motel. She was visibly getting tired; however, we had arrived for the next eight days and our pace could now be customized to match fatigue or energy levels.

Although she had volunteered to do most of the city driving, I wanted to be independent for the next few days. San Francisco can be a challenging city to drive, and I had planned to enjoy driving my van wherever I wanted to spend the day. Chelsea knew that she would be free to accompany me, take public transit to her own destinations, or stay at the motel to "veg out" at the pool. If we planned a separate day, she would be responsible merely for meeting me back at the hotel at night so I could get into bed.

In theory, we had the elements of an ideal vacation for each of us. However, as "PA wise" and experienced as I have become over the years, I had no prior indication of what was about to happen next.

As we initially arrived at our hotel and began to unpack my van on that first evening of our Bay Area arrival, Chelsea simply lost her composure and became a totally different person than I had ever known her to be.

It was as though a program switch had suddenly been flipped somewhere in her brain or physiology. Within two or three hours of our arrival, she suddenly became angry, disagreeable, and contrary to all the vacation plans to which we had previously agreed. For the next several hours that night, she ranted and raved about a variety of topics. In her opinion, my driving had been too slow (I drove at speeds less than 80, while she preferred 80+). She cited that the decisions about the trip had not been sufficiently democratic (yes, I had done most of the planning for the trip that I had initiated and was financing). Additionally, she found it unfair that I was refusing to completely relinquish my van for half of our week in and around the city.

Although confused, I recognized a potential crisis and flipped my own switch to cool, composed, and logical. My primary objective for now was to quietly observe her, let her vent, and not add any heat to the near-combustion, strange person who was barely providing assistance to me. I was over a thousand highway miles from any of my other PAs. I was in a survival mode and wanted to be sure I would have help with my basic ADLs for the next few days. Although I was naturally curious about the possible cause of Chelsea's dramatic personality change, I vowed to myself not to become emotionally involved or to try to assign blame or guilt. To survive in this situation, I would have to think clearly while making very logical—and intuitive—decisions. If I let my emotions take control, I would drown in overwhelming confusion.

That night, I excused myself, went down to the motel lobby, and made a long-distance call to my most dependable PA at home. I told Mariah simply that we were in San Francisco and Chelsea was not feeling well. I asked Mariah about her schedule for the next few days. I asked whether she would be available to suddenly drop her schedule, fly out, and take over if I found it necessary. In her sharp assessment of reading between the lines, and realizing that I was in potential trouble, she loyally replied, "Of course, Skip, call me day or night and I will be there in a few hours." I then gave her our motel address, room number, and phone number, just in case.

Chelsea and I made it through the rest of our trip, one day and night at a time. My key to keeping everything together was to quietly observe, allow Chelsea to vent, and have no interest in verbally defending myself or replying to her variety of disagreements. I slept lightly and within reach of the room's phone, having memorized Mariah's number.

The stress and uncertainty of that trip made it a hell at times, but I learned a lot from it. I will never know what happened inside Chelsea. As I dropped her off on our return back home, I thanked her for her assistance and wished her well. I have heard since then that she has many personal problems and addictions of which I was unaware during her months as a PA in my home.

This extreme will probably never happen to you, and you should not let it deter you from travelling with paid aides. My travels long before, and since, this extreme example have been very satisfactory.

So, my parting advice about the sudden discovery that your Dr. Jekyll traveling companion has turned into Mr. Hyde:

- Keep cool, composed, and quietly observant.

- Keep your emotions in storage, and maintain a clear head.

- Let go of any impulse to defend yourself, assess guilt or wrongdoing, or set the record straight. Only your survival matters, and not the senseless accusations that your PA is yelling in the attempt to get you angry.

- Remember the potential, through either long-distance PAs at home or a local home health aide agency, for an emergency fill-in aide if something suddenly incapacitates your one-and-only travel PA.

- If your travel PA becomes physically abusive, get out and away while ignoring your possessions. Call a local friend, an available contact back home, or the police.

- Trust that no matter how bad the current situation is, and how far from home you are, the nightmare will eventually end and you will survive.

- Whenever possible, travel with more than one PA, and be very careful in selecting those providers.

What to do when your PA—

- Fails to want merely a help recipient/help provider relationship, and instead wants an additional kind of relationship?

It is not uncommon for help providers to be attracted to your PA job notice because they are seeking a secondary relationship or benefit that is not part of your traditional job description.

These side agendas can come in a wide variety:

- Sexual favors
- A platonic but romantic relationship
- The desire to be needed
- The desire to have someone dependent on them
- A hassle-free haven for substance abuse or dealing
- An easy source (and a constant potential for loans) of money, food, clothing, medications, or your other possessions
- A hideout from the police, bill collectors, subpoena servers, boyfriends, or girlfriends

Indications to you that there is a side agenda seldom come up during the job interview. This type of provider is often, though not always, looking for a live-in position, for two reasons. They usually want as much privacy as possible, to permit hassle-free living with their personal idiosyncrasies. Second, they are attracted to living alone with you, being your one-and-only PA, and enjoying the personal power and control of having you dependent only on them.

Because these PAs are often desperate for a place to live, some money, and who-knows-whatever-else, they will frequently try to sell themselves during your job interview by promising to far exceed your basic expectations. If you routinely shower three times weekly, they might be willing to provide daily showers. If you mention having mechanical problems with your wheelchair, they might claim to be able to fix anything—if you hire them. If your live-in situation consists of two room-mate PAs, the questionable PA might encourage you to hire only him, so he can have your place to himself when you are away.

As the help recipient, you have three basic courses of action if you discover that your recently hired PA wants more benefits than you usually offer:

- If the side agenda is desirable also to you, you can tell the provider and live together as two happy clams—or can you?

  Relationships with side agendas tend to be unstable and often volatile. In addition, help recipients usually end up as losers. The PA's provision of disability help sooner or later becomes very undependable. After all, the recipient is seeking dependable help from a weak person with poor self-esteem who often has a substance addiction, needs money, and is already looking for another place to live. How long will this probably last, and how much will it cost you?

If you want to try life on the wild side for a while, please be careful. As a '60s buddy told me, "I used to hire cool PAs because they drank beer and scored good pot. Now, I hire them only if they don't."

• If the side agenda is not what you want, you might be able to straighten out the PA's expectations and salvage the work relationship. Whether this approach will work and is desirable for you depends on the ability of the provider to respect your standards and set aside his original intentions.

This approach takes considerable diplomacy and careful timing. You cannot be sure of the provider's reaction, so it is best to wait until you are out of bed for the day and independent before discussing your topic. The reaction to your being maturely assertive might be well received, or the provider might become angry, walk out, and not return.

Be direct and tell the help provider what actions or habits you have observed, state that these are not of interest to you, and you would like to know the provider's preference between changing his expectations or moving out. If the provider cannot respect your objectives and lifestyle, try to work out an easy separation and have the PA move out.

• If the agenda is not what you want, and you are not interested in saving the work relationship, then your objective is to fire the salaried aide or evict the live-in.

Once more, as you cannot be sure of the provider's reaction, it is best to wait until you are out of bed and independent before bringing up your topic. The reaction might be well received, or the provider might go ballistic.[7]

---

7. Further details about evicting an undesirable live-in PA are offered in chapter 📖 3, **"Live-In Aides and Other Residence Options."** In any case, you will want to quickly recruit a replacement, and you will find strategies for advertising in chapter 📖 8, **"Where and How to Advertise for Your Own PAs."**

Part VI

The Costs of Your Personally Employed PAs

Part VI

The Costs of Your Personally Employed PAs

The previous Part V advised you on strategies for being a good manager Several management tips focused on your earning the respect of your PAs by routinely showing them appreciation. You then were advised to divide your help needs among several providers, and you were given a procedure for having them assign themselves to work shifts. Part V wrapped up with hints on maintaining a clean, well-stocked work area, and for ways to cope with and react to several typical disappointments and failures from PAs.

This Part VI is about the costs of the help you routinely need. Chapter 📖 **19, "Your Costs of Recruiting, Training, and Keeping PAs Happy,"** begins by discussing the cost of recruiting each help provider whom you employ, from newspaper ads through training. Another section of the chapter compares the costs of using agency aides and personally employing your own. The chapter ends by reminding you that the most powerful means of keeping PAs happy—so they will work harder and remain employed longer—costs you nothing. It's called appreciation, and you are shown powerful ways to express it.

The second chapter, 📖 **20, "Paying Salaries: Cash, Non-cash, or Both,"** discusses three ways of paying the salaries of the help providers whom you personally employ. The first method, cash salaries, is traditional and straightforward: you calculate the gross salary ('hours worked' times 'hourly rate'), calculate and deduct the employment taxes, write the paycheck, and store these financial records. The second, non-cash salary refers to living space, goods, services, or travel benefits that you can offer to providers in exchange for their help to you. Here, you calculate the cash value of the salary you would traditionally pay, and then research an equivalent value of non-cash items that you can substitute. In a third alternative, it is often necessary to combine non-cash and cash salaries to fully compensate providers. The importance of considering a non-cash salary is because its cost to you is usually less than its cash counterpart. For example, if your residence has unused living space, you can offer the space as a non-cash salary and consequently have a free live-in aide. This chapter tells you how to do this, as well as how to set up a system of documents to record, calculate, report (to tax authorities), and store your payroll data.

The last chapter, 📖 21, **"Tax Obligations, Deductions, and Publications for PA Employers,"** introduces tax concerns—the obligations that must be met before employer-taxpayers can benefit from deductions. Although it concentrates on U.S. taxation, this introduction does not provide detailed analysis of policies, because of the date-sensitive content of frequently revised tax laws and regulations. If details were provided about tax obligations to be met, forms and documents to be completed, and deadlines to be observed, they would typically become both outdated and misleading sometime between the print date of this reference and the date you read the details. Consequently, this chapter tells you what tax-related topics should be of concern to you, and where you can find current policies and regulations. Employers and help recipients outside the United States may have very similar tax concerns, and should consult with local authorities or tax professionals for country-specific advice.

The next part, Part VII, discusses feelings, concerns, and remedies for everyone involved in receiving and providing personal help with dependent needs. The premise of the first chapter is that the help recipient, family caregiver, and paid help provider each have human rights that should be respected by the other two parties. In addition, each party has concerns and needs that relate to the interdependent relationship of receiving and providing assistance. The help recipient has concerns, needs, and consequent feelings related to receiving help, just as the family caregiver and the paid provider have the same related to providing help. To maintain a caring, appreciative, and enduring three-way relationship, each party should take equal responsibility for understanding, respecting, and accommodating these factors for his or her colleagues. The remainder of Part VII extensively lists and discusses concerns, needs, and suggested remedies for each of the three parties. The objective of these lists is for each party to better understand, respect, and honor the others—as well as themselves.

Part VII *"I Understand How You Feel"—Concerns Heard from You as a Recipient, Family Caregiver, or Paid Provider*

Chapter 19

Your Costs of Recruiting, Training, and Keeping PAs Happy

Ben and Jerry have often recounted the day when they finally realized they were actually running an ice cream business. In the mid '70s, the two former schoolmates had reunited in Burlington, Vermont, to make ice cream. Setting up shop in an abandoned gas station on Cherry Street, each took turns at arm-cranking a salt-and-ice ice-cream maker. In the afternoon, they would open the front door and sell ice cream cones to passersby. The cash from sales was tossed into a shoebox.

"We stayed closed one day," Ben once told me, "and put a sign on the door that said 'closed today to count our money.' We knew we were selling out of ice cream each day, but we didn't seem to be making any profit. It was on that day that we started listing all of our expenses, and it suddenly struck us that we were *really running a business!*"

An example of the time and financial costs of recruiting

One of your current aides tells you he must resign. He gives you the traditional one-month advance notice. You have had a very smooth working relationship and he assures you that he will stay on until you have a replacement in place.

Resignations are seldom delivered at convenient times. However, you use college students from the nearby campus, and a fruitful time in the campus recruiting calendar happens to be at hand.

You are very active each day, your personal calendar is filled with a busy mix of career and leisure appointments. Your appointment book comes out and you scan the next three to four weeks of activities. Each new recruiting period requires an investment of time and consequent schedule planning. There are costs to your appointment book as well as checkbook.

For the first years that you recruited new help, you just squeezed the extra activities into your already busy, routine schedule. Consequently, each three or four weeks of recruiting were really stressful. You were uptight and angry, and the interviewing PA applicants as well as your family all felt it. On the nights that you first phone-replied to inquirers, or later met candidates for interviews, you sometimes did not make the greatest first impression. In fact, you suspect that you might even have lost a few good applicants who decided there was too much stress in the job.

Now, after a few years of getting this recruiting thing down to a science, you are smarter. You pace yourself and allow for the extra time and energy that the upcoming recruiting will require from your schedule. Each night of answering phone inquiries, describing your routine, and interviewing candidates now gets the extra personal resources it deserves. You are less stressed, PA applicants see a cool guy who might be fun to work for, and your family no longer avoids being around you while you are hiring!

So what will be the costs both to your check *and* appointment books?

Here is an example of the typical time and financial costs of recruiting, interviewing, hiring, and training for one or more new, college-student PAs from a nearby campus. The costs for recruiting from a general community are almost identical to these.

Please remember that this chapter addresses costs and not step-by-step procedures. For detail about the procedures, please see one of the three, ten-step chapters (5, 6, or 7) on finding your help from family caregivers, agency aides, or personal employment.

- You begin running an ad in the campus paper. The cost is $12 per day for about 8 lines in the classified section, or $60 for the five-day, weekly rate.

- On each evening of that week, as you return home at 6 P.M. from your office, you have dinner and then check your phone answering machine for inquiries. From the facts stated by each person, as well as their tone of voice and attitude, you and your intuition decide which inquiries to screen out and which merit your calling back. Of the five people who saw your ad and left a message, four initially sound like good candidates. You erase the one reject and write down the details from each good prospect, perhaps with help from a current PA.

- You are tired from a long day, but you spend 15 minutes in calling back the four applicants. Two are not at home, so you leave a voice-mail message to ask that they call again with some windows of time when you might reach them. You speak with the other two. After you describe the nature and schedule of the work, one of the two is still interested. You schedule a night and time for her to visit you for an interview and demo of the routine. It's 9:15 P.M., and you have processed the inquiries from the first day of your newspaper ad. Your ad will run for five days, but you will typically get inquiries over seven or eight days, as people read yesterday's paper. One day down, and six to go!

- For the next six nights, you listen to fresh inquiries on your phone voice mail. The first string of undesirables is screened out from the content and attitude of their recorded messages. You call back good candidates to describe the routine, listen to their responses, and screen out a second group. For the survivors of these first two screenings, you set up interviews. Of 19 voice-mail inquiries over 7 nights, you drop 5 as being undesirable.

- Of the remaining 14 whom you call back, some fail to show up for your interview and demo, some fail to call you back on the day after the interview-demo, and you reject 2 others. You are finally able to hire one new PA!

If you personally hire PAs, you will be repeatedly conducting this *RISHTMP cycle* of recruiting, interviewing, screening, hiring, training, managing, and parting ways with your providers. Each time you run through this cycle of tasks, the mathematical results of your efforts will usually be different. For example, if you recruit new PAs in March, July, and September, you will find variances each time in the number of people who inquire about your PA ad, those who show up for the interviews, and those whom you finally hire.[1]

In this example, 19 initial inquiries yielded a single new hire—a ratio of 19 to 1. The next newspaper ad might pull in 10 inquiries and yield 3 new aides—a ratio of 10 to 3.

Because there are so many variables in each cycle, there is no firm inquiries-to-hirees ratio.

Combining my own recruiting and hiring experience with those of other PA managers, I would estimate that an overall, average, rule-of-thumb ratio might be 5-to-1 of received inquiries to hired PAs. As a very active, independent C 5/6 spinal-cord-injured quad (tetraplegic), I use a weekly average of 30 hours of assistance. I try to continually employ a team of five or six part-time PAs at any one time—an intentional diversification of college students and people from the general community. These 5 PAs divide my 30 weekly hours of need, for a weekly workload of about 6 hours to each provider.

Within hours of an aide informing me of an upcoming resignation, I fax my standard PA ad to the campus or community newspaper. Since the newspaper staff hears from me five or six times each year, I can sometimes just call the classified ad office and recite that famous line from the movie classic, *Casablanca*: "Play it again, Jennifer" They often have my ad on disk from its previous running.

To maintain a continuous staff of 5, I hire about 10 to 12 PAs each year. A rare few aides last only two weeks, most work for six to nine months, and a frequent few will stay on board for a year or more. That means running my ad about 5 times each year, totaling perhaps 50–60 initial inquiries on my phone answering machine.

In my 30-plus years of recruiting and hiring, I guess I have listened to more than 1,800 initial inquiries in order to hire a bit more than 350 PAs! That sounds like an overwhelming amount of work. However, the alternative would have been to use whatever aides an expensive agency would have assigned to me—and to almost double my out-of-pocket expenses. I am a firm believer that maintaining control over the quality, schedule, and expense of my daily lifestyle is well worth my time and effort.

The following listing recaps the time and financial costs for our example of a typical recruiting cycle.

---

1. If you follow the eight-opportunity screening process outlined in chapter 📖 7, **"Ten Steps to Getting All or Some of Your Help from Personally Employed Aides,"** you will notice varying numbers of applicants being filtered out by each screening step each time you use the process.

Your typical costs for each RISHTMP cycle of recruiting new PAs

Over seven nights, the scoring of costs—in your money and time—for the "PA recruiting game" (for recruiting from the campus or area community) might look like *Figure 19-1*.

Figure 19-1: **Typical costs for each RISHTMP cycle, from advertising through training**

- Days of newspaper ads...5
- Nights spent listening to phone-message callers, doing initial screening, and calling back respondents..7
- A typical total of inquiries 19
- Undesirable inquiries initially screened out..5
- Desirable respondents you called back 14
- Desirables who were not at home, you left a message 4
- Of the 4 with whom you left messages, those who called you the second time 2
- Of the 12 desirables you spoke to, those who weren't interested due to the nature of the work, schedule, or undisclosed reason 3
- Total whom you scheduled for an interview-demo evening at your home 9
- Of the 9, those who called in advance to cancel.......................................1
- Of the remaining 8, those who failed either to show for the interview-demo or to cancel by calling in advance 3
- Of the 5 who interviewed and who agreed to call back the next day with their job decision, those who failed to call back 2
- Of the 3 who called back, those who declined the job...............................2
- Of the 19 original inquiries, those who accepted the job and you hired 1
- Your total financial cost for hiring one new PA; week-long newspaper ad $60
- Total hours of your time for each recruiting cycle
  - ▶ 7 telephone nights x 20 mins. ....2+ hours
  - ▶ 4 interview-demo nights x 3 hours ....12 hours
  - ▶ Training demos and instructions for the 3 different parts of your routine, 3 parts x 5 hours each............................15 hours
  - ▶ Your total time, from interviews through training.................29+ hours

Estimated, typical annual costs of employing your own PAs

Let's apply these costs to an annual expenditure (see *Figure 19-2*).

Figure 19-2: **Typical annual costs of personally employing PAs**

- Total number of annual recruiting, hiring, and training (RISHTMP) cycles required to maintain your continuous supply of PAs ....5+

- Total personal hours spent during the several days of each PA recruiting, hiring, and training cycle ....29+

- Total annual personal hours spent during the 5 annual cycles of approx. 29 hours each 145*

- Total annual cost of newspaper ads for recruiting your PAs...............$300.00

- A typical weekly need for PA help, in hours 30

- A typical annual need for help, in hours, 30 x 52 weeks 1,560

- Hourly rate paid for personally employed PAs (Midwest example) as of this book's 2002 printing $8.00

- Annual gross salaries paid in this example, $8.00 x 1,560 hours $12,480.00

- Annual social security (FICA) tax, costs contributed by the employer, 2001 effective rate, 7.65% of $12,480 ....$954.72

- Sample state unemployment tax $25.00

- Worker's compensation insurance cost (varies depending on whether it is provided by a homeowner's policy or a special WCI policy; the higher $1,500 cost is used in the total below)....$500–$1,500.00

- Accountant fees for calculating and filing employer's quarterly and annual reports $350.00

- Annual total cost for 1,560 hours of help at $8.00 per hour + (above) costs $15,609.72

- Average of all hourly costs for personally employing 30 weekly hours of help at an $8.00 hourly rate ($15,609.72/1,560 hours) ....~$10.01

* or about 18, 8-hour days

For more details on the cost comparisons of personally employed and agency employed aides, please see chapter 📖 1, "Beyond Family Caregivers: Options and Settings for Finding Outside Assistance." On page 56, you will find comparisons of the hourly and annual costs of personally and agency employed aides, including an example of the annual savings of using your own PAs.

Chapter 20
Paying Salaries: Cash, Non-cash, or Both

There are three primary ways to pay the help providers whom you personally employ.

The traditional way is to write a paycheck for a cash amount, and then to record, report, and store that data. When a personal cash budget is insufficient, and third-party funding is either also insufficient or undesirable because of restrictions, a second, non-cash type of salary is often an attractive alternative. With a non-cash salary, you would substitute services, goods, rent-free living space, or travel benefits of equal value to the forgone cash paycheck. In certain circumstances, such as offering live-in space within your house or apartment, a non-cash salary might actually cost you nothing. A third option is to combine the cash and non-cash alternatives.

The chapter covers the basics about paying salaries. Within the topic outline of those three salary alternatives, you will first be provided with step-by-step methods for recording salary-related data about your PAs. This data storage includes initially logging their names and social security numbers and then routinely recording their work shifts on time sheets.

You are then introduced to the use of either a pencil-and-paper or a computerized spreadsheet to record time-sheet summaries. If using a computer spreadsheet, you will see how a few minutes of programming will enable that sheet to calculate salary-related withholdings and the net paycheck amount for you! Finally, you will write the PA paychecks and record them in a computerized and categorized checkbook register.

If you are personally employing your aides in the United States, you will have quarterly and annual payroll documents to complete and send to tax authorities. Your new payroll summary spreadsheet will calculate the data required for these reports, so you or your accountant can complete and file the reports.

If you opt for the non-cash salary—and perhaps getting some of your PA help without cost!—you will find a six-step process that enables you to assess the value of non-cash salary items. Consequently, you will be able to offer a non-cash (or a combination cash and non-cash) salary that is clearly fair to both you and your help provider.

If all of this sounds terribly complicated, then you have come to the right chapter—it is about to become very clear and easy! As your author, I have employed my own PAs by using cash, non-cash, and combination methods. In addition, I have personally developed these systems for recording, calculating, reporting, and storing my own salary-related data.

However, you might be asking, "Will these records get me through an IRS audit of the medical deductions that I claim on my income taxes?" Once more, I am proud to tell you that the recordkeeping system outlined here actually earned me an auditor's compliment when I was audited a few years ago. Although the system is certainly not guaranteed to successfully sail you through your own tax audit, it will at least enable you to present a well-organized set of salary records as an opening argument.

Before embarking into the databases and spreadsheets of this chapter, or before proceeding into the next chapter that discusses tax obligations, you are urged to seek the professional advice of a local certified public accountant (CPA). Your personal accountant will probably find the information in these two chapters useful, but he or she should have the final word about how you should set up and maintain your own salary records.

Bookkeeping and salary differences between using agency aides and personally employed PAs

There are two primary sources of aides who are paid a salary. Either an agency employs the PAs you use, or you personally employ them. Let's look at the advantages and disadvantages of each of these approaches when it comes time to pay salaries and maintain financial records.

An agency employs the PAs you use

If you are unable or unwilling to manage and employ the PAs you use, then it's best to let an agency do the work. The agency takes care of all management and employment, and then takes care of you. It recruits, interviews, screens, generically trains, manages, and pays the PAs you use.

In return for the services you receive, you or your funding source will get a routine bill from the agency. You do not pay the aides directly, but instead pay the agency. The agency bill will include the hourly salary the agency pays its aides plus an hourly administrative fee that the agency charges for its management services and other office overhead.

When using an agency, you simply pay their bills. You have no responsibilities for calculating and paying salaries directly to PAs or for filing employment forms and taxes to federal or state agencies. You can usually deduct the total paid to agencies as a medical expense on your personal income taxes, if the funding has come from your pocket and not from another source. You might be able to recover some or all of these expenses from your health insurance or other funder.

In addition to your preference for having an agency coordinate the financial billing, another reason to use an agency can be your receipt of outside funding. Are you using outside or personal funding to pay the aides you use? If you are eligible for outside funding, that funding source usually requires the use of agency aides. In contrast, if you will be using personal funds, can you afford the extra cost of agency aides?

The cost of agency providers is often two to three times that of personally employed help. That is acceptable if you receive outside funding. However, if you are paying for help from personal funds, the savings of employing your own aides year after year can be significant.

For example, at a time when both personally and agency-employed aides actually receive an $8.00 hourly salary, the bottom-line agency billing to you or your funding source could typically range from $18 to $25 or more per hour. In contrast, the typical hourly total when you personally employ your own aides (at the same hourly rate, plus costs for advertising, taxes, insurance, and other related items) will be about $10!

You personally employ the aides or PAs you use

If you are able and willing to manage the PAs you use, and you are paying salaries from personal funds, then you might want to employ them directly. When you directly employ PAs, you perform all the management tasks. You recruit, interview, screen, hire, train, supervise, pay, and part ways with the PAs you use.

Unlike using agency-supplied PAs, you as the employer have complete control over whom you employ, the list and schedule of help that PAs provide, and the quality of help you receive. If any PAs develop problems in their quality of work, their dependability of arrival or departure, their attitude toward you or your work, or any aspect of their trustworthiness, you have complete control to correct the problem or fire the person. In addition, let's not forget the biggest benefit of directly employing the PAs you use: You save money!

However, as experience has taught us, there is a cost to every freedom in life. These freedoms of personal employment come with a nonmonetary cost: the extra time and effort you spend in managing your own aides. Your extra time and effort, with regard to this current topic of bookkeeping and paying salaries, means maintaining weekly time-sheet records of how many hours each PA worked, and then calculating employment taxes before signing actual salary checks.

Your signature on an aide's salary check—and the absence of an agency's—significantly contributes to your power and control in the eyes of your PAs. "Who is my boss, who is in charge here?" The person who pays me, that's who.

As you will see in each section that follows, these payroll tasks will vary according to whether you pay your aides by cash, non-cash, or a combination of the two. You will also see that the accountant who might already do your annual tax reports can usually be enlisted to advise you on the design of your bookkeeping system. In addition, she can complete and file the quarterly and annual payroll reports that federal and state governments require.

The remainder of this chapter explores the three types of salaries you can pay PAs whom you personally employ: cash, non-cash, and a combination of the two.

Paying cash salaries: outside, third-party funding or personal funds?

There are two main sources for paying a cash salary: outside, third-party funding or your own personal budget.

Sources for outside, third-party funding

The good news is that there are a few funding agencies that will pay all or part of PA expenses. The downside is finding them, proving eligibility for the funds, and then accommodating the restrictions and routine paperwork that are required for using it.

I wish I could provide you with a simple chart that listed scores of funding agencies, and then the eligibility criteria and toll-free phone numbers for each one. However, this is another type of data that would be outdated by the time this book was printed and distributed. Instead, this reference identifies the agencies with the best potential for PA funding, so you can research up-to-date policies and eligibility criteria that apply to your personal financial situation.

Generically, the professionals who might best assist you in identifying funding agencies are the counselors at disability-related consumer organizations or independent living centers (ILCs). Of consumer organizations, many states sponsor a chapter of ADAPT (American Disabled for Attendant Programs Today). ADAPT's main Web site is www.ADAPT.org.

In addition, you might contact social workers and case management staff at hospitals and rehab centers. If your community includes a college campus, check with its disability services center. Charities like the United Way or one of their sponsored agencies sometimes fund personal aides or know of agencies that do provide funding. Look them up in the phone book, tell them that you are researching potential funding sources for health aides, and go from there.

Additionally, the following agencies have been known to directly or indirectly sponsor funding programs. Contact your nearest chapter for up-to-date policies and eligibility criteria:

- Medicare is a federal program that provides assistance primarily to people over the age of 65 and those with disabilities.

- Medicaid is a federal and state program that benefits those with low incomes and disabilities.

- Veterans Affairs will often fund health aides for eligible veterans of military service.

- Vocational Education is a federal and state program in most states that will consider health aide funding when it is a required part of a client's educational program.

- Some states provide assistance that is specially earmarked for PA funding. Try calling your state's vocational rehabilitation office, or departments of human services or public health services.

- Private insurance occasionally funds in-home health aides; however, most limit coverage to a temporary period of recovery from a hospital stay. Few will fund ongoing needs due to a lifelong disability.

Disadvantages of outside, third-party funding begin with your time and effort at establishing and maintaining your eligibility for receiving the funds. If you are dependent on third-party funding for the PA paychecks that you issue, inquire about the usual schedule for your routinely receiving funds. Paychecks that come from a funding source are often delayed. Be sure to discuss this schedule with the PAs, and prepare them not to be disappointed when delays occur that are beyond your control.

Three ways for funding sources to pay your PAs

Once you are eligible for funding, there are several possible ways to receive it. Third parties use at least three common routes for paying PAs. You should know the advantages and disadvantages of the route assigned to you. The actual restrictions and step-by-step route to be used by a source are purely their decision. After all, they believe that if they are giving you money, they should have the right to stipulate how you shall receive and spend it.

The funding source pays your aides. In this first method, you are instructed by the funding source to directly hire PAs, and then to sign and submit time sheets that request the funding source to process paychecks. The funding source will process checks made out directly to each of your PAs. It will then either send you their checks for you to hand to PAs, or send the checks directly to your PAs.

If you are given a choice of either having checks sent directly to PAs or receiving checks that you hand to PAs, there are at least two advantages to choosing the second method. When agency paychecks pass through you and you hand them to your PAs, you will be able to monitor whether the checks are arriving on schedule, and whether your PAs are receiving them. In addition, the mechanical process of your handing each check to the PA gives you an added image of authority for controlling the schedule and quality of services you receive. PAs will realize that their checks are not automatically mailed to them, and that you have the final say in whether they are given their checks. There are also a few rare instances, when a PA has turned ugly, in which you can use to your advantage the extra power that comes with "delaying" a PA's check or checks. The more money you hold for a PA, the more respectful and accommodating an otherwise uncooperative PA can be!

This method gives you many of the same advantages as paying by personal funds, except that the paychecks are sometimes delayed in arriving from the funding source. The source will also usually dictate the salary rate, as well as whether and when merit increases can be given.

From a tax standpoint, there is a distinct advantage to this system of a funding source issuing checks directly in the name of the PA. Federal and state tax authorities will almost always consider the PA employer to be the funding source, and not you. This usually means that the funding source will be responsible for filing and paying employment taxes. If your funding source uses this direct-payment system, be sure to ask it or your accountant whether you have any responsibilities for the employment taxes.

The funding source pays you, and you pay your aides. In a second example, the third party gives actual money to you, and you deposit it into your personal bank account. You hire and pay PAs with checks from your own account. Periodically, you supply the funding source with the items of documentation it requests, such as signed forms or copies of canceled checks, to prove that you are indeed paying your PAs.

You should ask your accountant whether these funds are considered taxable income, even though you receive them for a dedicated purpose and then spend them for that purpose. You might have a tax liability for these funds.

The funding source works through an agency. A third and quite common funding route is characterized by a set of severe restrictions. The funding source requires you to get your aides through a home health aide agency. The agency hires, pays, and schedules PAs to provide you with assistance. The funding source then directly pays the agency for the aide services that you use.

This method is frequently used by governmental funding agencies. It is the least desirable method for those who are able and willing to independently manage and otherwise maintain quality control over the PAs they hire. An increasing number of disability consumer groups are rightfully protesting this requirement to use a home health aide agency. They understandably cite, as a primary grievance, denial of the right to directly employ the PAs they use. However, for those who are unable or unwilling to manage PAs, the required use of home health aide agencies is welcomed.

Using your personal budget for cash salaries

A cash salary is, in fact, seldom paid to a PA in actual green cash; instead, it is by written checks. You should be paying by personal check all salaries, medical expenses, household and personal bills, and any bills you send through the mail. By paying salaries and bills by check, and not in actual currency, you will always have proof of having made a payment, and your paid expenses are easy to record and categorize.

The cost of a personal checking account is usually only that of having checks printed. You can actually make money if you use an interest-bearing checking account. The use of money orders purchased at places like a bank or post office is an expensive, band-aid alternative to using personal checks. When the term *cash salary* is used in this section, it is referring to paying PAs by checks that they can readily convert to cash.

By the way, cashing a PA's paycheck is the PA's responsibility, not yours. Occasionally, aides who lack their own checking accounts, and who therefore might have difficulty cashing their own paychecks, sometimes balk at being handed a salary check. Ninety-nine percent of all bona-fide employers pay salaries by check, not in actual cash. Point these disorganized aides toward the nearest bank and tell them to grow up and open their own account.

In addition, you might also be wary about a PA applicant who lacks a personal checking account. There is often a shady reason for someone not to have established a bank account, a street address, and a long-term job. If somehow you learn this fact about an applicant who has come into your residence for your job interview and demo, keep an eye on her. Of course, it is never a good idea to allow any interviewing applicants to wander around your residence by themselves.

Calculating the cost of cash salaries

What will your paid PAs cost you? How much weekly, monthly, and annual budget should you dedicate to provider salaries? The answers to these basic budget questions are essential to your personal financial planning. If you have reviewed one or more of the three, ten-step chapters for finding your help, you know that these calculations are in **Step ❷** of each chapter's planning steps ❶ through ❸.

> *Cash salaries and most routine bills should be paid by personal check, not in actual green cash.*

Here is that calculation procedure plus explanatory detail:

① **Total up the weekly hours of help that you need, for both routine and unforeseeable needs.**

- From your list and schedule of help needs, add up the weekly hours for your routine needs.

- Then add another 25 percent for unforeseeable (but predictable and frequent) special needs.

- Use this total when calculating a budget for personal or outside funding.

> Your total hours of need =
>   Routine, predictable needs
> +   25% allowance for sporadic, unpredictable needs
>
> Example:
> Your weekly total =
>   32 hours of routine needs
> +   8 hours of unpredictable needs
> =   40 total weekly hours, or 160 monthly hours

If you have reviewed any of those ten-step chapters on finding the help you need, you know that **Step ❶** of each chapter addresses creating your list and schedule of needs.[1] As a result of creating this list, you should know both what help needs you have and approximately how much time you require help.

---

1. Additional pointers on creating your list are included in chapter 📖 **13, "Defining and Describing Your Help Needs."**

Unless you are especially detailed in knowing and listing your needs, there will be additional non-routine needs that occasionally occur. These sporadic needs can include (depending on your disability) cleaning up from bowel or bladder accidents, extra help for treating temporary skin breakdowns, or repair help to your mobility aid. Although these do not occur every day, they do present themselves with sufficient frequency to merit adding an allowance to your budget calculations. This is the 25 percent allowance noted here.

② **Calculate an estimate of the salary cost for your help.**

- If using personal funds and personally employing PAs, research the hourly salary rate that other help recipients are paying their PAs in your community.

- Multiply the total hours of your needs by this going salary rate.

- If using personal funds and personally employing PAs, please note:
  Total cost = (Salary cost) + (Employment taxes) + (Accountant services-optional)

Your total cost of personally employed aides or PAs =
  Total hours of help need
x   Hourly salary rate

Example:
Your weekly cost =
  40 total hours
x $8.50 per hour
= $340.00 weekly, or $1,360.00 monthly

Once you have calculated the weekly and monthly total of hours, you will probably want to additionally figure the cost of these hours. Your first step is to research the "going rate" of hourly salary that other employers are paying their aides. If you create an arbitrary rate out of thin air, you risk not paying enough, and thus having trouble attracting and keeping good aides, or needlessly paying too much. Ask other help recipients, an aide agency, or already employed aides about what salary rate aides expect to receive.

If there are many help recipients in your area, and there is consequently competition for good providers, you might decide to offer $.25 to $.50 more per hour than the most common rate. If you can afford to do this, it will make your job more attractive and you will have an easier time recruiting good help and keeping it longer.

I have repeatedly seen the wisdom of paying a slightly higher salary than other employers around me. I have a choice of either paying a slightly higher salary, or paying the same lower salary as my competitors and consequently attracting fewer applicants and having more frequent resignations. By attempting to save money in paying a lower initial salary, I would ultimately incur higher costs for more frequent advertising. In addition, I would annually spend more of my personal time and effort in recruiting, interviewing, screening, hiring, training, and counseling a series of unhappy help providers. Consequently, I usually find that the slightly higher salary provides me several categories of savings!

When you have identified the hourly salary rate that you will offer, the remainder of this process is the number-crunching of multiplying total hours times hourly salary rate, as illustrated earlier.

③ **You decide whether to use personal funds or outside funding for your help.**

- Personal, out-of-pocket funds

- Federal or state agency or assistance program

- Accident or insurance settlement

- Other

If using personal funds and personally employing PAs, use your cost estimate to plan your personal budget. If the cost exceeds your personal funds, you will need to research some sources of outside money.

If using outside funding, identify the source(s), research the eligibility criteria, and apply for the funding. Be sure to note if the funding source places any restrictions on the type of help you can hire.

Paying cash salaries, and maintaining records

What follows is a well-designed system of five documents for recording PA work-shift data, calculating and issuing paychecks, and keeping simple financial records that satisfy both your budget planning needs and IRS audits.

④ **You hire as many PAs as you need and your budget allows**
It is wise to divide your needs among as many part-time aides as possible, for several reasons.[2]

⑤ **You record some basic employment data for each PA**
Each time you hire new aides, you should record some basic data that you will need for your own salary records and for filing reports required by tax authorities. Your records of the aides you employ should include name, address (current or parent's permanent address, if the PA is a student), phone number, U.S. social security number, and date of birth. Because the address will be used for mailing end-of-year tax forms to the aide, you might ask for a permanent address if the aide is a student living in temporary housing. A parent's address can usually be used. It is a good idea to store contact data for both current and previous PAs; several times I have had to contact aides who helped me several years ago.

---

2. For more details about hiring, managing, and using several PAs, please see chapter 📖 **16,** "Dividing Your Needs, and Assigning Work Shifts, Among Several PAs."

You could use handwritten formats like index cards to store these data. However, it is much more efficient to use a computer for this biographical data, as well as for salary records. According to your preferences (and the software available to you), the format of this PA data storage can be as simple as an ongoing series of bullet entries within a word-processor file, or as fancy as a specially created database.

In the following example, Sam stores his provider data in his PC, in a simple text or spreadsheet file that he has entitled "PA Contact Data." His current PAs are listed first, and the previous PAs are listed next, in reverse chronological order with the most recent aides at the top. (See *Figure 20-1.*) When a current PA resigns, Sam cuts and pastes that data to the top of the "previous" list. Sam writes paychecks to his PAs and maintains these salary records, and also provides printouts of the current records to his CPA. The CPA, in turn, completes and files the federally required quarterly and annual tax reports on Sam's behalf.

Figure 20-1: **Employment data for all PAs**

Name	Address	Phone	SS #	DOB
Kim Johnson	123 Laurel St, Carbondale, IL 62901	555-8239	123-45-7890	5-11-77
Betty Laramay	110 Pierce Hall SIU Campus Dr,	907-555-3721	012-34-5678	2-1-75
	Albany, NY 12222			
Jennifer LaBarge	403 S Williams St, Carbondale, IL 62901	555-2140	345-38-9149	11-13-77
	(parent's permanent address)			
Previous PAs				
Megan Burris	408 Pleasant St, Brookline, MA 02146	617-555-7033	074-38-3721	6-5-75

⑥ **You assign each PA a blank time sheet**
When initially setting up your recordkeeping system, you should create a format for some sort of time sheet that PAs will use to record their work shifts. As shown in *Figure 20-2*, Sam uses an 8-1/2" x 11" plain sheet of paper with the headings illustrated. He stores this template as another text file, so he can easily computer-print a dozen new time sheets whenever old ones are filled.

Figure 20-2: **Assign a blank time sheet to each PA**

Work Log

Name_____

Date	Time In	Time Out	Total Time (Use decimal totals, please)

It is important that the time sheets stay at your place; PAs should not take them home. As your author, I have dedicated a small area of my kitchen counter to the stack of current time sheets. This area is next to the refrigerator, where I also post the master calendar of the month's work shifts.[3]

As PAs complete work shifts, they are responsible for hand-writing their shift data on their individual time sheets. Each shift gets a one-line entry. Later, when you process paychecks, your first step is to total the time-sheet entries for each PA.

Sam needs about 35 hours of help each week. He employs three part-time aides who each work about 12 hours per week. To enable his PAs to maintain accurate records of work shifts—so he can accurately pay them—he keeps a stack of the three active time sheets on the corner of his desk. At the end of each work shift, the working PA completes a one-line entry on his or her sheet. Each two weeks, when Sam processes paychecks, he totals the data on each PA's sheet. *Figure 20-3* is a sample time sheet that Kim Johnson has been using for about two weeks. She recorded each of these entries as she finished each work shift.

---

3. For detail about this master calendar of work shifts, please again see chapter 📖 16, "Dividing Your Needs, and Assigning Work Shifts, Among Several PAs."

Figure 20-3: **Time sheet, showing the PA's handwritten entries for each work shift**

Work Log

Name____Kim Johnson____

Date	Time In	Time Out	Total Time (Use decimal totals, please)
5/3	6:00 am	7:30 am	1.5
5/5	8:00 pm	10:45 pm	2.75
5/5	Grocery shopping and errands		2.5
511	8:00 pm	9:30 pm	1.5
5/14	6:00 am	7:45 am	1.75
5/17	6:00 am	8:00 am	2.0

⑦ **You process paychecks on a routine schedule**

As early as the interview stage, you should clearly state the hourly salary rate you are paying, what taxes you will be withholding, and on what schedule you process paychecks. You can offer to have checks available each week, or you can cut your work in half by paying each two weeks. Whatever your decision, don't exceed it. You can delight PAs by occasionally having checks ready ahead of schedule—especially just before a vacation period—but don't disappoint them by becoming lax.

Each two weeks, I grab an available aide and take 15 minutes to do the payroll. I do the computer recording and check signing while she totals time sheets and fills in the rest of each check. The steps to processing your own payroll are pretty straightforward.

You (or a PA) gather the time sheets, a calculator, and a red pen. First, add up the "Total Time" column (if you are using the time-sheet format shown in *Figure 20-3*). If aides have been using blue or black pens to record their hours, you might consider writing each total in red so that the end of each pay period is easy to spot. I would suggest having aides use a decimal format (instead of fractions) when recording partial hours, so that your use of a calculator will be easier.

In *Figure 20-4*, Sam has summarized Kim's "work dates" to show the actual range of dates that she worked during this two-week pay period. Additionally, he has totaled the "Total Time" column.

Figure 20-4: **Time sheet, showing Sam's handwritten total for this pay period**

Work Log

Name___Kim Johnson_____

Date	Time In	Time Out	Total Time (Use decimal totals, please)
5/3	6:00 am	7:30 am	1.5
5/5	8:00pm	10:45 pm	2.75
5/5	Grocery shopping and errands		2.5
511	8:00 pm	9:30 pm	1.5
5/14	6:00 am	7:45 am	1.75
5/17	6:00 am	8:00 am	2.0

5/3-5/17/01   12 Hours

Once you have totaled these two items on all the time sheets, the next step is to record these pay-period summaries on one master spreadsheet. If you are taking the advice about computer-storing these salary records, a spreadsheet format is tailor-made for the columns of data you will be recording, calculating, and storing. A spreadsheet program will do all of this for you, if you initially perform some very simple, one-time setup and programming activities. You do not have to record each shift from the time sheets, but only the two data items for the current pay period for each PA.

In these examples, Sam created this spreadsheet with his PC's spreadsheet program. Maintaining a separate, blank template is not necessary, because this ongoing record of all the PA time sheets will be stored in the computer. When it is time for Sam's CPA to file quarterly or annual reports for him, Sam can select and total the most recent pay periods before printing them.

Figure 20-5 shows the bare-bones format that Sam created before entering the PA data:

Excel File: PA Salaries Spreadsheet
Beginning May 2001

Figure 20-5: **Spreadsheet summary format, ready for payroll data
from time sheets**

	A	B	C	D	E	F	G
1	PA Name	Work Dates	Total Hours Worked	Gross Pay	FICA Withheld	Net Pay	Check #
2							
3							
4	Kim Johnson						
5							
6							
7							
8							
9							
10							
11	Betty Laramay						
12							
13							
14							
15							
16							
17							
18	Jennifer LaBarge						
19							
20							
21							
22							
23							
24							

Here are definitions for each of the column headings. After you have typed them in,
you will probably want to program the mathematical relationships among three of
the columns. This simple programming will enable the spreadsheet to perform the
salary calculations each time you enter the two items of data from the PA time sheets.

PA Name—   You enter the names of all your PAs under this heading, in
                         this one column. Each name is separated from the next by
                         about six blank rows. These blank rows for each PA will be
                         used for recording future pay periods.

Work Dates—   From each PA's time sheet, you enter the one- or two-week
                         range of dates (according to how often you process
                         paychecks) that the PA worked during this pay period.
                         This specific range of work dates will usually be a bit
                         different for each PA.

Total Hours Worked—   To complete this entry, you begin with each PA's time
                         sheet. First, total the hours that the PA worked during this
                         one- or two-week pay period, and write this total directly
                         on the time sheet. Next, copy this total from each time
                         sheet to this space on the spreadsheet.

Gross Pay—	This is equal to "Total Hours Worked" x the hourly salary rate that you pay. It would be nice if this could be the amount used for the paycheck; however, U.S. employers must first deduct a FICA percentage from this gross total. If your spreadsheet is programmed correctly, this calculation should appear as soon as you enter the "Total Hours Worked." [Please see the spreadsheet program later in this section.]
FICA Withheld—	U.S. employers are required to deduct a specified percentage from an employee's gross pay before writing a paycheck for the amount of the "Net Pay" (see the next in this list). As of this book's printing, this is 7.65 percent. If your spreadsheet is programmed correctly, this calculation should appear as soon as you enter the "Total Hours Worked."
Net Pay—	This final, paycheck amount is equal to "Gross Pay" minus "FICA Withheld." If your spreadsheet is programmed correctly, this calculation should appear as soon as you enter the "Total Hours Worked."
Check Number—	You manually enter the number of the paycheck used for this PA.
Gross Pay	(Column D) = Column C x The hourly salary rate that you are paying [For $8.50, you would enter 8.5, or "C*8.5"]
FICA Withheld	(Column E) = Column D x The current percentage specified by the U.S. tax authorities [If 7.65%, you would enter .0765, or "D*.0765]
Net Pay	(Column F) = Column D - Column E

Now that your summary spreadsheet is ready for entries, here is how it is used:

- With your spreadsheet ready, enter the names of all your PAs under the "Names" heading, skipping about six rows between each name. These blank rows for each PA will be used for recording future pay periods.
- Once the PA names have been entered, copy the range of "Work Dates" and the end total of "Total Hours Worked" for this pay period from each time sheet. If the remaining spreadsheet columns have been properly programmed, the calculated figures should appear in the columns "Gross Pay," "FICA Withheld," and "Net Pay."

To illustrate these entries, *Figure 20-6* shows is Sam's spreadsheet after he has entered the time-sheet data for his three aides. For each aide, he entered only the range of dates (column B) and the total hours (column C); the programmed spreadsheet performed the consequent calculations and automatically entered the dollar figures in columns D, E, and F.

Excel File: PA Salaries Spreadsheet
Beginning May 2001

Figure 20-6: **Summary spreadsheet showing entries for three PAs, one pay period**

PA Name	Work Dates	Total Hours Worked	Gross Pay	FICA Withheld	Net Pay	Check #
Kim Johnson	5/3-5/17/01	12	$102.00	$7.80	$94.20	5432
Betty Laramay	5/2-5/13/01	19.25	$163.63	$12.52	$151.11	5433
Jennifer LaBarge	5/1-5/12/01	10.5	$89.25	$6.83	$82.42	5434

- After a PA's "Net Pay" calculation appears, you can write the paycheck and enter the check number in column G. When writing the paycheck, use the same data from the summary spreadsheet. To be consistent, use the last date that the PA worked—from the range of dates—as the check date. Use the spreadsheet's "Net Pay" for the check amount. The range of dates and the total hours worked can be recorded on the check memo line. (See *Figure 20-7*.)

Figure 20-7: **Paycheck, data taken from summary spreadsheet**

John Smith   3001
123 1st Street
Denver, CO 70123
303-303-0303   Date 5/17/01

Pay to the order of Kim Johnson $ 94.20

Ninety four dollars and 20/100   Dollars

For 5/3-17/01: 12 hours   John Smith

:123456789012: 1234567890123" 3001

Before you let go of the paychecks, you should record them in your handwritten checkbook register or in your computer's checkbook register program. Programs like Quicken® and M.Y.O.B.® ("Mind Your Own Business") provide for very easy entries and categorized recordkeeping (see *Figure 20-8*). If you are using such a program, each PA should be set up as a "recurring transaction." Consequently, the next time you begin to enter an aide's name, the computer program will recognize it and automatically enter the rest of the name. You should create a category for "PA Salaries" so the total for these paychecks can be included with other tax-related medical deductions. The "memo" window could include the same data as the check memo line: the "Work Dates" and "Total Hours Worked."

Figure 20-8: **Using a computer checkbook register for each PA paycheck**

Date	Number	Payee/Category/Memo		Payment	Clr	Deposit	Balance	
5/7/01	2997	LePeep		17.50			4,033.69	
		Dining	Breakfast					
5/9/01	2998	Qwest		75.27			3,958.42	
		Utilities	Phone-Home					
5/12/01	2999	Public Service		127.39			3,831.03	
		Utilities:Gas & Electric	Monthly					
5/14/01	3000	DSRM		113.20			3,717.83	
		Auto:Fuel	Monthly					
5/17/01	3001	Kim Johnson		94.20		*Deposit*	3,623.63	
		Medical: PA Salaries	5/3-17/01; 12 Hours			Split	Shortcuts ▼		
5/17/01								

Record   Restore   Sort by: Date ▼   Balance Today: $3,623.63 ▼

After all spreadsheet and checkbook register data have been recorded, you can enclose each paycheck within its folded (in half) time sheet. The sheets can be stacked and returned to their area, where the checks will be found by PAs at their next shift. If you use the 8-1/2" x 11" time-sheet format recommended in this chapter, PAs can resume writing in their work shifts for several weeks until a time sheet is filled on both sides. You should encourage PAs to compare, for accuracy, each paycheck to their handwritten time-sheet data.

⑧ **Maintain these employer records to monitor your budget and fulfill tax requirements**

In the United States, you will be totaling the summary spreadsheet data at the end of each three-month calendar quarter. These three-month quarters are:

- January 1 to March 31
- April 1 to June 30
- July 1 to September 30
- October 1 to December 31

Certain reports that must be completed and sent to federal and state agencies.[4] If you use the summary spreadsheet format described here for recording and storing PA salary data, you will additionally need only to total this data at the end of each quarter for the quarterly data required for the reports.

---

4. These are briefly described in chapter 📖 21, "Tax Obligations, Deductions, and Publications for PA Employers."

At the approximate end of each quarter's data, create a separate row in the spreadsheet for totals. Because the data on time sheets will probably not end exactly on the last day of a calendar quarter, it is okay to declare the end of your calendar quarter within a week or ten days on either side of the exact end date (please see the dates in *Figure 20-9* for an example). Just be sure to begin your next quarter where you ended the previous one.

- First, in the column for "PA Name," type in a notation like "Totals 1/1-3/31/01."

- Next, use the spreadsheet program to total these columns:
  - ▾ Total Hours Worked
  - ▾ Gross Pay
  - ▾ FICA Withheld
  - ▾ Net Pay

To illustrate these entries, *Figure 20-9* shows Sam's summary spreadsheet after he performed the second-quarter time sheet summaries (April 1 through June 30). Please note that Sam began employing his own aides, and created this spreadsheet, around May 1st.

In addition to doing this quarter's summaries, Sam has also set up the spreadsheet for the next quarter (July 1 through September 30). Like many of us who lack a passion for completing tax forms, Sam contracts a local accountant to complete quarterly and annual employer documents for him. Sam's responsibility is to select, total, and print the quarter's payroll summary from his spreadsheet. The only additional data needed by the accountant are the PA contact data (names, addresses, etc.) for his current PAs.

Figure 20-9: **Spreadsheet summary showing the totals for paychecks in a calendar quarter**

	A	B	C	D	E	F	G
							Book Spreadsheet Example C1
1	PA Name	Work Dates	Total Hours Worked	Gross Pay	FICA Withheld	Net Pay	Check #
2							
3							
4							
5	Kim Johnson	5/3-5/17/01	12	$102.00	$7.80	$94.20	5432
6		5/18-29/01	10	$85.00	$6.50	$78.50	5468
7		5/30-6/11/01	11.35	$96.48	$7.38	$89.09	5487
8		6/12-6/26/01	11.35	$96.48	$7.38	$89.09	5518
9		6/27-7/6/01	10.1	$85.85	$6.57	$79.28	5528
10							
11	Betty Laramay	5/2-5/13/01	19.25	$163.63	$12.52	$151.11	5433
12		5/14-5/28/01	7.25	$61.63	$4.71	$56.91	5469
13		5/29-6/10/01	20	$170.00	$13.01	$157.00	5488
14		6/11-6/24/01	18	$153.00	$11.70	$141.30	5521
15		6/25-7/6/01	9.75	$82.88	$6.34	$76.54	5527
16							
17	Jennifer LaBarge	5/1-5/12/01	10.5	$89.25	$6.83	$82.42	5434
18		5/14-5/28/01	12.92	$109.82	$8.40	$101.42	5470
19		5/29-6/10/01	3	$25.50	$1.95	$23.55	5489
20		6/11-6/25/01	5.75	$48.88	$3.74	$45.14	5519
21		6/26-7/4/01	6.5	$55.25	$4.23	$51.02	5528
22							
23	Totals 4/1-6/30/01		167.72	$1,425.62	$109.06	$1,316.56	
24	Second Quarter 2001						
25							
26	Kim Johnson						
27							
28							
29							

So there you have it: a five-part system for calculating and paying PA salaries, and then storing and periodically reporting the data. I created this system many years ago. I have subsequently refined it over three decades, even from the time before personal computers were available. (I won't even begin to relate how this system looked before the PC!)

It has worked well for me and for many others. It has also earned the praises of an IRS auditor. One year, I was audited for medical expenses. For a quadriplegic, the documentation for 12 months of medical expenses can result in quite a pile of paperwork. When the auditor arrived at my PA expenses, he randomly checked three or four salary payments, tracing each payment from my summary spreadsheet, to my Quicken® printout, and finally to my stack of cancelled checks. After I passed with ease, his only comment was "nice recordkeeping." From an IRS agent, *that* was a huge compliment!

Figure 20-10 is a flow chart that summarizes this five-part system.

Figure 20-10: **An integrated system for recording, calculating, paying, storing, and reporting PA salaries**

PA Personal Data File
Soon after you hire each new PA, record the types of personal data that you will need for your own salary records as well as for quarterly and annual salary reports to federal and state tax and business agencies. These records might be handwritten, with one PA on each 3" x 5" index card, or computerized, in an informal text file or a dedicated database. The data you will need for each PA includes name, address, phone number, U.S. social security number, and date of birth.

Individual PA Time Sheets
At the end of each work shift, each PA hand-writes a one-line entry onto his/her time sheet. At the end of each one- or two-week pay period, when you process paychecks, you total the hours of each PA's sheet and write that total on the sheet. The PA can continue to use his/her time sheet, pay period after pay period, until both sides are filled. After you record the last pay period of a filled time sheet onto the computerized spreadsheet summary, the time sheet can be tossed and a new one started.

Computerized Spreadsheet Summary of the Time Sheets
This one, master spreadsheet calculates the net pay for each PA's paycheck and permanently stores the data for all of your PAs, month after month, year after year. Each time you process paychecks, type in a one-line summary for each PA from his/her time sheet. This summary has two items: the range of dates and the total hours that a PA has worked during this pay period. If the computer spreadsheet is programmed correctly, it will then automatically calculate the amounts of gross pay, FICA to be withheld (for U.S. employers), and the resulting net pay as soon as you enter each PA's total of hours. The calculated net pay is the amount to be entered on the paycheck.

Written Paychecks
From the data calculated by the spreadsheet, you can write each paycheck. The spreadsheet's "net pay" amount is the amount of the check. The range of dates and total hours can be recorded on the check memo line. You should next record the data for any check you write in your check register; this certainly applies to PA paychecks.

Computerized Checkbook Register
If you use a computer, consider using Quicken®, M.Y.O.B.® ("Mind Your Own Business"), or similar software for maintaining your checkbook register. Create a new, tax-deductible category of "PA Salaries" for recording all the paychecks. The register memo line for each check entry can be the same as the check memo line: the range of dates and the total hours for each PA (in our example, "5/3-17/01: 12 hours").

Paying non-cash, or combination cash and non-cash, salaries

Many help recipients who must pay for assistance from their pocket have found that they could not possibly afford all of their PA help without using non-cash salaries.

Defined

You might consider using non-cash salaries when third-party funding is not available, or is not desirable because of its restrictions.

A *non-cash salary* is personal payment in a form other than the money of a salary check. The basis of a non-cash salary is usually your paying PAs with one or more of the following in exchange for their providing an equally valued amount of help to you:

- Rent-free living space, sometimes with your additional provision of utilities, food, or transportation

- Services, such as your providing educational tutoring, child care, clerical help, computer-based tasks, financial accounting, or tax preparation

- Material goods, such as your home-cooked meals, artwork, or merchandise from a business or retail store that you own

- Your provision of transportation, room, or meals, for PA help during business or vacation travel.

In addition, it is common for the value of help needs to exceed the value of solely non-cash items. Consequently, non-cash items must often be combined with personal or third-party cash salaries.

Calculating the value

Initially, a non-cash form of payment might seem too difficult to quantify. If somehow you were able to decide how much of a non-cash item to offer, how would you be able to objectively convince a PA that your valuation was fair?

Actually, assessing how much help you need, in non-cash terms, is a straightforward, objective process, as shown in *Figure 20-11*.

Figure 20-11: **Calculating the fair value of non-cash salaries**

❶ Determine the hourly salary that you would otherwise offer a PA for providing assistance.
For example, $8.50 per hour.

❷ Determine the average number of weekly and monthly hours of help you need.
For example, 30 hours weekly or 120 hours monthly.

❸ Multiply ❶, the hourly cash salary you would be paying, times ❷, the weekly and monthly hours of help you need. These figures will indicate the weekly and monthly cash salaries you would otherwise be paying.
For example, $8.50 per hour x 30 hours weekly and 120 hours monthly = $255 weekly and $1,020 monthly cash salaries.

❹ List the possible non-cash living space, services, material goods, or travel expenses that you could offer a PA—and that your potential PAs would want, need, or enjoy.

❺ Next to each possible service or item, list its weekly or monthly monetary value.
For example, the live-in space in your home, with bed, bath, kitchen access, and paid utilities, would be worth $400 in monthly rent, according to a realtor friend of yours.

❻ Compare those estimates of ❸, the weekly and monthly value ($255 and $1,020) of the help you need, with ❺, the value of the non-cash item you can offer ($400 monthly). Be creative in imagining some way to pay for all— or at least some—of your needs with non-cash items. You will often have to accompany a non-cash item with a complementary cash salary to provide a fair, total salary.

You probably do not—or certainly should not—employ only one PA to provide all 30 hours of help each week. If you employ college students, you probably divide your needs among at least three aides. Your $1,020 of monthly needs, when divided by three, means that each PA is assuming about $340 worth of work. Your live-in space with side benefits is worth about $400. Consequently, you could offer the space to one of the three aides you will employ. To closer equate the $400 value of the space with the $340 value of one-third of your work, you could shave off one or two side benefits to reduce the value of the $400 space, or add more work to the $340 work load.

So, you will be getting one-third of your needs provided without cost. To pay for the other two-thirds, you could find additional non-cash items, find an outside funding source, or dip into the cash in your personal savings.

Often a non-cash salary will not cost you anything, because you are sharing something valuable that you already own. Here are two examples.

Tutoring local college students. You determine, for your locale, that the hourly cash salary rate for a PA is $8.00. You calculate that you need an average of 3 hours of help per day, or 21 hours weekly. This amounts to $168 per week (plus employment taxes) that you would otherwise be paying as a cash salary. Because you hire primarily college students from the local campus, and you are skilled in several academic areas, you decide to advertise free tutoring in exchange for PA help. The local rate for tutoring is $15 per hour. This means that you can fairly offer a PA about 12 hours of free tutoring each week (worth $180) in exchange for 21 hours of assistance to you.

Live-in space in your residence. Using the same figures from the preceding example, you have calculated that you have a weekly, average cash value of $168 weekly, or $672 monthly, in required PA assistance needs. You have decided that you have extra space in your apartment, condo, or house that you could offer an aide. Your newspaper or Internet ads could be headlined "Free Furnished Room."

In one case, you might have a two-bedroom apartment for which you already pay rent of $800 monthly. If two people were to share this apartment, each would pay $400 per month. You could offer the spare bedroom plus $272 cash salary in exchange for PA help. In another scenario, you pay the mortgage on a house that has two spare bedrooms. By inquiring with a local realtor, you have found that each room, with kitchen access and paid utilities, could rent for $350 per month. In the house example, you could offer the two rooms to two students and receive $700 worth of monthly assistance for free.

In the previous section on paying cash salaries, we proposed a five-part system for neatly recording PA personal data, as well as calculating and paying cash salaries. In addition, the system provides a way for reporting quarterly and annual tax documents and then storing all of these data.

However, the circumstances around valuating and paying non-cash (or combination cash and non-cash) salaries are usually not as clearly definable in dollars and cents.

- What records should be kept when paying non-cash or combination salaries?

- From a tax viewpoint, how should the rent-free living space that the PA receives be reported as income?

- If you were paying a cash salary to a help provider, you should be able to claim this amount as a medical expense. Can you do the same when providing a live-in PA with a rent-free residence in exchange for her help?

In summary, I suggest that you take advantage of offering a non-cash salary, especially if doing so would provide you with free PA help.[5] When you get to the stage of asking these questions about maintaining salary records and filing tax reports, you should consult a local CPA. This accountant can advise you on setting up your own recordkeeping system, can turn your quarterly salary records into the tax reports that you are required to file, and can accompany you to a tax audit if your lucky number comes up in the IRS lottery.

---

5. Be sure to check out the additional examples and discussions about the advantages of live-in help in chapter ▢ 3, **"Live-in Aides and Other Residence Options."**

Chapter 21

Tax Obligations, Deductions, and Publications for PA Employers

In the United States, it is important to understand and fulfill your federal and state tax obligations when you directly employ PAs. These obligations include completing and filing reports about your employment of PAs, as well as computing and paying actual taxes. On a positive note, when you pay help provider salaries or health agency fees from your personal budget—without funding from an outside source—you are usually entitled to deduct a percentage of these costs as medical expenses from your income tax.

If you are like most of us, your reaction to reading the somewhat dry, boring title of this chapter has been one of concurrently feeling increased stress while your eyes glaze over! With these humanitarian concerns in mind, your author has written this chapter from the simplified perspective of his personal experience, plus advice from the pros.

The preceding chapter addressed different ways to pay salaries and how to keep salary records. This complementary text introduces you to using those salary records to meet your employer tax obligations—and take advantage of any tax deductions and credits to which you might be entitled.

The intentionally limited detail of this chapter does not provide step-by-step guides to paying employment taxes and realizing deductions. If this chapter tried to cover detailed IRS policy and legal interpretations, you would have out-dated information by the time this reference was printed and you obtained a copy.

Instead, the scope of this text provides you with a basic outline of PA-user concerns, as well as reference to a list of (usually) free and (sometimes) up-to-date IRS policies and interpretive publications. Most importantly, you will be given a strong recommendation to at least initially consult with a local accountant who knows your personal situation and can get you started.

This discussions, strategies, and references presented in this chapter will help you answer this question: *"What strategies should I follow, and what records should I maintain, for my personal way of employing PAs—so I can either do my own filings and payments, or provide adequate data to a CPA who does these for me?"*

Cautions about the information in this chapter

Please note that the topics of this chapter merely constitute an introduction to tax information about employing medical aides for personal needs. The information is intended only as a guideline and not as professional accounting or legal advice.

Before personally employing your own aides, you should obtain professional advice from a certified public accountant (CPA) or attorney about:

- How you intend to pay your aides—by a cash, non-cash, or combination salary

- How you are planning to set up your employment, salary, and tax records, including categories of gross salaries, employment taxes, and net salaries

- What employment forms and payments are due to the various federal and state agencies, and the scheduled due date for each

- How to calculate medical deductions, as they relate to your PA expenses, on your federal income tax forms

- Whether you, yourself, should be responsible for filing and paying these obligations in a timely manner, or you should contract a CPA to perform these tasks on your behalf

This chapter includes a list of free publications available from the U.S. Internal Revenue Service (IRS). Although free tax assistance and technical information are also available from the IRS, you are advised to consult with a CPA or tax preparer who is familiar with your personal situation. A CPA can advise you on the best financial strategy for paying your PAs, and on how to keep salary and tax records. This professional can also interpret IRS information for you, and will advise and accompany you through any IRS audit.

Tax differences in paying agency aides and personally employed aides

There are two ways to employ PAs, and each carries a different set of tax obligations. Either an agency employs them, or you employ them.

An agency employs the PAs you use

As discussed in the previous chapter, if you use agency-employed aides, you have no employer responsibilities. From a service point of view, the agency employs and provides its aides for your use. It claims to do its own recruiting, interviewing, screening, hiring, training, and managing so you will not have these concerns.

In keeping with this full-service concept, the agency handles all the employer and tax-related obligations for the help providers that it employs and provides. Help recipients, or their funding source, in turn receive comprehensive bills from the agency. The bottom-line total of these bills includes the salary paid to the aides, as well as costs of employment taxes and the agency's operating expenses.

If you, as the help recipient, pay the entire agency cost from personal resources, then these total agency costs are often eligible, as a medical deduction on your income tax. Since you are obligated to pay the end total of each agency bill, it is this total that might be eligible without regard to whether some cost lines are attributable to aide salaries and others to agency operating expenses.

What percentage of an eligible cost is actually deductible from your tax bill? That depends on your level of income and the total amount of medical expenses. If you are not familiar with the calculation of medical deductions, then check with a tax preparer or CPA.

In contrast, if you receive third-party funding for some or all of an agency's billing, the portion that is paid by outside funding cannot be eligible as a medical deduction. If payment for a cost did not come out of your pocket, you cannot deduct it.

> *If payment for a cost did not come out of your pocket, you cannot deduct it as a medical expense from your taxes.*

You employ the PAs you use

If you are able and willing to manage the PAs you use, then you might decide to employ them directly. When you directly employ PAs, you perform all the management tasks. You recruit, interview, screen, hire, train, supervise, pay, and terminate the PAs you use. The bad news is that you are also usually responsible for filing tax and employment documents, and paying taxes and fees. The good news about your personally employing and funding your own PAs is that this route is less expensive than using agency aides, and the costs are usually eligible as medical deductions from your income taxes.

These medical expenses can include the provider salaries as well as the related costs, such as newspaper advertising and accounting fees directly related to PA employment.

Again, in contrast, if you receive outside funding for any part or all of these costs, then the funded portion is not eligible as a medical deduction.

As you know from the previous chapter, when you personally employ your aides you can often choose whether you pay a cash, non-cash, or combination salary. The remainder of this chapter addresses tax obligations when you personally employ the PAs you use.

Two funding sources for paying the PAs you employ

When you directly employ the PAs you use, there are two primary funding sources. Either a third-party funding source pays your PAs, or you pay your PAs from your personal funds.

A third-party funding source pays your PAs

You might be eligible for funding from federal, state, or local agencies. The bottom line is that one of these parties agrees to partially or totally pay for your PAs.

The previous chapter, discussed three ways in which funding sources pay your PA expenses: the funding source pays your aides; the funding source pays you, and you pay your aides; or the funding source works through an agency. Within these three ways are two primary ways for you to receive the funds: the funding source gives you money for paying your PAs, or it pays them directly.

In a few cases the funder might decide to provide money to you; you deposit its checks into your private account, and then you pay your PAs. Avoid this situation if you can. Here, you are technically the employer who calculates PA salaries, writes them checks, and additionally is responsible for employment taxes. Because you are supplied with the funding, you might or might not be able to deduct salaries on your income tax as a medical expense. However. you might still have to pay employment taxes, so be sure to negotiate with the funding source about receiving additional funding to cover these additional costs.

In the second, more common third-party scenario, the funder pays your PAs directly. You supply the funding source with the names of your PAs, as well as weekly time sheets. The funding source then issues checks directly to the PAs. Here, you usually have no tax obligations because the source is "employing" (paying) your PAs; they calculate PAs' salaries, issue the paychecks, and should also be responsible for all employment tax documents and payments.

I have two pieces of advice when using this second procedure. First, confirm with the funding source that it will indeed be responsible for all employment tax issues. Second, if possible, arrange for the PA paychecks to be sent to you, so you can personally hand them to the PAs. This might seem to be a minor point, but the act of your handing checks to your PAs provides you with a significant image of authority. You can still maintain considerable authority and control without this procedure; however, it does bolster your image in some cases where it is needed.

You pay your PAs from personal funds: cash and non-cash salaries

There are three primary ways to pay the PAs you directly employ from personal funds: cash salaries, non-cash salaries, and a combination of the two.

As an employer paying cash salaries, you are responsible for:

- collecting PA time sheets
- calculating salaries and employment taxes
- writing paychecks
- keeping records of the salaries and employment taxes
- periodically filing federal and state employment tax forms
- paying employment taxes
- issuing employment tax summaries at the end of each year to employees and federal and state agencies
- maintaining records of these documents and payments in case of a tax audit.

As discussed in a previous chapter, a non-cash salary can include rent-free living space, services, material goods, or travel room, board, and transportation that you exchange with the PA for the help you receive. The calculation of how much of a commodity you offer should equate with the monetary value of the salary you would otherwise be paying.

Strictly speaking, the PA is receiving a non-cash income and you are paying a non-cash salary. The IRS might be interested in knowing about both transactions. Consulting an accountant is especially important in these situations. Your CPA can advise you on whether the value of the services you provide and the help you receive should be reported to the government, and how to maintain adequate records.

Two alternatives for filing and paying tax obligations

For either cash or non-cash salaries, there are good reasons why I will not attempt to provide how-to, step-by-step, detailed instructions for meeting tax responsibilities. Again, too many policies, interpretations, current calculation percentages, and payment due dates would become outdated too soon to provide you with a reliable, printed reference. Instead, the approach of this book for these areas is to list a bibliography of resources that you can research for the most recently revised and updated data. In addition, only you can best interpret these data to determine which are relevant to the specific way you employ help providers.

When it comes to your fulfilling your own employer tax responsibilities, quite simply, either you can do your own filings and payments, or you can hire an accountant to routinely do them for you.

The first route requires that you collect the appropriate IRS and state publications, study and map out the requirements for paying your PAs, and routinely file all the employment documents and payments on schedule. The IRS publications are available free by visiting IRS offices, by phone (check your local phone book in the section for United States Government), and through the Internet (www.IRS.gov). To answer your questions about the requirements cited in these documents, the IRS also provides free technical assistance at IRS offices; the locations include federal buildings and major post offices.

There is an alternative way to getting set up as a do-it-yourselfer. You might make a one-shot appointment with a local accountant, explain how you intend to employ PAs, and get your questions answered. For a nominal fee, your consultation with an accountant will usually get you a much more personalized prescription for a recordkeeping system than time spent with an IRS clerk. To get even more out of your CPA meeting, you might decide—in advance of the meeting—to gather several IRS publications as references. Your CPA will be able to mark these publications for the specific sections that pertain to employing your PAs. To get you started, at the end of this chapter is a glossary of employment terms and a list of IRS publications pertinent to your employing PAs in different situations.

The second route is to hire an accountant (CPA) to routinely perform the filings and payments for you. You would initially meet with the accountant, explain how you intend to employ your PAs, and decide with the accountant on a routine schedule and procedure for his or her processing of the salary data that you provide. The accountant will advise you on how to pay the salaries and keep records, as well as what details he or she needs in order to file your paperwork. The accountant fees for these services vary, and are usually quite reasonable. If you are either unable or unwilling to become your own tax pro, these services are essential. If you are a career professional who already hires a CPA to file your annual taxes, then simply use that same person for this additional service.

A glossary of tax terms

To help you further, here is a list of topics that are related to some, but not all, PA employment situations. You should have this list handy when researching IRS publications, or when consulting with an IRS technical assistant or your personal accountant.

- Social Security (FICA) and Medicare payments: FICA (Federal Insurance Contributions Act) payments are a percentage of each salary amount and made jointly from an employee and employer. As of this book's printing date, you would calculate a PAs gross pay (hours worked x hourly salary rate) and then deduct 7.65 percent. The result is the net pay, and this is the amount that you use for the PA's paycheck. In the previous chapter, the "summary spreadsheet" that is described will automatically perform these calculations and dollar displays for you. Throughout the year, you must carefully safeguard these deductions. At each year's end, you (or your CPA) must total these deductions from PA salaries and combine them with an equal amount from your own pocket. This double deduction of 15.3 percent of all gross salaries is sent to FICA authorities.

- FUTA and SUTA payments: These employer payments are made for federal and state unemployment taxes. You should consult your CPA regarding the applicable rates and filing deadlines.

- Income tax withholding: In some situations, an employer withholds a percentage of each salary as a contribution toward an employee's personal income taxes. Since you probably use your PAs primarily at home, you are termed a "household employer," and you are usually not required to withhold federal income tax from each PA paycheck. Be sure to tell your PAs that you are not withholding taxes although you do withhold FICA contributions. Your PAs will still be taxed on the salary income you pay them, and they might elect either to make voluntary quarterly payments on their own, or—if they have another job—they might ask their other (non-household) employer to make an extra deduction from their other paychecks.

- Identification numbers: To report taxes, pay taxes, and otherwise communicate with the government, employers need an EIN (employer identification number). Each employee must have a social security number.

- Medical deductions: As an employer, you might be able to deduct a portion of the PA salaries you pay—and related expenses, such as newspaper ads and accountant fees—as medical expenses on your personal income tax.

- Independent contractor: This is a category of employee within some professions. Common examples of independent contractors include architects, accountants, lawyers, carpenters, or painters. You pay these people and yet you are not responsible for any employment taxes. Why not your PAs? Nice try; however, independent contractor status can rarely be applied to any PA or any other employee whom you directly employ, train, and supervise.

- Household employee: The IRS defines this category of employee as "persons you hire to perform services in and about your private home." If someone qualifies as a household employee, they are exempt from some employment taxes. This status often applies to personally employed PAs, and makes your life easier as an employer.

- Family members as paid help providers: Under certain circumstances, paying a family member for PA work can exempt you from some tax requirements, and might provide you with some tax deductions or credits.

- Employment eligibility verification: This form (I-9) is obtained for each employee from the Immigration and Naturalization Service (INS) office of the Department of Justice. As each employee is hired, this one-page form must be completed and kept in your files. The form verifies that each employee is eligible to work in the United States. If you are ever audited by the INS or IRS, you must have a completed I-9 form for each previous PA whom you employed.

- Worker's compensation and disability insurance: PA employers are being increasingly required to provide worker's compensation (WC) insurance for their help providers. This is insurance that you purchase, like home or car insurance, from an insurance company. The WC regulations in some states allow PA employers to purchase a rider to their renter's or homeowner's insurance policy, whereas other states require purchase of a special WC policy. Consequently, the annual insurance cost of your WC requirement might range from $100 to more than $1,500.

IRS publications of interest to PA employers

Here is a partial listing of publications that are available free for the asking at most offices of the U.S. Internal Revenue Service. You might also be able to order them by phone; look in the phone book under U.S. Government. If you have an Internet connection, check for these publications and other resources at www.IRS.gov.

- "Guide to Free Tax Services"
- "Employer's Tax Guide – Circular E," Publication 15
- "Medical and Dental Expenses," Publication 502
- "Child and Dependent Care Expenses," Publication 503

- "Credit for the Elderly or the Disabled," Publication 524
- "Taxable and Nontaxable Income," Publication 525
- "Record keeping for Individuals," Publication 552
- "Tax Information for Older Americans," Publication 554
- "Taxpayers Starting a Business," Publication 583
- "Tax Highlights for Persons with Disabilities," Publication 907
- "Taxpayer's Guide to IRS Information, Assistance, and Publications," Publication 910
- "Employment Taxes for Household Employers," Publication 926
- "Employment Taxes: Employees Defined, Income Tax Withholding, Social Security Taxes (FICA), Federal Unemployment Tax (FUTA), and Reporting and Allocating Tips," Publication 937
- "Identification Numbers under ERISA," Publication 1004

Part VII

"I Understand How You Feel"—
Concerns Heard from You
as a Recipient, Family Caregiver,
or Paid Provider

Part VII

"I Understand How You Feel"– Concerns Heard from You as a Recipient, Family Caregiver, or Paid Provider

In Boulder, Colorado, the Peace Park hugs the curving shoreline of the scenic Boulder Creek. A small monument bears the inscription:

Peace Through Respect,
Respect Through Understanding

This reference book recognizes that there are three primary parties involved in the process of receiving and providing personal assistance: help recipients, family caregivers and other family members, and paid providers.

Although these participants share many common concerns, each also has unique, individual ones. Before being able or willing to provide help to another, each party must be mentally and physically strengthened by first satisfying his or her own needs. As other chapters have shown, when a caregiver or even paid provider is not sufficiently strong before attempting to assist another, premature fatigue and depression create needless crises that could have been avoided.

Of the strategies successfully used to avoid crises, two are perhaps paramount: careful advance planning and continually open communication. As you might have noted, a variety of topics dedicated to both strategies are discussed throughout this book.

The four chapters of Part VII focus—one by one—on opening and building communication and understanding among all three parties. Therapists and counselors often say that two of the most frequent complaints heard from clients in troubled relationships are founded in that client's belief that he or she is not being heard or understood.

"He never *listens* to me."

"She simply doesn't *understand* what I'm going through."

When these three parties enter into a relationship to provide years of daily, uninterrupted, personal assistance to a help recipient, their ability to hear and understand each other is essential. And, as pointed out earlier before one can be able or willing to hear or understand another, one must be accomplished at having heard and understood one's own concerns.

437

At first glance toward the "caregiving ball field," it would seem that the objective of the game is for two of the parties—the family caregivers and paid providers—to be united in providing assistance to the third, help recipient, party. However, in the opinion of more experienced providers and recipients, caregiving teams are most successful and longlasting when all three parties, including the designated help recipient, are equally engaged in providing and receiving assistance and support to each other.

More than three decades ago, when I first began receiving assistance from my own family caregiver, I quickly realized that with the family assistance I received also came family disagreements. No matter how many times I told her or how angry I became, my mother could not seem to hear how important it was for me to routinely get out of bed on a 6 A.M. schedule. Similarly, my 50-year-old mother could not get me to understand that she was becoming chronically exhausted from attempting to single-handedly accommodate an 18-year-old's fast-paced activity level.

As I struggled through more and more of these emotional exchanges, I became aware that each of us had valid concerns. Our attempts to communicate would continue to be unproductive—and, indeed, destructive to our relationship—as long as our ego-centered objective was to identify who was right and wrong. Instead, each of us could at least partially receive what we needed if we first heard and understood the other, and then worked toward mutually beneficial compromises.

With daily experiences of hearing, understanding, and analyzing exchanges with my mother, I got better at negotiating each individual compromise, in a sort of microcosmic approach. With time, I acquired a more comprehensive, macrocosmic understanding of the concerns and needs of help providers in general.

This "big-picture" understanding of help providers as a culture provided a couple of advantages. First, it was easier for me to understand and accommodate their opinions in individual situations. In addition, I was often able to predict their concerns and needs, thereby heading off potential misunderstandings. This provided me with a head start toward totally avoiding some misunderstandings and providing early accommodations.

I became convinced of the advantages of better understanding the culture of each type of provider who routinely helped me. Consequently, for years now, I have been taking notes on the recurring concerns and needs of help recipients, family caregivers, and paid providers. The notes for these chapters have come from personal experiences, interviews and counseling sessions, classroom observations, and literature reviews.

I encourage you, whether you are a help recipient, family caregiver, or paid provider, to read through the four chapters of this Part VII. First, you might begin by reviewing the sections that describe your own role, to better understand your own concerns. This might initially seem to be a waste of time, but you could consider these sections to be your peer support groups. These sections speak your language, have walked in your paths of experience, and might offer you some new advice for coping with old issues.

Second, you will be wise to review the chapters that address the concerns and needs of the other people in your life. Whether a recipient or provider, you are dependent on them, and you want them to care about what is important to you. The best way to get them to care about what is important to you is for you first to care about what is important to them. To do this, you could spend many months or years in observing and taking notes, or you can spend half an hour reviewing these chapters.

If you prove to them that you care enough to learn about their concerns, they will want to learn about yours. This is the mutual respect that is so important between recipients and providers.

Part VII consists of four chapters. Each chapter provides a specialized list. The first chapter lists human rights for help recipients, family caregivers, and paid help providers. The second and third chapters list common concerns of help recipients and caregivers. The fourth contains two lists for paid providers: ten reasons why providers quit their jobs, followed by ten reasons why they are often fired.

My original intention for the first part of each chapter was to provide the numbered list of items, followed by a discussion of each numbered item. However, it soon became obvious that the available space in this reference would not be large enough to house the detailed discussions that I had researched.

This book's next part, Part VIII, is my parting advice to you. These short chapters address topics that you would hear as I wrapped up a "how-to" seminar, workshop, or 16-week course. This is where you'll get some summary advice, after faithfully reading through the chapters of this reference; or some generic reassurance, because nothing seems to be working and you doubt you will have help to get into bed tonight. In yet a third instance, perhaps you are sitting in a bookstore and reviewing each of these introductory sections before deciding whether to purchase this book.

In any situation, pour yourself some herbal tea—or take this book to the store's espresso bar—and join me for these parting chapters!

Part VIII *Parting Advice for You*

Chapter 22

A Bill of Rights for You
as a Help Recipient, Caregiver, or Paid Provider

Regardless of your dependence on help from others, you have some very special rights. Your dependence should never make you feel subordinate to your help providers, with a mindset of "be not critical—but instead grateful—for whatever help you receive." Instead, you have a right to be in control of the quality of *help* you receive as well as the quality of *help providers*.

In return, and in fairness, the people who help you also have rights. They retain the right to put their own needs ahead of yours and should be encouraged to do so for their own health. Balance and coordination are required to respect the rights for each of you, while not compromising the what, when, and how of the dependable help you need.

This chapter is about identifying the rights that are inherent in the help recipient and provider. Consequently, each of you can feel assured about your own rights while respecting those of the other.

When rights are mutually respected, your relationship with help providers tends to be harmonious and reciprocal. In contrast, when parties get greedy about rights, the overall relationship becomes competitive, inflexible, and often angry. Contrary to the culture that predominates in military service, in which respect is demanded, the recipient-provider culture is one where respect should be earned.

This chapter has three sections: a three-way statement of overall humanitarian rights for you and your providers, and then two additional lists of more specific rights for each of you. These lists are original and appear here for the first time. I have compiled them over the years from many interviews. When asked to summarize the humanitarian wishes, needs, and intentions of help recipients and providers, I provide these lists.

Please note, due to space limitations in this book, that a detailed discussion of the needs and suggested remedies for each listed concern could not be included here, but is available in another of our publications.

A three-way statement of basic humanitarian rights

To introduce this chapter's theme, the following three-part section is the foundation for your right to determine your own lifestyle as well as to manage your help providers.

As the recipient of help, you have the humanitarian right to maintain your body in the ways that you prefer. You first have the right to choose to live or die, and then to pursue your choice with respect and dignity from both yourself and others.

With the objective to either live or die, you have the right to accommodate your body's functions and needs according to the methods and schedule that it requires—and you prefer—for your physical and mental health and safety. You have the right to control the quality of help you receive as well as the quality of help providers.

If you are unable to directly manage your help, your agent—usually a family caregiver or agency—has the obligation to represent your values and lifestyle choices as accurately as possible in directing the ways you receive assistance.

You have this right regardless of who provides you with assistance or where that assistance is provided. If you choose to live, and your physical or mental health and safety are being reduced because of how your help is provided or who provides the help, then you have the right to make necessary changes. In a similar way, if your right and desire to die are not being respected with dignity, then you also have the right to make necessary changes.

Caregivers and aides have the right to receive your respect, unless they fail to respect you and your rights.

These family caregivers and paid providers who help you are entitled to receive your appreciation for the help they provide you. When they care about your welfare, they are entitled to receive your caring about theirs. When they accommodate your limitations, they are entitled to have you accommodate theirs in appropriate ways you are able to do so. They have the right to set personal boundaries and limitations about the help they provide without feeling or receiving shame or guilt.

Help recipients and providers each have the right to consider their own needs first, and then to negotiate a working relationship so that each person's needs are reasonably accommodated.

Rights of help recipients

You, as a recipient of help, have the rights:

1 To employ an adequate number of PAs for several objectives: to meet your variety and schedule of needs, to provide for substitutes and backups, to reduce provider burnout and keep people longer, and to avoid a single PA from taking unfair advantage

2 To maintain ongoing control over the dependability and quality of help you receive

3 To identify your own needs for help, and to train PAs for what help you need, as well as how you prefer them to provide it

4 To schedule dependable and punctual help around your own daily lifestyle, and not primarily around that of your aides

5 To have your aides communicate in a clear, direct, assertive manner that is neither weakly passive nor abusively aggressive, and to be reasonably free of receiving any of their personal anger, stress, or depression

6 To receive personal respect and dignity as an individual who, regardless of physical impairments, has a mind that is fully capable of knowing your needs, making decisions, and managing the help that your body—and not mind—requires

7 To receive an employer's respect and appreciation from PAs, in return for your providing respect and appreciation to them

8 To receive confidentiality and privacy from PAs for your personal thoughts, values, beliefs, relationships, medical concerns, and activities, regardless of their unavoidable physical presence while they assist you

9 To security and safety for your living quarters, personal possessions, food, medications, and financial assets

10 To receive help from providers who are physically, cognitively, and emotionally able to perform the duties, who are not under the influence of alcohol and drugs and who are reasonably fast and efficient while working

Rights of help providers

You, as a provider of help, have the rights:

1 To initially receive a clear, well-defined set of routinely scheduled duties, and then to receive requests for additional duties or schedule changes as much in advance as possible

2 To work in an environment that is safe and secure, reasonably clean, logically and efficiently organized, and adequately stocked with supplies

3 To hear your instructions and other communications delivered in a clear, direct, and assertive manner that is neither weakly passive nor abusively aggressive

4 To work with a person who is reasonably happy, and lacks the anger, depression, and "bad attitude" that some other persons with disabilities routinely display

❺   To set reasonable limitations and boundaries on the type, amount, and schedule of work that you as an aide are willing to perform

❻   To receive personal confidentiality, respect, and dignity as a human being who has personal thoughts, values, beliefs, relationships, activities, and a personal life that are rightfully held in a higher priority than providing the help recipient with PA assistance

❼   To receive an employee's due respect and appreciation from the help recipient, in return for your providing respect and appreciation to him or her

❽   When you are on of several PAs employed by a common supervisor, to receive respect and fair treatment equally, across the board. The supervisor should not:

- favor one aide over another
- tolerate one PAs routinely leaving unfinished duties for the next PA to complete
- tolerate the poor performance and habits of uncaring aides who have bad attitudes, while unfairly expecting different standards from other, quality aides
- speak unfavorably about one PA to the others,
- shame, harshly reprimand, or otherwise embarrass one aide in the presence of others
- tolerate or contribute to gossip, favoritism, unfair advantages, inequitable salaries, or other inequalities or injustices

❾   To make genuine mistakes in performing tasks within a human (and not perfect) standard, to periodically forget parts of the job routine, to have reasonable physical and cognitive inabilities, and to have limits to personal stamina—in short, to be respected as a human and not be treated as a robot or slave

❿   To periodically take off-duty, vacation, and sick times, to receive relief or replacement help, and to resign with appropriate advance notice—and for the recipient of help to be responsible for providing the relief and replacement workers

Chapter 23
Your Personal Concerns as a Help Recipient

Most of this reference coaches you in ways to find quality help and keep it longer. Inherent in keeping providers longer is the ability to better understand their concerns and keep them happy. Indeed, much of this book provides strategies about your accommodating caregivers and aides, so they in turn can accommodate you.

However, as the help recipient, you also have concerns. Some are related directly to your disability. Others occur in your relationship with both family caregivers and paid, outside providers.

We have all read those sterile generic descriptions of sterile, disability concerns that we are supposed to have. These textbook fillers are often created by a psychologist who has interpreted theories. In contrast, the concerns in this chapter have come right from the source: 30-plus years of my personal experiences, as well as my discussions with your peers during interviews, one-to-one counseling, and the formal, 16-week courses in PA management skills that I have taught.

There are many advantages to experiencing, learning, and growing from the consequences of the daily, year-after-year lifestyle of having a disability. These concerns describe those recurring experiences with which we cope in a variety of ways. Initially, we experience and survive them. If a concern occurs repeatedly, we devise ways to prevent its future occurrence, or (if unavoidable) to minimize its negative effects. Each time we succeed, we feel stronger for having conquered "another one."

This list is specialized. The objective is to share concerns related to our limitations and the help we require from others to accommodate those limitations. These are also the topics we would like our able-bodied peers to hear firsthand from us, and to better understand. The secondary benefit is for us to better understand who we are; perhaps to provide a new understanding of an old concern that results in that "ah-ha" enlightenment of an epiphany.

Family caregivers, paid help providers, and help recipients should be familiar with each other's concerns. You all work together, and your relationships will be smoothest when you better understand each other's concerns. Each of you might be surprised to learn how many concerns you have in common, though sometimes they come with slightly different labels.

In addition, if you have a disability, and would enjoy reading a list of "me, too" concerns, this chapter has been researched and written for you.[1]

Please note that space limitations in this reference book made it impossible to include a detailed discussion of the needs and suggested remedies associated with each listed concern here. However, this is an important topic, these discussions do appear in a separate publication also available from Saratoga Access Publications.

I invite you to share your own favorites, if they are missing here. You might therapeutically benefit from the journaling experience of recording them, and your peers will benefit when they appear in future editions of this reference. Please see the later section, which requests your advice, for details about where to send your contributions.

Your personal concerns as a help recipient

❶   I feel depressed about not being physically able to do as many things as my able-bodied friends can do, or that I was able to do before my disability.

❷   In addition to feeling sad about not being able to do many activities, I feel depressed and embarrassed about being so physically dependent upon asking—begging—other people for help.

❸   I especially feel like a burden when I have to ask for help from family caregivers, because I know that they are often tired, tight on personal time, or just dislike providing me with help.

❹   In addition to my feeling like a physical burden to my family caregivers, I feel like a financial burden because of the costs of my hired aides, medical supplies, and other expenses of maintaining my disability.

❺   I feel angry when outside, hired aides unavoidably intrude on my family or marital privacy.

❻   I get tired from all the basic energy and effort that I spend in managing my help providers, as well as special health needs and disability equipment.

❼   In addition to all the basic, essential energy and effort that I spend in managing my disability, I get really angry at the extra, unnecessary work that I am often caused by careless, lazy, and negligent people. Why can't family caregivers or paid PAs simply assume my responsibilities?

❽   I worry as I get older, and my dependence on help providers increases, that my energy and mental sharpness required to manage that help will decrease or fail.

❾   In addition to losing my mental sharpness for managing help providers, I also worry about losing my ability to think clearly for problem solving, managing my needs, and staying in control of my quality of life.

---

1. Please be reminded that there are two other lists in these parallel chapters: 📖 24, "Your Personal Concerns as a Family Caregiver," and 📖 25, "Your Personal Concerns as a Paid Help Provider, plus Ten Reasons Why PAs Quit and Are Fired."

⑩ I am afraid of losing the human resources that provide me with help; namely, my unpaid family caregivers, as well as the paid outside aides whom I know so well.

⑪ Even after years of hiring aides and seeing each one eventually resign, I still often get depressed when it is time to part ways.

⑫ Sometimes I am afraid, for my safety and possessions, to schedule aide applicants—complete strangers—to come into my place for an interview and demo.

⑬ As the years of hiring new aides go on and on, it seems to take me a longer time to trust and become comfortable with each new help provider. Why should I bother to get to know each one?

⑭ I get angry when an aide applicant who schedules an interview chooses not to show up, and also chooses not to call to cancel.

⑮ When I first came home from the hospital, my family and friends were so happy to see me and help me. Since then, I have been disappointed to see their attitude toward me change so much. I no longer feel welcome—I feel like a burden.

⑯ I get frustrated when I state my needs to providers and somehow they either do not understand what I need (although they smile and nod like they do), or they complain that I have a bad, angry attitude.

⑰ I worry about being assertive with my sole PA concerning the help I need, because I do not want him or her to get angry with me and suddenly quit.

⑱ I get frustrated and angry during hospital stays when (especially) nurses and aides accuse me of being too demanding, too detailed, or just having a bad attitude when I ask that they:

- provide me with help in personal, quite specific ways

- keep certain items in my hospital room organized and located in specific places where I can reach them

- assign me, as staffing permits, the same nurses and aides for my personal help on subsequent days.

⑲ It bothers me that I have PR and management responsibilities, and I usually have to appear to be happy whenever I am with an aide, regardless of how I really feel.

⑳ I am having a hard time deciding between the privacy of living alone with a degree of insecurity, and the security of living with an apartment/house mate without as much privacy.

㉑ I feel like I have been abandoned by my family and have lost control of my lifestyle and preferences. Instead of greeting my own family, I see an endless stream of uncaring health providers.

Chapter 24
Your Personal Concerns as a Family Caregiver

As a family caregiver, your own personal concerns are equally important to the disability needs of your loved one. Why? In contrast to him or her, there are *two* people dependent upon your well-being: you and the help recipient!

Unpaid, family caregivers are among the most generous, warm-hearted people anywhere. Most help recipients with long-term disabilities use a combination of family caregivers and paid, outside providers. It is not uncommon for a help recipient to think back several years to his first caregiver as the quality standard to whom all paid providers have been compared.

Many of their role-model qualities are due to their unlimited caring and commitment. These prompt their exemplary attention to detail, quality methods, and memory for the schedule of when periodic maintenance items should automatically be done.

Unfortunately inherent in their donation of seemingly limitless time and taking on of such comprehensive responsibilities are the negative consequences of chronic fatigue, sacrifices of personal and spiritual activities, and a high incidence of burnout and depression.

Typically, when a loved one comes home with a long-term disability, family members drop their own priorities to provide whatever help the recipient needs, whenever it is needed. The hope and intention are that after the help recipient's needs settle into a routine schedule, the care providers will be able to reclaim their own time and needs.

It is rare that the caregiver's day ever returns. The help recipient develops more and more needs, and the caregivers find it harder and harder to set limits on what they can and cannot do.

When the family caregiver and help recipient are out in public together, the caregiver too often becomes invisible, as family friends focus on how well the recipient is doing. The caregiver stands quietly off to one side and can think only about the caregiver help she now provides. So often, there is no longer time, energy, or financial resources for anything else. Her law studies have been put on hold, she hasn't sufficient time or energy for working out at the club any longer, and she finds it hard to think of herself as romantic or attractive anymore.

She is now solely a caregiver, one of the most honorable positions that too few people sufficiently understand. The irony is that the caregiver now needs help as much as the help recipient.

The following lists of frequent concerns have been compiled from one-on-one discussions as well as round table workshops involving many caregivers of both sexes and a wide range of ages.

Family caregivers, paid help providers, and help recipients should be familiar with each other's concerns. You all work together, and your relationships will be smoothest when you better understand each other's concerns. Read through these lists, and be reassured that you are not alone with your concerns. Literally, millions of other family caregivers have many of the same feelings and concerns as you.

Please be reminded that there are two other lists in parallel chapters.[1]

Space limitations in this reference book made it impossible to include a detailed discussion of the needs and suggested remedies associated with each listed concern here. However, this is an important topic, and these discussions do appear in a separate publication also available from Saratoga Access Publications.

Your personal concerns as a family caregiver

❶ My caregiver tasks and time requirements are increasing, my fatigue, stress, and depression are increasing, and I would like to know about my options for getting some relief—and then learn how to accept that help.

❷ I resent some recipient requests that seem to be unnecessary.

❸ I need to set some personal limits and boundaries on whether I continue to provide caregiver help, as well as within what conditions. I also realize that I might initially feel guilty about doing so.

❹ I need some relief help, but I worry about hurting the help recipient's feelings.

❺ I need some relief help, but I worry about appearing to be selfish and uncaring to my family and friends.

❻ I need some relief help, but I doubt that the quality of anyone else's work will equal mine—or even be adequate. I can't seem to let go of my responsibilities and entrust them to someone else.

❼ I need medical help for my physical illnesses as well as psychological counseling for my stress, chronic fatigue, burnout, depression, and grieving over so many sources of loss.

❽ I need some peer support—other caregivers who can listen and understand.

❾ I feel overwhelmed by my personal, family, and caregiver concerns, and I need a professional who can help me coordinate them all.

---

1. 📖 23 "Your Personal Concerns as a Help Recipient" and 📖 25 "Your Personal Concerns as a Paid Help Provider, plus Ten Reasons Why PAs Quit and Are Fired."

10. I feel responsible for providing the best possible care to the recipient, and therefore I feel liable if the recipient is not healthy and happy.

11. I feel hurt and angry when the help recipient and I appear together in public and people ask about his welfare while ignoring mine.

12. I feel sad that my identity and sense of worth are now completely centered around my caregiver role.

13. I feel that I am no longer an attractive person and romantic spouse, but only a working caregiver.

14. Why am I the only faithful backup to outside relief help?

15. I have lost my space and privacy within our home.

16. The costs of relief help are sometimes not worth the benefits.

17. I miss the joy of vacations—they have become too much work and expense.

18. I no longer enjoy being around the recipient of my help because she is so angry and stressed.

19. I really do need relief help now, in case something happens to me as the only caregiver.

20. On a positive note, I feel comforted when I read of, or remember, the side benefits to my being a dedicated family caregiver.

21. I need some relief help, and I—as well as several other types of caregivers— need advice about how to recruit, hire, train, and manage the providers.

22. I wish medical and disability-related equipment were better designed and easier to use.

23. I wish there were health and disability insurance programs that were specially designed—with discounted premiums—to meet the special concerns of family caregivers.

24. I wish there could be some tax relief for the respite and day-care services that both my help recipient and I require.

Chapter 25

Your Personal Concerns as a Paid Help Provider, plus Ten Reasons Why PAs Quit and Are Fired

As a paid help provider, you might work at a health care facility, and provide assistance to inpatients who reside there. You might work for an agency, and be assigned to work at health care facilities or private homes. As a third alternative, you might prefer working directly for private clients.

In your career, you have probably worked in all three situations, and know the advantages and disadvantages of each. Consequently, your provider concerns are different from those expressed by unpaid, family caregivers. You have often wanted to compare notes with help recipients, family caregivers, agency or facility supervisors, and your paid, professional peers.

The first section of this chapter enables you to do just that, with its list of typical personal concerns for paid help providers. This list will help you, as well as the family caregivers and help recipients with whom you work, better understand your own concerns.[1]

In addition, if you are a salaried help provider, you want to keep each good job as long as possible. You want to avoid being fired. If you are often "let go" from working in a nice home with a help recipient you like, or you are frequently transferred from one agency or facility to another, then you would probably like to know why. It is entirely possible that a disagreeable personal habit or work style has repeatedly been the cause. In contrast, if you are proud of being told you exemplify the habits of a model provider, you probably want to avoid any chance of unknowingly developing bad habits.

---

1. In addition, you can refer to their chapters to better understand them: 📖 23, "Your Personal Concerns as a Help Recipient," and 📖 24, "Your Personal Concerns as a Family Caregiver."

From a different viewpoint, if you are a help recipient or PA manager, you understandably want to hire quality aides and then keep this trained help as long as possible. You want to avoid unnecessary resignations from help providers. Although each aide whom you manage or employ will eventually resign, you work to minimize the chances that an unfavorable personal or management trait of yours is the recurring reason for the resignations.

Both employers who fire employees and salaried employees who quit jobs have at least one thing in common: they usually avoid expressing the true reason for their actions. People who fire employees as well as those who resign from jobs all want to avoid conflicts and lawsuits. They want to accomplish their objectives as easily and quickly as possible and go on with life. Consequently, both populations provide vague, impersonal, uninformative reasons for their actions.

Whether you are a salaried aide who is frequently fired, or a help recipient who frequently loses good-quality aides through resignation, how can you uncover the reason(s) if no one will tell you? How many times must this happen before reasons become self-evident and you can improve your style? How many months (years?) might this take?

Wouldn't it be nice if there were a quick-and-easy reference list available to advise you about which unfavorable personal habits and work traits most often cause problems? You could look through the list, identify any habits or traits that apply to you, change your ways, and reduce your future losses!

Well, wish no more. This chapter has the inside scoop that you need now, or will need in the future.

You can be a better paid help provider, or a better help recipient and employer, if you understand and respect concerns, as well as your personal concerns, the reasons why aides quit their jobs, and the reasons why employers sometimes must fire them.

You would be wise to review your personal concerns, and then both lists of why help providers quit and why they are fired. From the "why quit" list, become familiar with problems that have occurred for others, and will probably also happen for you. As a paid provider, whether employed by a help recipient or an agency, you should know what other aides often dislike about their jobs. You have rights regardless of how you are employed. You always have the right to request improvements in poor working conditions or, if your requests fail, to quit!

From the "why fired" list, know that these are situations that aide managers most commonly find intolerable. Quite simply, avoid adopting any of these traits while performing your duties. If you develop similar habits, your manager should first try to work through the problems with you. However, if your bad habits continue, you could be dismissed for good reason.

In this chapter, there are three lists:

- Your personal concerns as a paid help provider
- Reasons why paid help providers quit their jobs
- Reasons why paid help providers are fired.

Although these are not exhaustive lists, they do represent the most common personal concerns and frequently occurring reasons for employment changes. If you spot any significant omissions from any list, please take a moment and pass them along to me. They will be included in the next edition of this reference.

Please note that space limitations in this reference book made it impossible to include a detailed discussion of the needs and suggested remedies associated with each listed concern here. However, this is an important topic, and these discussions do appear in a separate publication also available from Saratoga Access Publications.

Your personal concerns as a paid help provider

❶ We see our job as a lifetime career, and it hurts that most agencies and health care facilities treat us as only temporary, part-time workers. More of us should be offered the full-time positions, salaries, and benefits that nurses get.

❷ Even some of our at-home patients and clients fail to respect us as professional medical providers. Their lack of respect is evident by the names they call us, the bottom-level tasks they purposely reserve or even create for us, and the sexist ways they treat us. These things never happen when our nursing supervisor comes with us.

❸ I love most of my patients, and that is why I get so angry at the agency, facility, and insurance regulations and policies that too often limit what I can do, as well as how much time I can spend.

❹ I feel that CNAs get the assignments that nurses don't want. Doctors give directives to nurses, nurses fulfill some of the tasks, and then they assign us whatever they don't want to do. This often happens when I am contracted by my agency to work briefly at a health care facility.

❺ I believe that our agency and hospital supervisors have little regard for our working conditions. Nurses have national unions and professional associations; however, we lack that bargaining power because no one represents our rights and concerns.

❻ I feel it is not fair that many agencies and facilities offer health and disability insurance benefits only to full-time employees, and then offer aides only part-time positions. Either offer us full-time positions, or offer us insurance with partially paid premiums for part-time workers. Aides are given the most hazardous tasks while getting the worst insurance coverage.

❼ I wish medical and disability-related equipment were better designed, safer, and easier to use.

❽ I love providing help to most of my patients and clients. It hurts me to see that so many of them cannot afford—and do not have insurance for—an adequate amount of help, or to receive that help in a clean, quality facility. We caring aides feel the effects of help recipients being denied the services and facilities they require.

⑨ For the most part, I wish we had better agency and facility supervisors and administrators. Too few of these people have the professional skills required for hiring and then retaining quality aides. These lazy supers hire anyone who applies, they unfairly practice favoritism to retain this low-quality help, and the patients receive poor-quality services. Too often, it is us—the quality aides—who resign because of this intolerable situation.

⑩ Those of us who work in communities for agencies wish that home visits were more carefully assigned. Agencies assign us to a series of home visits each day without much regard for the distance or travel time between sites, the dangerous neighborhoods where we have late-night assignments, or the agency refusal to reimburse us for mileage.

Reasons why paid help providers quit their jobs

❶ They receive an incomplete list of duties or instructions on being hired, and become frustrated as unexpected duties are added.

❷ The step-by-step order and methods for performing duties are not logical, and waste the time and effort of the PA.

❸ Their work area is unpleasant and frustrating because it is disorganized and dirty, or lacks adequate supplies.

❹ They perform high-quality work, but are not paid a sufficient monetary salary, and their supervisor fails to routinely express appreciation for their work.

❺ When more than one PA is employed, the supervisor:

- obviously favors one over another

- tolerates one PA routinely leaving unfinished duties for the next PA to complete

- tolerates the poor performance and habits of uncaring aides with bad attitudes, while unfairly expecting different standards from other, quality aides,

- speaks unfavorably about one PA's to the others

- shames, harshly reprimands, or otherwise tries to embarrass one aide in the presence of others

- tolerates or contributes to gossip, favoritism, unfair advantages, inequitable salaries, or other injustices.

❻ Their supervisor is angry, stressed, aggressive, and in general has a bad attitude.

❼ Their supervisor is dishonest regarding the PA's possessions, time worked, or salary owed, or has hidden expectations of the PA, such as unstated duties, extra work hours, sexual favors, or loans of money or possessions.

❽ The help recipient is abusive, unreasonable, and stressful in demanding that duties be performed that are inappropriate because:

- the help recipient could easily perform certain duties for himself, and should not be requesting PA help

- certain duties are not appropriate for the PA to perform

- there are too many duties for a specific period of work time (or not enough aides to do the work), and the duties must be performed with unnecessary speed, urgency, and stress

- the duties are to be performed in ways that are too detailed and exacting, without a good reason

- the duties are being performed under unnecessarily tight, stressful control, and supervision.

⑨ Their supervisor is intolerant of their making honest mistakes and having true inabilities, occasionally forgetting details, being unable to physically perform certain duties, or needing occasional sick or personal time off from duties.

⑩ Their supervisor fails to respect the aide's personal life, rights, time, or other concerns by assuming or demanding that job responsibilities and schedules take priority over the aide's personal life.

⑪ The aides or personal care providers are frustrated at the limitations imposed on them by agencies—types of care, time allotments, poor salary and benefits, and a lack of voice in policy decisions.

Reasons why paid help providers are fired

❶ Providers become undependable and uncaring about it. In contrast to the dependable, punctual, and conscientious people who were originally hired, these PAs begin arriving late for work without calling ahead, their sick days become frequent, and they routinely want to leave early. Overall, they seem not to care about the negative consequences of these habits for the help recipient or employer.

❷ They are not reasonably clean and professional in personal hygiene, clothing, language, or habits.

❸ They jeopardize the safety or health of the help recipient by

- performing a poor quality of work

- not observing the safe procedural methods requested by their employer;

- becoming physically or verbally abusive

- working while smoking or under the influence of drugs, medications, or alcohol.

❹ They have lost their previous sense of interest and efficiency, and are now physically, cognitively, or emotionally unable to perform some duties, or have become unreasonably slow or lazy while working.

❺ They are dishonest with the employer's work time, possessions, finances, medications, or food. In addition, they may be similarly dishonest with fellow PA employees by routinely not completing assigned duties and purposely leaving them for completion by the PA who has the following work shift.

6   They have a bad attitude, which can range from being subtly unfriendly to obviously arrogant or abusive toward the help recipient. They also fail to assertively communicate in a clear, direct, and pleasant manner. Instead, the aide is either weakly passive or abusively aggressive, and becomes angry when discussing standard needs, special needs, changes in duties or schedule, opinions, preferences, or feelings. The PA routinely mumbles partial communications while avoiding eye contact—classic symptoms of not wanting to be working at that job.

7   They have lost interest in performing the work according to the methods and schedule the employer requires and to which they originally agreed. They routinely show this declining interest by—

   • working slowly or sporadically with many rest periods and being easily distracted from work by TV, magazines, or phone calls

   • at other times, rushing to accomplish job duties as quickly as possible, with details left unfinished, in an attempt to leave before the scheduled departure time

   • having very little interest or pride in performing high-quality work or in meeting the help recipient's special preferences

   • having a declining interest in the help recipient as an individual, and seldom initiating and often refusing to participate in friendly discussion

   • saying little beyond a mumbled "See ya...," when leaving a work shift and seeming to be bothered by the painful thought of the next scheduled arrival for work.

8   PAs lack respect for the employer's and help recipient's rights and their need for confidentiality and privacy with regard to personal preferences, opinions, feelings, problems, values, beliefs, relationships, and activities.

9   They have an inappropriate attitude toward people with disabilities and lack respect for the employer or help recipient as an intelligent, decision-making person.

10   They try to take control of the employer's or help recipient's right to make decisions regarding:

   • the selection and number of employed PAs

   • the choice and schedule of specific duties to be performed

   • the preferred methods for performance of those duties

   • the quality and dependability of assistance that is required.

Part VIII

Parting Advice for You

459

Part VIII

Parting Advice for You

These four final chapters cover topics that you would hear if you were wrapping up one of my seminars, workshops, or 16-week courses.

Of the dozens or hundreds of help providers who assist you, some will have a contagious disease, the HIV virus, or symptoms of AIDS. Some of these PAs will know about their condition and some will not yet know. Of those who know, few will inform you. Indeed, perhaps you are a carrier yourself and have been thinking about the stance you will take with your providers: Will you inform them or not? The first chapter of this Part VIII helps you make those decisions about whether disclosure—by you or your providers—is important. What you will discover in chapter 📖 **26 "When You or Your Help Provider Has—or Might Have—AIDS"** is that identification and disclosure are not as important as adopting the healthful habits of common-sense self-protection.

The next chapter, 📖 **27 "Medical Monitoring Services: Your Push-Button Lifesaver,"** discusses the high-tech, in-home monitoring services that can be as useful to "twenty somethings" as they are to seniors. If you live at home, and feel unsafe when your PAs are not around, then a monitoring service might be beneficial. For many help recipients who are vulnerable to falls or sudden health crises, these push-button services can safeguard your privacy of living alone while providing the peace of mind that comes from being able to summon help when you need it.

Help providers unavoidably know a lot about your values, concerns, and problems, but you are still entitled to maintain your privacy. Chapter 📖 **28 "Your Discretion, Privacy, and Confidentiality,"** provides you with strategies for ensuring that what PAs overhear and learn while at your house will stay there.

Throughout this reference, you have reviewed the many hats you wear as you periodically run through the RISHTMP cycle of recruiting, interviewing, screening, hiring, training, managing, and parting ways with your help providers. These PAs come in all shapes, sizes, and capacities. Some barely have the abilities and desires to remember steps of basic tasks for getting the job done. In sharp contrast, others have the mega capacity of thoroughly learning your routine, analyzing what you tell them, and making constructive suggestions for improvements. Chapter 📖 **29 "Your Educational Role and Objectives..."** discusses the different roles you find yourself assuming with different providers. For those with only a double-digit IQ, you can only direct; for the average PA, you perform a higher role of teaching; and for a select few, you are an educator.

Chapter 26

When You or Your Help Provider Has—or Might Have—AIDS

Regrettably, a steadily increasing population of both help recipients and providers has the HIV virus or AIDS. This section is not about identifying the symptoms or what precautions to take. The symptoms and precautions are well documented in other information sources.

Instead, this chapter addresses a more difficult philosophical question of whether a party with AIDS should inform the other of the presence of the virus or condition.

The decision about "tell or don't tell" is highly individualized, based primarily on each person's ethics as well as practical experience. Consequently, we will discuss three approaches, which we will term *full disclosure, assured protection* (for someone else), and *self-protection*.

The *full disclosure approach* dictates that the help recipient or provider who is infected with the HIV virus has a moral obligation to fully inform the other party about the infection. Furthermore, proponents insist that this disclosure should take place at an early stage, such as a job interview, before an employment commitment is made or any possibly infectious physical contact can occur.

After the infected party informs the other, and assuming the other party is still willing to work with the former, it is usually the infected person's responsibility to provide a full list of necessary procedural precautions. The two parties next discuss who will assume the financial cost of providing the precautionary supplies (rubber gloves and any other equipment).

Within what might be termed the *assured protection approach,* the infected party does not believe it has an obligation to inform the other. However, in return for maintaining one's right to privacy, the infected person secretly assures ongoing protection to the uninfected party. He or she privately agrees to assume the complete responsibility and cost for assuring that the uninfected party will constantly be protected.

The third approach is one of *self-protection,* where people simply take common-sense precautions to protect themselves against everything from a common cold to full-blown AIDS. This is the approach that has been already mandated by U.S. federal law for health professionals who come in contact with the bodily fluids and waste of patients. This is why physicians, dentists, nurses, nursing assistants, and phlebotomists ("phlebes" or technicians who draw venous blood) usually wear protective gloves and facial masks.

This set of federal precautions was implemented more than a decade ago to protect both health professional and patient from both known and unknown contagious infections. The protection is in place for all three instances of infection:

- A professional or patient knows he or she is infected and possibly contagious, and decides to disclose the infection to other parties and then practice precautions

- A professional or patient knows he or she is infected, and decides to practice precautions but sees no need to disclose

- A professional or patient does not know whether he or she—or the other party—is infected, and disclosure is not an applicable topic.

So, why shouldn't persons who know they are infected and possibly contagious— whether help recipient or provider—be morally required to disclose their status? It would seem that everyone who came in contact with those infected, labeled people would clearly know the identity of the contagious disease and be best equipped to take precautions.

If the only reaction of an informed public were its adoption of appropriate precautions, it would seem logical to require knowing carriers to publicly disclose their condition. However, experience has proven that perhaps the majority of an informed public takes additional action toward carriers who disclose. They too often additionally avoid, discriminate against, and even attempt to banish known carriers.

Proponents of the *full disclosure approach* indeed include both those who fear acquiring a contagious disease and those who already have one. The rationale for the "have nots" to promote disclosure is obvious. They usually want to avoid the disease as well as the person carrying it. In addition, there is sometimes a self-righteous desire to assign blame to—and often punish—the infected person for the inappropriate activity that resulted in the infection.

Ironically, the rationale for those who are infected to promote full disclosure for themselves is often due to the discrimination they have experienced from others in the past, and want to avoid in the future. A quadriplegic help recipient with AIDS related this personal story to me.

"I have been HIV-positive for several years while being fortunate to be able to hide most outward manifestations to the help providers I employ. My initial strategy was to keep my infection a secret. However, when PAs did find out I had AIDS, they sometimes became furious and a couple of times walked out the door.

> *"Now, instead, I insist on self-disclosing at the initial interview stage. It is true that most PA applicants still categorically fear AIDS and anyone who has it. Most of the applicants politely disqualify themselves or find another job. However, for the minority to whom I disclose and who still want to work with me, I can rest assured that I will be accepted for who I am. These PAs know about my darkest side and still want to work with me. I am choosing not to hide my headline news, and it is a big relief to be able to discuss my personal concerns without the fear of repercussion."*

To summarize, let's cite our primary objective. Is the full disclosure approach important for its function of identifying who has AIDS and how they acquired it? Or, instead, are we more concerned with the other two approaches, for their protection against the spread of this and other contagious diseases?

In the interest of containing these diseases, the other two approaches of assured protection and self-protection seem to make more sense. With the assured protection path, those who knowingly have a contagious infection routinely take precautions so others will not catch it. This is nothing new. If you know you have a common cold, you respect others by taking steps to prevent their catching it from you.

Within the third avenue of self-protection, each person takes common-sense precautions to protect themselves and others from catching any infection—or that common cold—they may sporadically encounter. There is no need to know who is and is not infectious, especially since this absolute identification is impossible.

It might seem that someone who is taking precautions within the self-protection route, and asking PAs to put on gloves before applying antibiotic ointment to an open skin burn, might be worried about being mistaken for an HIV or AIDS carrier. However, there are many other reasons for asking a PA to "glove up" before treating an open wound.

One of those reasons reminds me of a story.

> *One evening, several years ago, I answered the phone to speak with a very concerned mother of a recently injured quad in a wheelchair. Her son, Gary, would soon head out to begin his freshman year at a college campus. He was planning to live in a campus residence hall and hire fellow students as PAs.*
>
> *She quizzed me about a long list of questions regarding how to recruit, hire, and manage college-student PAs. The last question addressed Gary's bowel routine. Gary's routine began with transferring from wheelchair to commode chair, getting undressed, and then being wheeled over the toilet. His PA then would use a combination of suppositories and digital stimulation to get things moving.*
>
> *This phone call occurred within a year or so of initial lectures from the medical world that taught us how the HIV virus and AIDS were contracted. As Gary's mom came to the end of her well-planned "how-to" questions, it became obvious that she was embarrassed about some part of this final topic.*

She had conceptually heard that the HIV virus could be contracted by unprotected anal sex. She knew that Gary's help providers usually would be male. In an indirect way, she was vaguely concerned that if Gary's male PAs provided his anal suppositories and digital stimulation without the precaution of wearing rubber gloves, Gary might contract infection!?!

I realized that my role was not to educate her in the difference between engaging in anal sex without using a condom and conducting a bowel routine without using a rubber glove. Instead, I assured her that of all the details Gary and his various help providers might occasionally forget, I could assure her—from personal experience—that forgetting to have Gary's PA wear a rubber glove during his bowel routine would probably never become a problem. I assured her that this was one detail that would always be remembered! Gary's mother was very relieved.

I am not concerned that any of my PAs might knowingly or unknowingly carry any contagious disease. Why? I have made a routine habit of taking self-protection precautions for my own health and that of my providers.

My health insurance policy provides non-sterile rubber gloves for reasons of general hygiene and disease protection. If AIDS did not exist, I would still equip my PAs with gloves for bowel routines, dressing of more serious wounds, and changes of my indwelling catheter. AIDS or no AIDS, these self-protection precautions still make sense.

As help recipients who will come in contact with dozens or hundreds of help providers, we will undoubtedly be assisted by people who knowingly or unknowingly carry contagious diseases. Instead of spending largely wasted effort in attempting to identify them, let's adopt the common-sense habits of self-protection. As a foundation of self-protection, everyone should know and use the basic precautions for preventing infection.

Chapter 27
Medical Monitoring Services:
Your Push-Button Lifesaver

Whether you and your car have broken down while exploring 120-degree Death Valley, or you have tumbled out of your chair in your air-conditioned home, your continuous ability to communicate is essential to your survival. *Continuous* means "wherever and whenever" you are: in bed, in the shower, out in your backyard, wheeling along a hiking trail, driving along a mountain top, or fumbling for your keys in a dark, downtown parking garage after closing a bar at 2 A.M.

If this means wearing a cell phone, get the best you can afford—perhaps with voice activation. Clip it to your belt so it will be within reach if you are suddenly on the floor; it will be worthless in your backpack if you can't reach it.

If there might be times when punching cell phone buttons won't be possible—as we quads well know from experience—then get a subscription call service for around the house.

You've seen them advertised in senior citizen magazines. The grey-haired grandfather or grandmother pictured in the ad is wearing a necklace or wristband that contains a push-button transmitter. The emotion-packed caption under the photo says, "My Med Access communicator gives me instant help—and peace of mind—in any emergency. Now, I seldom worry about my heart condition."

Is this a product only for seniors, or should "twenty somethings" who have certain disabilities also give its merits careful consideration? Is this type of product truly a potential lifesaver that can contribute to prolonging personal privacy and independence, or is it instead an electronic Big Brother monitor of the type predicted in the novel *1984*?

The question for this chapter is, "When should you consider a medical alert monitor?" As your author, I was in my forties and totally opposed—until a couple of personal experiences changed my stubborn mind.

I can comfortably categorize myself as among the most active and independent C 5/6 quads (tetras). My morning PA pops through my front door at six, and by seven-thirty I am in my van and heading down the road toward a cafeteria breakfast, my downtown office, and a full day of appointments. I am on my own all day until meeting up with my evening aide around eight o'clock.

During those times when I am at home, I am reasonably careful about my health and safety. My at-home safety record was unblemished until nine years ago. It was a typical Saturday afternoon around two-thirty, and I was wheeling down a hallway toward my bathroom when the joystick box on my motorized chair caught on the edge of a door jamb. The chair stopped abruptly, but I did not. My out-of-balance shoulders arched forward over my hips and knees. When the split-second action stopped, I was still seated in the chair, but I was bent over at the hips. My shoulders rested on my knees, my head was between my knees, and I was unable to return myself to a "full upright position."

Within a few minutes, my breathing became restricted and my face began to swell. I was living alone, and the next person scheduled to see me would be my eight o'clock PA. That was more than five hours away. I was in serious trouble.

To make a five-hour story much shorter, I knew that if I panicked and started gasping for air I would not survive. So, I summoned all the mental discipline and will power I had learned and turned my metabolism w-a-y d-o-w-n. My breathing became very shallow and I voluntarily entered a semi-conscious state. The house gradually became darker as the sun set, and my eight o'clock aide arrived and helped me sit upright again.

I was very fortunate to have survived, and was very successful in preventing any type of recurrence—until five years later.

> *A medical monitoring service might enable you to stay at home, maintain your privacy, and avoid hiring live-in help.*

On a Sunday afternoon, while editing this reference book on my iMac, I leaned toward my right to reach something on the desk. For whatever reason, I lost my sitting balance and fell over the right armrest of my wheelchair. Again unable to sit myself upright, I remained bent sideways over the side of my chair for the next six hours.

My PA found me unconscious, with my face and head very swollen. She and a neighbor got me to the hospital's ER. Four days later, when I regained consciousness, doctors informed me that I had temporarily succumbed to cranial edema. They also informed me that I was—a second time—very fortunate to have recovered.

As I was being discharged on the fifth day, a hospital case manager brought me the flyer for a company that provides "personal response services (PRS)." I had been fortunate to survive two nearly fatal accidents. Within my first 24 hours back at home, I had subscribed to the monitoring service, and I have faithfully worn their wristband transmitter ever since.

In each accident situation, I was initially clear thinking and well coordinated. However, my disability's paralysis prevented me from independently regaining my posture or reaching a phone to summon help.

The PRS company I now use offers several types of transmitters, including a necklace, wristband, sip-and-puff tube, and even a device that can be actuated by eyelid movement.

> *A monitoring service should not be used to replace routine PAs, but instead to summon help during true emergencies.*

The waterproof wristband I chose contains a push button. Pressing this button by any way possible (including perhaps whacking it against the frame of my wheelchair!) will transmit a low-powered signal from anywhere within my house or surrounding outdoor yard to a company-supplied combination radio receiver and speaker phone located in my kitchen.

The activated speaker phone automatically dials the company's 24/7 switchboard near Boston from wherever in the United States I reside. Within 60 seconds, a company operator very courteously responds, "Yes, Mr. DeGraff, how may I help you?"

- If I am testing the system (as the company encourages me to do on a weekly basis), or have mistakenly activated the system, I inform the operator that everything is okay. She thanks me for calling, invites me to call her again anytime, and hangs up.

- If I need help and am conscious, I inform her of the kind of help I need. I might have supplied her in advance with the names and numbers of my nearby relatives, neighbors, or PAs. If so, she consults this list from her computer screen and starts calling them for me. If I have not supplied her with an advance list, I might dictate some names and numbers from memory. Or, if I need an ambulance, police, or fire department, she will call them for me. In any event, she will maintain conversation with me until someone actually arrives.

- If I do not respond to her speaker phone answer, she automatically calls an ambulance and monitors the sounds in my house until they arrive.

For this 24-hour service, I pay a flat fee of about one dollar per day regardless of how much or little I use the service. A rental fee for the wristband and speaker phone is included in the monthly fee.

Without the benefit of this medical monitoring service, I would probably resign myself to hiring a live-in aide while forfeiting some of my privacy and independence. A live-in aide would be away from the house at times, and would not be as present or dependable as this service.

Currently, the push-button transmitter must be within range of its counterpart receiver, which is, in turn, connected to your phone line. In short, you must be at home and cannot be on a hiking trail. Consequently, I will personally look forward in probably a few months to having the technology of these services catch up with my active lifestyle. This will mean that my push-button will activate a GPS satellite tracker that will tell the monitoring service "Mr. DeGraff, who lives in Colorado, needs help at the top of Cadillac Mountain in Bar Harbor, Maine."

So, my personal experience prompts me to suggest that you consider a service like this if your disability and living situation warrant it. Don't make my mistake of associating these services with only a senior age bracket and grandparent status. I am told these companies serve clients with a wide range of ages, disabilities, professional careers, and lifestyles. The costs are sometimes covered by health insurance when prescribed by a physician.

There are several companies throughout the United States that provide services like the one I use. You are wise to call two or three services to compare monthly monitoring costs and types of service. Your local hospital should have brochures for those that serve your area; your phone book's Yellow Pages might list them under "Medical Alarms and Monitoring"; an Internet search engine might list them as "Personal Emergency Response Services." As a starting point to your researching these companies, the company I use is the Lifeline Personal Response and Support Services, 800.543.3546, www.lifelinesys.com. (This contact data is provided merely for your convenience without any expressed or implied endorsement.)

Chapter 28
Your Discretion, Privacy, and Confidentiality

Picture the following scenarios.

It's a bright, sunny day and you are sitting in your wheelchair, by yourself, at a restaurant's sidewalk picnic table, eating lunch and reading. You came here on your own, in part to blend into the able-bodied, public mainstream for an afternoon. Your reading is distracted when you overhear your PA's voice at a nearby table. Unaware of your presence a few feet away, she is conversing with some of her friends. You try to ignore the conversation and go on with your reading, but your subconscious alerts you to the topic being discussed.

Scenario I—You're a help recipient

"Yeah, I'm working for this guy in a wheelchair. It's a live-in situation where I live rent-free in exchange for helping him out with his personal needs. He's got a really nice house. A big stereo, tons of CDs, nice artwork, poshy furniture. Funny, all this stuff and he rarely locks the garage. Yeah, I begin each morning that I work by changing this gizmo he pees into all day. Then I help him get dressed and into his wheelchair. At night I care for his bowel routine. Not bad unless he has diarrhea. Next, he needs help with his shower and then transferring into bed. His commode and shower chair is weird—has a hole in the seat. His legs jump around a lot. I don't understand what happens, but they spazz a lot. Kinda pitiful, actually. Sorta like a pretzel."

Scenario II—You're a help recipient

"Yeah, I'm working for this guy in a wheelchair. It's a live-in situation where I live rent-free in exchange for helping him out with his personal needs. Rich, what are you up to this summer?"

    Each of these two scenarios portrays a different way for a PA to describe her live-in job to her able-bodied friends. However, if you were overhearing your PA in the first situation, how would you feel? Embarrassed? Violated? Angry? Would it matter whether the PA identified you by name? What would you do the next time you saw your PA?

Now, let's reverse the roles.

Imagine this time that you are an able-bodied help provider, and doing some reading in the library. Three or four people assemble at the next table and a familiar voice tells you that Amy, the wheelchair user to whom you provide assistance, is among them.

Scenario I—You're a help provider

"Hey you guys, I've got this new PA, Chastity. An odd name; must be some free-love thing with her hippie folks. Man, I'll tell you that good help is tough to get. She does the job okay, but she's a little strange. For starters she's a veggie, you know, doesn't eat meat. You should see the health stuff in her side of the fridge. At night she burns this weird incense in her room. I wish instead of incense she would pop once in a while for a stick of deodorant. Usually she needs a shower more than I do. It's no wonder she's a loner."

Scenario II—You're a help provider

"Hey you guys, I've got this new PA. She's a grad student at CSU and answered my ad in the campus paper. She'll be with me just through the summer. Anne, are you going to San Francisco this summer?"

If you were Chastity, how would you feel hearing yourself described in each of these scenes? In the second, Amy briefly describes you but doesn't violate your sense of privacy. In the first scene, she both reveals private things about you and is sarcastically critical.

The primary hurt that a person feels by being the subject of each "Scenario I" is a violation of trust and privacy. In the typical help recipient/provider relationship, each party is exposed to very private details about the other. Each person must be able to trust that discretion will be used in not publicizing inappropriate details.

> *"What you learn about me and my private lifestyle here at my home, stays here at my home. In return, what I learn about you will also stay here. These unavoidable-but-confidential details about either of us are no one else's business."*

In each Scenario II, the speaker changed the topic before the listeners either heard inappropriate details or could ask about them. Perhaps the key to discretion here is asking yourself, "If so-and-so were here next to me, would they be embarrassed or feel violated by what I am about to say?"

The bottom line is to be discreet and respect privacy about the personal details you learn and convey about other people.

My advice is to establish a firm policy with your help providers, whether they come from an agency or your own personal employment:

You are wise to include this policy with the others that you list during job applicant interviews, as well as to remind your PAs of it occasionally at staff meetings. As an example, you are looking for PAs who are responsible, rock-solid dependable, punctual, and confidential.

Often, a help provider who works with you will also be working with someone else. To impress you with their experience, these PA applicants tend to say things like, "Yes, I'm experienced and well qualified to work with you, because I already work with another quadriplegic. His bowel routine is almost the same as yours, except Phil uses..."

As soon as I identify this type of conversation coming, I abruptly interrupt the job applicant.

> *Laura, excuse me. With all respect to you and whomever he is, these details about him are none of my business—just as my details are none of his. In addition, if you are hired to work with me, I will never discuss elsewhere any personal topics about you and your lifestyle.*
>
> *Please do not be offended, because I know you are simply trying to make friendly conversation. However, you have entered into a very serious area that medical professionals refer to as "privileged conversation." Legally and ethically, the medical and personal topics we discuss here cannot be repeated to anyone else—not even my other aides—without my permission about a specific topic.*
>
> *Does this make sense to you, and do you have any questions? Thank you for understanding. By the way, I am bound by the same confidentiality for any topics you discuss with me about yourself.*

A word of special caution is warranted for family caregivers. These very giving family members often have a tendency to discuss very personal aspects of the help they provide and concerns they shoulder.

Is their intention to attract attention from neighborhood friends by discussing gossip about your current case of stomach flu? Do they enjoy embarrassing you in front of your friends by talking about the clumsy way you use a toothbrush?

Probably not. Instead of intentionally wanting to publicly display your private matters, they are often substituting inappropriate discussions with general friends for the appropriate, confidential sharing that they need, but currently lack, from a formal, peer, caregiver support group.

Most family caregivers need a formally structured, caregiver support group of peers with whom they can appropriately share, grieve, laugh, cry, and trade coping strategies. When caregivers lack routine access to and participation in such a group, they substitute informal sharing with common friends—yours and theirs.

However, this rationale is of little comfort to you while you become increasingly embarrassed with your friends at that restaurant table.

The remedy that cooled down my own mother and her discussions about my catheterizations and diarrhea, when I was a very sensitive 18-year-old, was ultimately to embarrass her as she had me.

First, I had to repeatedly tell her how embarrassing it was for her to discuss these disability-related topics—her tasks relating to my bodily functions. At first, I spoke with her alone, and she claimed that I was being too sensitive. "These are our friends, they care about both of us. They have first been asking about what kinds of tasks I do for you. So, understandably they would feel hurt if I told them I couldn't talk about these issues."

She continued to red-face me to our mutual friends, until one day around a neighbor's pool party, I briefly took her on in front of her friends.

Excuse me, everyone. Mother, I have politely asked you at home not to discuss embarrassing details about my disability, my urinary catheter, my diarrhea, and other really embarrassing things about my care in front of our friends. Since you still don't seem to understand how badly I feel when you do this, I'm asking you again—in front of our friends—not to discuss these topics. I am very sorry if this embarrasses you; however, I believe you all understand my point of view. Thank you for understanding.

Not asking for a response, I promptly wheeled away from the group. I knew I would catch hell when I got home, about embarrassing my mother, but I knew her friends would validate my concerns. Surprisingly, I was not punished later, and she ceased her conversations—or at least the ones I could overhear.

The bottom line here is to respect others in your life with discretion, privacy, and confidentiality—and to insist that they also respect you! You will find that few people—if anyone—will ever object.

Chapter 29

Your Educational Roles and Objective: Direction, Training, and Education

> *To direct some;*
> *To teach, instruct, and train most; and*
> *To educate a select few.*

As a lifetime trainer and manager of the people who help you, what exactly are your role and objectives? To each temporary provider, you convey the hundreds of details of the what, how, and when about the help that you require.

Why do some PAs remember so few details, and require a great many prompts from you during every work shift, whereas others enthusiastically soak up your instructions with 99 percent retention of those tasks? There are several variables at work. The level of training you provide to caregivers and PAs will vary according to the person and circumstance. In addition to the skills and benefits they receive, there can be personal and sometimes even spiritual fulfillment for you.

Training can be an art form, and defined in several ways. Check out these definitions of verbs from the Random House *Webster's College Dictionary* (1992):

- To *direct* means provide instructions as to the steps necessary to accomplish a purpose—*He directed me to organize the files*

- To *teach* is the most general of these terms, referring to any practice that furnishes a person with a skill or knowledge—*to teach children to write*

- To *instruct* usually implies using a systematic, structured method of teaching—*to instruct paramedics in first aid*

- To *train* stresses the development of a desired proficiency or behavior through practice, discipline, and instruction—*to train military recruits*

- To *educate* stresses the development of reasoning and judgment; it often involves preparing a person for an occupation or for mature life—*to educate the young*

From my years of experience, I can apply these dictionary definitions to managing caregivers and PAs with some interesting comments:

- If you are grocery shopping or attending a concert and you drop something onto the ground, you might enlist very brief, temporary, volunteer help from strangers or passersby. You would *direct* them, or provide them with *directions*, on how to pick up the dropped object and either hand it to you or put it into your backpack. Your objective is to quickly tell someone what you need, with little or no emphasis on detailed ways for or reasons behind doing the task. The strangers who help you in the street for 30 seconds, as essential as they are to supporting your independence, have no desire to receive more detailed and time-consuming instruction or training. You will, however, also frequently give caregivers and PAs directions for one-shot tasks that are not routine.

- When you have just hired a new aide or PA, you use a combination of *teaching* and *instructing* in conveying the what, how, and why for the routine tasks that will be done repeatedly. These *instructions* are more complex than the simpler *directions* given to a stranger for a one-shot task. These tasks are part of your daily lifestyle, and there are reasons why you want them done in certain ways. For these folks, from the previous definitions, you are using "a systematic, structured method of teaching." Indeed, that method is what this reference is all about. There would be less need for this comprehensive reference and its methods if PAs were merely given directions. This minimum learning stage from teaching and instruction is as far as some PAs ever get, and that is okay because this basic instruction will get you in and out of bed.

- As better PAs spend more time with you, and learn more about your preferences and values, they become *trained* beyond the basics. These are the 18-karat, sharper PAs who could make a professional living from doing quality aide work. Each of these folks thoroughly understands your preferences. These are the aides who take the initiative to help you problemsolve, and who take a bit more pride in their work than those who have been taught and instructed.

- For most professions, there is a hall of fame for the truly distinguished. These PAs have been *taught, instructed,* and *trained*, and have learned everything you can convey about being a top-notch aide. In addition, there are a distinct few who additionally learn a lot about what it is like to live with a disability and to accommodate it. These 24-karat people have become *educated* through their experiences with you. These hall-of-famers are often college students on their way to becoming OTs, PTs, and other medical professionals. If not college material, they are especially caring, compassionate people—and very appreciative to be working with you.

The monetary salary you pay is secondary to the *knowledge* and *education* you have contributed to their upcoming medical careers. In return for the education you give them, this class of PAs provides you with a way of giving back to the medical professions that initially helped you with your own disability. It is my firm belief that each of these gems was *meant* to meet and experience one of us on her way through life. What each of these current PAs learns from you or me will in turn benefit one of her future clients or patients. If this PA is not to become a medical professional, then her education from you is meant to benefit a friend, family member, or perhaps even a personal need.

And *that* is one of the primary reasons why some of us have proposed that perhaps we chose—or were chosen by a higher power—to have our disabilities: to share our experiences and growth, to give back to society, and to make life a little easier for the next person who follows us!

Appendices

MiCASSA, Olmstead, and ADAPT— Your Medicaid Rights to and funding for PA Services

A primary mission in my researching and writing this reference book has been to provide you the skills to control the quality and schedule of your daily lifestyle. This is accomplished, in part, by your taking charge of the quality and schedule of the *assistance* you receive, and that is made possible by your directly selecting and supervising the *people* who provide that help.

Although these management skills can be used while living in a health care facility, I hope instead that they will contribute to your living at home. No facility can provide the comfort, security, and privacy of living in your own castle.

While some of us have concentrated on publishing and teaching management *skills*, others have dedicated themselves to ensuring your management *rights*. Disability advocates have spent years negotiating with administrators so that children and adults of any age who have a long-term disability or illness, and who require Medicaid funding for housing and support services, have rights that include the following:

- being able to remain at home, and avoid being institutionalized against their will
- having sufficient funding for personal assistant (PA) services
- being able to select and supervise those funded PAs who help them, and avoid being assigned agency aides who are selected and supervised by the agency administrators
- having access to rent subsidies and affordable mortgages that enable community living for low-income families

- having access to educational services, counseling, and transitional community programs that enable taking advantage of these freedoms and funding

- involving program beneficiaries and their families both in planning these programs and in disseminating information about them

- having easy access to information about services, funding, and the right to obtain them.

Medicaid is the main source of health care, housing, and PA services for people with disabilities and low incomes. Therefore, a primary strategy of disability advocates and activists has been to negotiate how beneficiaries receive Medicaid's "long-term care expenditures." There have been two main options. Institution-based services, which are planned and controlled by administrators, are available only while living in nursing homes and intermediate care facilities. In contrast, community-based services, which include the options of home health care and managing one's own PAs who are funded by the program, are available to people living "at home."

In federal fiscal year 2000, 73 percent of Medicaid long-term expenditures went to people living in institutions, and 27 percent to people living in the community. Though this is an improvement over the 85:15 percent ratio of fiscal year 1992, disability advocates have a long way to go to better balancing—and tipping—the scale in favor of self-determination. As we will see, *disability advocates* is a term that should include all of us.

At home refers to people receiving services in "the most integrated setting appropriate to the individual." This terminology came out of a Supreme Court ruling in *Olmstead v. L.C. & E.W.,* in which the Court affirmed that the ADA (Americans with Disabilities Act, 1990) requires states to avoid discriminating against people with disabilities by keeping them segregated in nursing homes. Beneficiaries of Medicaid services cannot be forced to live in institutions in order to receive services.

The primary advocacy group behind this and other progress has been ADAPT. The group was formed as American Disabled for Accessible Public Transit when its goal was disability access to public transportation. When ADA mandated public transit access, ADAPT's national and state chapters next poured efforts toward CASA, the Community Attendant Services Act.

ADAPT gave Speaker Newt Gingrich the CASA wish list in 1996. In 1997, Gingrich introduced it as the MiCASA bill (the Medicaid Community Attendant Services Act); however, it died at the session end in 1998. ADAPT has since renamed MiCASA to be MiCASSA (the Medicaid Community Services and Supports Act), having added "supports" to include people who are eligible for Medicaid's institutional services.

As this book goes to press, ADAPT is continuing its push both for the passage of the MiCASSA legislation and for the adoption of the "Olmstead Plan" by individual states. It is hoped that President Bush will sign an Executive Order calling for "swift implementation of the *Olmstead* decision" by each state. According to New Mobility,[1] "to ADAPT, the push for MiCASSA, implementation of the Olmstead ruling, and activism for more community services are all part of what is called 'the real choice campaign,' enabling PA services for anyone who needs them.

As your author, I urge you to consider yourself a "disability advocate" merely because of your dependence on physical assistance from others. Regardless of whether you are personally eligible for Medicaid services and funding, you have brothers and sisters with disabilities whose lives depend on them.

I urge you to accomplish at least three objectives.

First, keep up with the news and progress regarding the MiCASSA legislation, the availability of federal funding to states for their implementation of the Olmstead Plan (and the progress of states toward that implementation), and the progress of formal disability advocacy groups like ADAPT. You can monitor ADAPT's national and state-level actions at <www.adapt.org> and other advocacy efforts at <www.newmobility.com>.

Second, monitor whether your state has applied for the available funding for its adoption of the Olmstead Plan and similar community-based programs. Then, support programs where people with disabilities design and deliver the services. It appears that the Health Care Financing Administration (HFCA) is leading the way in making "starter grants" available to states that apply for them. Has your state made itself eligible yet? Check out <www.hcfa.gov/medicaid/systemchange> and <www.freedomclearinghouse.com>.

Third, petition your state's legislators and Medicaid officials to initiate and support community-based programs *for* people with disabilities that are planned and operated *by* people with disabilities.

The PA management skills outlined in this book are useless unless people have the financial resources to hire the PAs they require as well as the right to select and supervise them. The programs and people outlined here have the potential to facilitate some of those goals for a large segment of our population.

Selected Resource Bibliography

The primary resources used in writing this reference book were experiences of the author and those of scores of help recipients, family caregivers, and paid help providers who were interviewed over 30-plus years. Although this reference is quite comprehensive in presenting "how-to" strategies, it is far from exhaustive.

The following books were selected because they provide additional details on specialized topics, usually addressing coping skills for family caregivers. The disability-related magazines, short publications, and videos either specialize in caregiver issues or periodically offer articles on managing help providers. Please excuse the occasional omissions of bibliographic data; some secondary sources were deficient. ISBN identifiers have been included in some citations due to their increasing use during computer searches.

Books

Brandt, Avrene L. *Caregiver's Reprieve: A Guide to Emotional Survival When You're Caring for Someone You Love.* Atascadero: Impact, 1997, ISBN 1-886230-06-4.

Burger, Sarah Greene, et al. *Nursing Homes: Getting Good Care There.* Atascadero: Impact, 1997, ISBN 0-915166-97-6.

DeGraff, Alfred H. *Attendants and Attendees: A Guidebook of Helpful Hints.* Washington, DC: College and University Personnel Association, 1978.

DeGraff, Alfred H. *Home Health Aides: Managing the People Who Help You.* Saratoga Springs, NY: Saratoga Access Publications, 1988.

Hammond, Marilyn, et al. *Personal Assistance Services Guide: A Guide for Hiring, Management and Conflict Resolution.* Logan, UT: Center for Persons with Disabilities.

Holicky, Richard. *Taking Care of Yourself While Providing Care: A Guide for Those Who Assist and Care for Their Spouses, Children, Parents, and Other Loved Ones Who Have Spinal Cord Injuries.* Englewood, CO: Craig Hospital, 2000.

Ludlum, Catherine D. *Getting from Here to There: A Manual on Personal Assistance.* Storrs, CT: A.J. Pappanikou Center, U-CONN.

McLeod, Beth Witrogen. *Caregiving: The Spiritual Journey of Love, Loss, and Renewal.* NY: John Wiley & Sons, 2001.

Navarra, Tova. *Wisdom for Caregivers.* Thorofare, NJ: SLACK Inc., 1995, ISBN 1-55642-288-1.

Price, June. *Avoiding Attendants from Hell: A Practical Guide to Finding, Hiring and Keeping Personal Care Attendants.* Chesterfield, MO: Science and Humanities Press.

Shatto, Michael E. *Optimum Independence Through Self-Managed Attendant Care: A Guide Both for Persons with Disabilities and Professional Case Managers.* Sorrento, FL: Michael E. Shatto and Associates, Inc.

Sherman, James R. *Conquering Caregiver Fears.* Golden Valley, MN: Pathway Books, 1994.

Sherman, James R. *Creative Caregiver.* Golden Valley, MN: Pathway Books, 1994, ISBN 0-935538-17-8.

Sherman, James R. *Preventing Caregiver Burnout.* Golden Valley, MN: Pathway Books, 1994, ISBN 0-935538-16-X.

Susuk, Helen. *Hiring Home Caregivers: The Family Guide to In-Home Eldercare.* San Luis Obispo, CA: American Source Books, 1995, ISBN 0-915166-91-7.

Whiteneck, Gale G. *Aging with Spinal Cord Injury.* New York: Demos, 1993, ISBN 0-939957-48-5.

Wildenberg, Stacey. *The Resourceful Caregiver: Helping Family Caregivers Help Themselves.* St. Louis: National Family Caregivers Association, Mosby Lifeline, 1996, ISBN 0-8151-55565.

Magazines, journals, short publications, and videos
Abilities: Canada's Lifestyle Magazine for People with Disabilities. 489 College Street, Suite 501, Toronto, Ontario M6G 1A5, www.abilities.ca.

Accent on Living Magazine. P.O. Box 700, Bloomington, IL 61702, (309) 378-2961, fax (309) 378-4420, e-mail: acntivng@aol.com.

Active Living; The Health, Fitness & Recreation Magazine for People With a Disability. 2276 Rosedene Road, St. Ann's, Ontario LOR 1YO, Canada. (905) 957-6016, e-mail: activeliv@aol.com.

Alert. Association on Higher Education And Disability (AHEAD), University of Massachusetts Boston, 100 Morrissey Boulevard, Boston, MA 02125-3393, (v) (617) 287-3880; (fax) (617) 287-3881; (t) (617) 287-3882; e-mail: ahead@umb.edu, www.ahead.org.

As the Years Go By: Accepting New Help and Caregivers. RRTC on Aging with Spinal Cord Injury, The Research Department, Craig Hospital, 3425 South Clarkson Street, Englewood, CO 80110. (800) 5REHAB8.

Attendant Care Services. Arkansas Spinal Cord Commission, 1120 Marshall Street - #207, Little Rock, AR 72202.

Careers & the Disabled. 445 Broad Hollow Road, Suite 425, Melville, NY 11747, (631) 421-9421, www.EOP.com.

Caregiver Bereavement Kit. NFCA.

Caregiver Survivor Kit (for caregivers of people with Alzheimer's disease). NFCA.

A Caregiver Guide to Information and Resources; A Path for Caregivers; Caregiving; The Source for Consumer Information; Miles Away and Still Caring; Staying at Home; and The Eldercare Locator: A Way to Find Community Assistance for Seniors (800-677-1116). American Association of Retired Persons (AARP), 601 E Street, NW, Washington, DC 20049. (202) 434-2277, www.aarp.org.

Caregiving Across the Life Cycle (June 1998). NFCA.

A Checklist for Evaluating Personal Care Assistance Services. Center on Human Policy, Syracuse University, 200 Huntington Hall, Syracuse, NY 13244-3420.

Exceptional Parent Magazine. 555 Kinderkamack Road,. Oradell, NJ 07649. www.eparent.com.

Long-Term Caregivers: For Better and For Worse. RRTC on Aging with Spinal Cord Injury, The Research Department, Craig Hospital, 3425 South Clarkson Street, Englewood, CO 80110. (800) 5REHAB8.

MSFocus. Multiple Sclerosis Foundation, 6350 North Andrews Avenue, Ft. Lauderdale, Fl 33309-2130. (800) 225-6495, www.msfocus.org.

A National Report on the Status of Caregiving in America (November 1999 and December 2000). NFCA (National Family Caregivers Association), 10400 Connecticut Avenue, Suite 500, Kensington, MD 20895-3944. (800) 896-3650, www.nfcacares.org; CareThere.com.

New Mobility. No Limits Communications, Inc., PO Box 220, Horsham, PA 19044. (888) 850-0344, www.newmobility.com.

Outreach to Faith Community Kit and Supporting Caregiving Families: A Guide for Congregations. NFCA.

Paraplegia News. 2111 East Highland Avenue, Suite 180, Phoenix, AZ 85016-4702. (888) 888-2201, www.pn-magazine.com.

Personal Assistant Recruitment (video). Marianjoy Rehabilitation Hospital, 26W171 Roosevelt Road, Wheaton, IL 60189-0795.

Personal Care Assistants: How to Find, Hire and Keep Them. RRTC on Aging with Spinal Cord Injury, The Research Department, Craig Hospital, 3425 South Clarkson Street, Englewood, CO 80110, (800) 5REHAB8.

Quest. Muscular Dystrophy Association, 3300 East Sunrise Drive, Tucson, AZ 85718-3208. (520) 529-2000, www.mdausa.org.

SCI Life. HDI Publishers, Houston, TX, 77219. (800) 321-7037.

Take Care! NFCA.

Today's Caregiver. P.O. Box 21646, Ft. Lauderdale, FL 33335. (800) 829-2734, www.caregiver.com.

Total Access. Canadian Paraplegia Association, 1101 Prince of Wales Drive – Suite 230, Ottawa, Ontario K2C 3W7, Canada. (613) 723-1033, www.canparaplegic.org.

Your Advice Is Requested and Please Register for Your Free Newsletter— May I Have Your Comments, Strategies, and Advice, Please?

If you have appreciated this comprehensive, detailed reference, you may thank your peers more than me. Without the hundreds of comments, strategies, and advisories from PA managers like you, this reference would not have been possible.

Please contribute to your free, periodic e-newsletter and to the next edition of this reference. All comments are significant, and none is too big or too small.

At last, as help recipients, family caregivers, and paid help providers, we now have our own e-newsletter for sharing ideas and concerns! Here is your chance to make receiving, managing, and providing quality personal assistance easier, less stressful, and more efficient.

- What is working well for you, and what is not?
- What recent crisis have you experienced that you want to share, so others can avoid it?
- With what recurring problem would you like advice from others?

Regardless of whether you have ideas to share, you are invited to sign up for your free, internet e-newsletter. Simply send us an e-mail with "Newsletter" in the subject line. We will register your e-mail address as it appears in the sender line unless you provide a preferred e-mail address in the message area. You may also provide e-mail addresses for friends who want to subscribe. Recipients can cancel their subscriptions at any time.

In addition to the newsletter, please contribute to the next edition of this reference. If I use your suggestion, you will be listed in the book's "Acknowledgments" and be eligible for a complimentary copy.

With regard to your personal privacy, I am proud to state that I have not shared a single name or phone number in the entire 20-plus years I have been writing on these topics. I have no intention of starting a policy change if we hear from you.

Please let me know about the methods you use to work in harmony with the people who help you, and to control the quality of help you receive. In addition to wanting to hear from help recipients, I am also very interested in the special needs and concerns of family caregivers and paid providers.

- As you review and use the topics of this reference, please comment about which ones worked well for you, and about any that did not

- As you use this book as a reference, please note whether its structure, organization, table of contents, or index could be improved for easier use

- As you develop new "how-to" strategies of your own, please take a moment to share them with us, so we can share them with others

- As you think of new ways that we could be sharing these ideas—CD ROM innovations, heavy-traffic Web sites, "how to" videos, an annual conference you usually attend—please pass along your advice.

By postal mail

Saratoga Access Publications, Inc.
P.O. Box 1427
Fort Collins, CO 80522-1427 USA

By fax

970.484.5531

At our Web site

www.saratoga-publications.com

By e-mail

Please use this address to sign up for your free e-newsletter!
caregiver@saratoga-publications.com

How to Order Additional Copies of This Reference

- Need an extra copy for your family?
- Would you like to gift a copy to a friend, library, hospital, or health care facility? (It's a tax-deductible donation when given to an eligible organization!)
- Instructors, do you need multiple copies—at a discount—for an upcoming class, seminar, or workshop?

If your local bookstore is temporarily out of stock of this reference, we invite you to consult our Web site for access to our current supplier and for special details about quantity discounts.

Postal inquiries: Saratoga Access Publications, Inc.
P.O. Box 1427
Fort Collins, CO 80522-1427 USA

Fax inquiries: 970.484.5531

Web inquiries: www.saratoga-publications.com

E-mail inquiries: caregiver@saratoga-publications.com

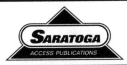

SARATOGA ACCESS PUBLICATIONS, INC.
FORT COLLINS • COLORADO • USA

Index

Your Author

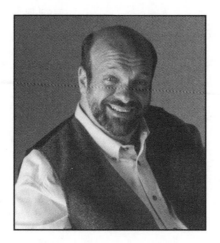

Alfred H. "Skip" DeGraff
Currently resides in Colorado where he personally employs a continuous team of five or six part-time college student PAs.